Advance Reviews for
Having Your Baby through Egg Donation

Having Your Baby through Egg Donation is an indispensable resource for all parties involved in reproductive medicine: married couples, single individuals, gay and lesbian couples; donors and gestational carriers; medical personnel; and friends and family who need to understand and provide support to all considering and/or choosing egg donation as a means of creating their families.

Its examination of the multiple and complex issues that are a part of both anonymous and known egg donation is thorough and includes the psychological, medical, legal, and ethical concerns of this process. Even an interesting history of egg donation is included as well as the various ways it is practiced in other parts of the world.

A very important theme in this book is the need for all of us "to think outside the box" as we examine egg donation and to remember that "reproductive medicine is a changing field." The personal stories within its pages help the readers to understand the tangible losses that precede the use of egg donation. Congratulations to Ellen Glazer and Evelina Sterling on their accomplishment.

Patricia Mahlstedt, Ed.D
Psychologist, Private Practice
Houston, Texas

At long last there is a *comprehensive* guide for those considering ovum donation. This amazing book, chocked full of information and resources, covers the medical, ethical and psychological aspects of this family building option more completely than anything previously available.

Beginning with helping an individual or couple to make the decision to use donor eggs, the authors take the reader on a journey through every aspect of this choice. It includes who to share the information with, how much it will cost, how to proceed with the legal contracts, how to talk with kids and the importance of resolving infertility before moving on.

This book portrays families created through ovum donation in the positive light it deserves, reminding readers that our families are joyous, honest and grateful and very much like all families, but with a difference.

I will definitely be recommending this book to all my clients who are considering pursuing ovum donation as a path to parenthood.

Carole LieberWilkins, M.A.
Marriage and Family Therapist
Los Angeles

Having Your Baby Through Egg Donation is the first book that offers a thorough exploration and discussion of the major issues relevant to individuals and couples considering egg donation. In very basic language and terminology, Glazer and Sterling guide the reader through the maze of feelings and considerations. Using a tremendous amount of empathy and support, the authors offer the first real support in print for potential egg donor recipients. This book is a "must have" for those beginning the journey of egg donation.

Andrea Mechanick Braverman, Ph.D.
Director of Psychological Services
Pennsylvania Reproductive Associates of the Women's Institute

This is an important event. At last we have all in one place a book that addresses the emotions, ethics, psychology and practical tasks faced by any woman (and her partner) contemplating building a family with the help of egg donation and then raising those children.

Ellen and Evelina write from long experience of supporting families using donated gametes. They clearly listen to what people say and the book is full of lively case studies illustrating the varied situations and feelings of individuals and families. Although they recognise and respect difference, they also give clear guidance, for instance about the importance of openness with children, when they believe the issue is a key one.

Although there are parts of this book that are not relevant for the UK reader, all the ethical and emotional issues are familiar and addressed in depth. Indeed there are some assumptions and practices that challenge current thinking in the UK and provide a fresh perspective. I will be very happy to recommend this book to our members.

Olivia Montuschi
Founder Member Donor Conception Network UK
Mother of two donor-conceived young people

This valuable book draws out the range of issues to be faced by anyone involved with egg donation. Even when raising ethical controversies and medical challenges, the authors offer an optimistic and reassuring view.

Carol Frost, LICSW
co-author of *Helping the Stork*
Infertility Counselor in Woburn, MA

Having Your Baby Through

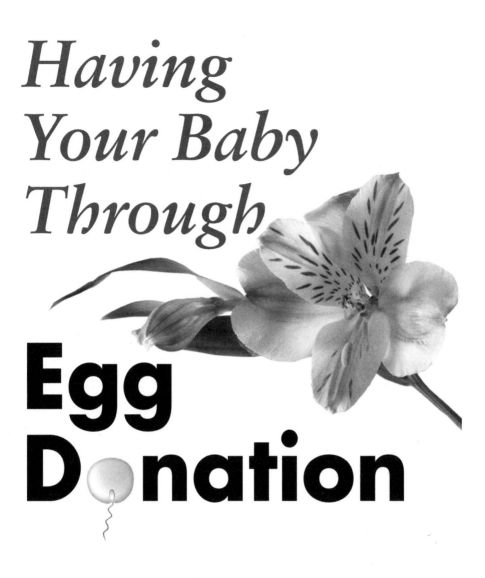

Egg
Dnation

ELLEN SARASOHN GLAZER
EVELINA WEIDMAN STERLING

Perspectives Press, Inc.
Indianapolis, Indiana

Prespectives Press, Inc.
The Infertility and Adoption Publisher
P.O., Box 90318
Indianapolis, IN 46290-0318, USA
(317) 872-3055
www.perspectivespress.com

Cover and interior design by Bookwrights.
Manufactured in the United States of America

Library of Congress Cataloging in Publication Data

Glazer, Ellen Sarasohn.
   Having your baby through egg donation / by Ellen Sarasohn Glazer and Evelina Weidman Sterling.
      p. cm
Includes bibliographical references and index.
ISBN 0-944934-32-3 (alk. paper)   ISBN 978-0-944934-32-6
   1. Human reproductive technology—Popular works. 2. Ovum—Transplantation. 3. Infertility—Psychological aspects. I. Sterling, Evelina Weidman, 1970- II. Title.

RG133.5.G56 2005
618.1'78—dc22

                                                     2004063517

This book is dedicated to the loving memory of Dr. Susan Cooper, who taught me all I need to know about life, love, motherhood and new ways of building families. Her life was a blessing.

EG

I dedicate this book to my children, Benjamin and Elena.

ES

Contents

Some Introductions

Most of us grow up expecting that we can and eventually will become parents. We know how it's done—you find a partner you love, make love, get pregnant, and nine months later you have a baby. Few people give any thought, initially, to the possibility that their own experience in family building may not be quite that simple. But things happen. Life intervenes. And, if you are reading this book, you have already come to understand that becoming a parent will not be as simple and straightforward as you once thought it would be.

You are not alone in finding your journey to parenthood and, subsequently, your parenthood experience, "different" from what you expected it to be. Although the "differences" others experience may not be the same as yours, those who parent with a difference have much in common. In 1987, Emily Perl Kingsley wrote of her own "different" experience in the essay below. She became pregnant. Her child was born with Down Syndrome.

"Welcome to Holland" by Emily Perl Kingsley

I am often asked to describe the experience of raising a child with a disability—to try to help people who have not shared that unique experience to understand it, to imagine how it would feel. It's like this...

When you're going to have a baby, it's like planning a fabulous vacation trip—to Italy. You buy a bunch of guidebooks and make your wonderful plans. The Coliseum. Michelangelo's David. The gondolas in Venice. You may learn some handy phrases in Italian. It's all very exciting.

After months of eager anticipation, the day finally arrives.

You pack your bags and off you go. Several hours later, the plane lands. The stewardess comes in and says, "Welcome to Holland." "*Holland??*" you say. "What do you mean, Holland? I signed up for Italy! I'm supposed to be in Italy. All my life I've dreamed of going to Italy."

But there's been a change in the flight plan. They've landed in Holland and there you must stay. The important thing is that they haven't taken you to a horrible, disgusting, filthy place, full of pestilence, famine and disease. It's just a different place.

So you must go out and buy new guide books. And you must learn a whole new language. And you will meet a whole new group of people you would never have met. It's just a *different* place. It's slower-paced than Italy, less flashy than Italy. But after you've been there for a while and you catch your breath, you look around, and you begin to notice that Holland has windmills. Holland has tulips. Holland even has Rembrandts.

But everyone you know is busy going to and from Italy, and they're all bragging about what a wonderful time they had there. And for the rest of your life, you will say, "Yes, that's where I was supposed to go. That's what I had planned."

The pain of that will never ever, ever go away, because the loss of that dream is a very significant loss. But if you spend your life mourning the fact that you didn't get to Italy, you may never be free to enjoy the very special, the very lovely things about Holland. [1]

Your own experience is not Emily Perl Kinglsey's, but your journey to parenthood has also taken a twist. You have found that you will not be having a baby in the "conventional way," and we offer you a guide to making decisions about whether or not to choose one particular alternative path to parenthood: using donated ova.

Introducing Us—Ellen and Evelina

Before we introduce you to other people whose personal and/or professional lives have been touched by ovum donation, we want to introduce ourselves and to say something about how we came to write this book together…

Ellen is a clinical social worker and writer who has been helping people build families for nearly 25 years. She has a private practice in Newton, Massachusetts, where she sees a variety of people, most of whom are struggling, in one way or another, around family building concerns. Ellen has special interests in adoption, pregnancy loss, gestational care and parenting after infertility, as well as in egg donation. She is the author of two books, *The Long Awaited Stork: A Guide to Parenting after Infertility* and *Experiencing Infertility: Stories to Inform and Inspire* and the co-author, with Dr. Susan Cooper, of *Choosing Assisted Reproduction: Social, Emotional and Ethical Considerations*. In addition to her clinical practice and professional writing, Ellen is an essayist and a feature writer for the *Newton Magazine* and other publications.

Evelina is a public health specialist with over 12 years working in the field of reproductive and women's health. She is currently a doctoral student in the Department of Sociology at Georgia State University in Atlanta, Georgia. Her research interests include issues related to gender and sexuality, as well as the long-term impacts of infertility. She is the co-author, with Angie Best-Boss, of another book, *Living with PCOS— Polycystic Ovary Syndrome* and has written several articles specifically addressing infertility.

Although this is our first book together, we are each authors or co-authors of several books and articles on reproductive medicine. We are also mothers—Ellen has two grown children and Evelina is busy parenting little ones. We met through our editor and publisher, Pat Johnston at Perspectives Press, Inc.: The Infertility and Adoption Publisher.

As we write, we will most often speak as "we," and when we do, we are expressing shared views. That is not to say that we agree on everything, but for the most part, we have tried to present material from a shared perspective. However, since we come from different professional backgrounds—clinical social work and public health—there are times when we do bring different perspectives. At those times, when we feel we must say "I" and not "we," we follow the "I" with the speaker's first name (Ellen or Evelina).

The Purpose of this Book

Not long ago, it was unimaginable—the idea that oocytes (eggs) could be transferred from one woman to another. Today it is common. Throughout the world thousands of women have become—and are becoming—mothers through oocyte donation. Perhaps one day you will be among them?

Egg donation is one of several paths to parenthood that require the use of a third party's reproductive capabilities. These collaborative reproductions include using donated sperm, using donated eggs, surrogacy, using a gestational carrier and embryo adoption. For some time these options have been lumped together in both consumer and professional thinking as extensions of medical treatment. In this book we are endorsing a change in perspective. While it is true that medical techniques (insemination, IVF or perhaps other ARTs) are required for conception in collaborative reproduction, conception is far from the end of the journey when families are extended by collaborative reproductive options. We believe that it is vital that families making these choices not consider them extensions of treatment, but that they understand that in choosing a collaborative reproductive option, they are embarking on a psycho-social and emotional journey with life-long consequences for all involved—would-be parents, third party participants, and, most of all, the children brought into the world as a result of collaborative reproduction. We believe that collaborative reproduction must be thought of more importantly as a psycho-social issue than as a medical issue

For this reason we want to make clear that, unlike many books about the infertility experience, this is not a book centered on medicine and treatment. While we will offer limited medical information that would-be parents need to have to make informed decisions, our basic focus in *Having Your Baby Through Egg Donation* will be on the psycho-social ramifications of having and parenting a baby using the ova of a donor. While the book presents many facts, it does not claim to be objective. Our book contains the strong, experientially-informed opinions of its authors.

We have written this book as a guide to your journey toward making decisions about whether or not to use donated ova. Whatever brings you to consider oocyte donation, we assume that the experience has not been easy. We hope that this book will offer you comfort, guidance, information and support as you make your way. We hope, also, that it will remind you that you are not alone. Others have traveled this path before you, and many women and men traverse it now.

Throughout this book we will be introducing you to people whose lives have been touched by oocyte donation. We include their stories and their voices not only to make you more familiar with egg donation, but also to offer you a sense of companionship. You will see, again and again, that egg donation touches the lives of a wide range of people who turn to it for varied reasons.

Here, in the introduction, we introduce you to one family—the Gordons. We have selected them for our introduction because their story and their perspective cover the central themes in this book. As with all the families who have shared their stories with us, we have changed their names, geographical location and occupations in an effort to respect their privacy. We have not changed key facts central to their story.

Meet Carla, Rob, Rebecca, Jennifer, Jake and Matt

A visitor arriving at Carla and Rob Gordon's home has an immediate reaction: **KIDS!** The Gordons' spacious front porch is filled with bikes, sporting equipment, a double stroller. A glance to the back yard reveals a swing set and a trampoline. *This is a busy family,* one thinks. *This is a home filled with kids.*

And indeed it is, but it was not always this way. Fifteen years ago, when Carla and Rob bought an old colonial farmhouse in what was then a quiet, rural town about 65 miles north of Boston, they were looking forward to having a child. Then, another. They were 26 years old, recently married, newly minted master's-trained teachers who chose to buy in "Rutherford," MA (we are changing all names.) because it was affordable, had good schools and seemed to be an all around fine place to raise a family. First came love, then came marriage, then came the house and now for the baby carriage.

Like many couples who come upon infertility unexpectedly, Carla and Rob were initially baffled when Carla did not conceive. After all, they were young, led very healthy lives, had no family history of infertility and had been dutifully using birth control since first they met. *Who us?* they thought. *Not us. We were made to have babies.*

And they certainly were, but not yet. When they had been trying to for a year, Carla sought medical attention, assuming that the problem was hers. Fortunately, her physician did not make the same mistake and told her that before he did any testing on her, he wanted Rob to do a semen analysis. "After all," Carla's physician said, "It is the man about half the time."

And indeed it was, but not entirely. Rob was tested and the couple was told that he had a very low sperm count—so low, in fact, that it was "fruitless" for the couple to try to conceive with Rob's sperm. The Gordons were stunned and upset that anyone could dismiss Rob's paternity so cavalierly and usher them on to donor sperm "as if it were nothing."

In fact, thinking about donor sperm was hardly "nothing!" Carla and Rob remember spending several months thinking about DI, all the while "hoping the doctor was wrong and that we'd get pregnant on our own." But that didn't happen, Carla and Rob spent a good deal of time talking about what it would mean to have a child who was genetically connected to Carla but not to Rob, especially since Carla would carry the child for nine months. After a time, the Gordons realized that they were beginning to feel receptive to the idea of using donor sperm. It was time to pick a donor.

When they made the decision to use donor sperm, Carla and Rob felt a sense of relief. "We'd done all the hard work—or so we thought." The couple felt certain that deciding on donor sperm was the difficult part and that picking a donor would be an easier task. The process of decision-making had brought them closer together, and both approached donor selection with optimism. "We'd have some fun with it. We'd look at profiles closely. We'd find someone we really wanted to have as a part of our family."

The Gordons' sense of fun and optimism carried them only so far and lasted only so long. The couple, who had expected to conceive easily on their own, now anticipated conceiving immediately with the first donor they selected. Neither could ever have anticipated trying with three donors and going through a series of fertility treatments all the way up to IVF.

"Eventually we did conceive, and by that time, it practically didn't matter that it was with donor sperm," says Rob. He remembers just wanting a baby and not caring so much how the baby came. But for Carla, it was different. She recalls being pregnant with the couple's first daughter, Rebecca, and worrying that Rob wouldn't love this baby. When Rebecca was born and Rob was not as involved and attentive as Carla was, she worried that her fears had come to pass. It was not until one day—a week or two into motherhood—that she burst into tears and said, "I'm so sad that you don't love her." What a relief it was for Carla when Rob looked at her, baffled and confused, and said, "Of course I do. Of course I do."

And of course he did. Rob and Rebecca were close from the start and remain so, even as Rebecca, now eleven, heads towards adolescence. For Carla, watching her husband and their first-born share such a strong bond has been a source of great joy and relief. Her pleasure has increased all the more since the couple's second daughter, Jennifer, came along. Jennifer was not conceived with donor sperm: Rob is her biological father.

So how did that happen, you ask? Thrilled with Rebecca, Carla and Rob returned to the fertility clinic that had "given us our daughter" and requested "the same again." They wanted the same donor, the same treatment and hoped for the same outcome. To their surprise, the physician responded to their request with a very different recommendation, "I know that we told you something different a few years ago, but with the use of ICSI—intracytoplasmic sperm injection—we believe that you can probably conceive with Rob's sperm."

This news startled Rob and Carla as much as the original bleak pronouncement had a few years earlier. They were, however, happy to take the doctor up on his offer to try IVF with Rob's sperm. Fortunate to live in Massachusetts, which has enjoyed an insurance mandate since 1985, the Gordons did not have to worry about the cost of treatment. Insurance would cover IVF and ICSI, and if treatment didn't work, there was nothing ventured, nothing lost financially. They would simply turn to DI again. DI had blessed them with a wonderful first child, and Rob and Carla were certain that it would work again.

This time around it wasn't going to be quite so difficult. The first IVF cycle didn't bring a pregnancy, but it did bring nice evidence of fertilization. The same thing was true the second time around. "We were a little discouraged, but our experience trying to get pregnant a few years earlier had taught us that patience and fortitude pay off."

And indeed they did. Carla was pregnant on the third IVF-ICSI cycle, and she gave birth to Jennifer nine months later.

"Was it amazing for you to be the biological father to your child?" we asked Rob.

"No," he replied. "What was amazing was to see her born at home. Rebecca was there and she was very much a part of things."

A home birth is hardly something that most infertile couples aspire to. "Give me the lights, the instruments, the cast of thousands and all the machines," many veterans of infertility declare. Many—but not Carla Gordon. For Carla, who "hates to take so much as an aspirin," the whole high tech trip through infertility had been difficult, "something I had to cope with because I wanted a baby so much." Now, with a healthy, uneventful pregnancy, she was determined to have as natural an experience as she could—a home birth followed by a long period of nursing.

When Jennifer was 4 years old, baby fever struck again. Although Carla and Rob had initially anticipated having two children and had felt prepared to "bargain for one" before

Rebecca was born, their struggles with infertility had altered their sense of family. "We had come to appreciate what an incredible miracle every child is and we wanted more. The only problem was that I had just about aged out of the picture."

Carla, 26 when it all began, was 40 when she and Rob returned to the fertility center for yet another try. "By this time they had declared that Rob was just fine, but I could see that the doctor was worried about my eggs. He did an FSH and a clomiphene citrate challenge test and came back with news that was remarkably similar to the news we had gotten about Rob nearly fourteen years earlier. 'You are wasting time to try on your own. You should use donor eggs.'

"Donor eggs? When I heard the words, I wasn't the least bit upset—I was ecstatic. The recommendation sent my heart soaring. After all, we'd long ago made peace with the idea of having a child through donor gametes. That work had been done, and we had a wonderful child to show for it. What sent my heart soaring was the news that ovum donors were now available. When we had gone through donor sperm I remembered hearing that women were on waiting lists for years for donated eggs."

"'No, it's become easy to locate a donor,' our doctor told us. He put us in touch with a lawyer who specializes in finding donors and helps match them with recipients. We made an appointment and eagerly piled the girls into the car for what would be the newest Gordon family project," Carla continues. "The lawyer was lovely but when he saw the children, he seemed a little surprised and confused. He pointed to them and asked how we could look at donor profiles when our children were with us. 'Oh, they came to help us,' I explained. Then he looked really surprised."

Indeed Rebecca and Jennifer were there to help their parents select a donor. Needless to say, the real choice would be the parents' decision, but Rebecca and Jennifer, who have both known about their own origins for as long as they can remember, wanted to be part of things. For them, it is entirely natural for families to be created in all sorts of ways and for parents to talk openly and honestly with their children about assisted reproduction and gamete donation.

Carla and Rob found a donor they liked. They were pleased to find that egg donation—at least with their lawyer—was more open than sperm donation had been for them. They were able to talk with their donor and to exchange letters and pictures in a non-identifying way. The process was set in motion, and to

Carla and Rob's surprise, she was pregnant on the first cycle. But there was to be a bigger surprise up ahead.

When Carla and Rob learned that she was carrying twins, they were stunned. Having spent over a decade in reproductive medicine, they were well aware that twins were always a possibility, but as Rob put it, "We weren't surprised, we were shocked."

Last year Carla gave birth to baby boys, Jake and Matt. When asked how this—her donor egg pregnancy—felt different from the others, Carla comments first on the fact that it was twins, then on the fact that she felt like an "old mother," and only then on the fact that the twins came from a donor.

"I felt that if I couldn't give them my genes, I could grow them as best I could. I did everything I could to eat well, rest well, take care of myself and to carry them as long as I could." Carla goes on to add that she carried the twins until 39 weeks and gave birth to them vaginally. And if that is not remarkable enough, the twins weighed 8 pounds 3 ounces and 6 pounds 13 ounces at birth!

And so that is how the Gordons' front porch came to exclaim, "Kids!" It doesn't announce "Donor Sperm" or "Donor Egg" or "IVF" or "ICSI". The bikes and sporting equipment and the double stroller, like life inside the home, say that this is what it is—a normal, natural, content and thriving family.

But what do the kids think? you might be thinking. *How do the children cope with information about donor insemination or egg donation? And how could the parents have been brave enough to tell them? I wouldn't be that brave,* you fear.

Carla and Rob do not see themselves as brave, nor do they see their children as suffering, in any way, from knowing how their family came to be. Rather, the Gordons feel that the topic is one to be handled honestly and openly with their children. Moreover, they are happy to tell all of their children how much they wanted them, how hard they worked to have them, how grateful they are to the donors who helped them and above all, how thrilled they are to be their parents. It is a joyous story, and one that is revisited in different ways, at different times.

As open as the Gordons have been at home, both are clear that the story of how their family came to be is a private matter. Beyond their minister, their reproductive endocrinologist, their obstetrician and Rob's mother, who learned because Rebecca told her, almost no one knows what Rob and Carla did to create their family. "We feel it is the children's private information and it is theirs to share, as they wish, when they wish." Thus far, Rebecca, the only Gordon child really old enough to talk about donor conception with others, has chosen to keep her story private.

When asked if they have any regrets, the Gordons smile and say, "No, only gratitude." But then Carla pauses for a moment and speaks a truth about the legacy of infertility. "I have a terrific family. I'm having a blast. I couldn't be happier, but I'll admit, I still wonder what it would be like to just find myself pregnant. I know it is a pipe dream at this point, as my eggs are old and I know that our lives are full with children, but how amazing, how wonderful it would be to just one day wake up and find myself pregnant." With this Carla pauses for a moment and then jumps up, one of the twins is crying and it is time to pick up Jennifer from school.

We thank the Gordons for introducing several of the themes that run through this book.

Reproductive Medicine Is a Changing Field

When I (Ellen) first called Carla Gordon and asked her to be interviewed for this book, she responded "Sure. Our family spans the history of modern infertility treatment."

Indeed, this is a changing field. Rob Gordon, the biological father of three children, was once told he would never father a child. Carla Gordon, in her mid-twenties when she first attempted pregnancy, never anticipated she would be turning to an egg donor as she neared 40. We cannot begin to fathom the changes that will occur between now and the time the Gordon children are ready to start families of their own.

On March 11, 2004, just days after I met with the Gordons, Dr. Jonathan L. Tilly, a researcher at Massachusetts General Hospital in Boston, announced findings that could revolutionize the treatment of female infertility. In a paper in the journal *Nature*, Tilly reported studies of mice that found their eggs dying off much more rapidly than assumed. However, in mice, the ovum supply was quickly replenished by stem cells. At this time, these findings are considered controversial and have yet to be replicated, but if they are eventually proven and can be applied to humans, there is the possibility that stem cells could be preserved and used when a woman wanted to have a child.

Another promising technical advance which, as we were writing, seemed to be moving rapidly from the strictly experimental toward more widespread application was the successful thawing and insemination of frozen eggs, followed by successful pregnancy and birth.

These and other rapidly changing technologies are examples of the snowballing effect of technical research on family building. As we watch these growing options that move well beyond the traditional use of eggs and sperm of a couple committed to parenting together we have come to believe that something else needs to change, too: in collaborative family building alternatives, mental health must now trump medicine. This conviction is another element that makes this book so different from previous books on infertility.

People Make Decisions Based on Their Changing Reality

We acknowledge throughout this book, yours is an unexpected journey. Although there are those among you who have anticipated egg donation for many years, the majority of women who conceive through donated ova never expected to travel this path. We know of no little girls who play with dolls and say, "Someday I am going to be a mommy with someone else's egg."

People come to egg donation after loss. You learn you were born without ovaries; you learn your eggs are "old" (even if you are not); you lose your ovarian function because of chemotherapy. Things happen. Your reality changes, and as it does, you come to see your options through a different lens.

Throughout this book, we will remind you repeatedly to "never say never."

Again, the Gordons' story is illustrative. When I (Ellen) first met Carla and Rob, they had just learned of Rob's infertility. As a couple, they were first grappling with questions of donor sperm. If someone had told them then that even with donor sperm, they would have to try IVF three times, they would have exclaimed "Never." Surely, if someone had told them that Rob's sperm would be capable of fertilizing an ova, they would have exclaimed "Never," in total bafflement. And, no doubt, the information that their third and fourth children would be conceived through egg donation would have startled them. You get the picture: their reality changed, and with it, their perspective.

The Importance of Truth Telling

Carla and Rob Gordon are open, honest parents who speak comfortably with their children about how they came to be a family. Unfortunately, not all parents through gamete donation speak with such honesty and confidence. Ironically, the very people who worked so hard to be parents and who should be able to proudly tell their children how deeply they wanted them are sometimes afraid to do so.

Thanks, in large measure, to the outspoken voices of people born through both adoption and sperm donation, attitudes are changing. Nonetheless, there remains a notion among some that ovum donation should be a secret. If you attend a talk on egg donation or read materials from an egg donor program, you will repeatedly hear or see the word *disclosure*. The use of this word—even by those who advocate disclosure–implies that there is a secret and a choice about whether it will remain a secret.

We do not see it that way, and we will not try to be objective on this point. We see no reason why egg donation should ever be something to be cloaked in secrecy and in the shame that inevitably attends a secret. You will hear this again and again from us throughout the book: this should be a proud and happy story. Plain and simple, **our belief is that there is no reason to lie to your children.**

Acting in the Best Interests of Children

Reproductive medicine exists to create children for people who want to parent them. These would-be parents are the "clients" of reproductive medicine centers and, in many instances, of gamete donation programs. Nonetheless, the primary concern should not be to please would-be parents nor the women who offer to help them. Rather, attention should always be paid—first and foremost—to the well-being of children. In the case of egg donation, we are often talking about unborn children.

Throughout this book, we pay close attention to the best interests of children. Adults, whether they are recipient couples or egg donors, should be capable of making informed decisions for themselves. But who speaks for the children? Their rights must be attended to and protected. Among these rights we include the right to know the truth about their origins, the right to information about their genetic ancestry, the right to privacy, and the right to parents who are of childrearing age.

This last right is increasingly difficult to define. We see from Carla Gordon's story the impact of age. Although Carla was in her mid-20s when she and Rob first attempted pregnancy, she was in her late-30s when the couple was ready for a third child. Age took its toll, and like so many older women, Carla was grateful that egg donation was available. She is an older mom for her twins, but she will still be in her 50s when they graduate from high school. Although there are couples in their late 40s, even over 50, turning to egg donation, we have serious questions about what it will mean to their children to have parents on Social Security during the children's teen years.

People Feel Differently about Genetics and Gestation

Women who donate eggs, whether to family members, friends or strangers, are able to do so because they do not see an ova as "their child." When asked what the oocyte means to them, they will often liken it to blood—a valuable and useful part of their bodies that they can give to someone else because they do not need it.

Not everyone feels this way. There are many women who say they "could never give away my genetic material." Often these same women can say with confidence, "I'd be happy to carry someone else's baby for them, but I could never give them my eggs."

Our point is that people feel very differently about genetics and gestational ties. For some, all that really matters are the genetic ties— these are the links to generations past and future. To others, it is the act of pregnancy—of gestating a child and giving birth—that really matters.

It is important, as you read this book, for you to think about how you feel about genes and gestation. There is no "right" or "wrong," "better" or "worse." We are simply acknowledging the natural differences among people. You need to understand where you are on the genes-gestation spectrum *and* where your partner is. Only then can you face decisions about egg donation clearly and honestly. If genetic ties are crucial to you, you may be most comfortable with an intra-family donation if one is available to you. Or you may decide to pursue adoption, feeling "it is only fair that if one of us cannot have a genetic tie to our child, neither of us can."

The Gordon family represents a spectrum of genetic and gestational bonds. Carla has gestational ties to all four of her children but genetic ties to two. Rob, who was prepared to parent without any physical ties to his children, ended up with genetic links to three or his four children. The parents and the children are aware of the differences that exist in the family, but, as Carla explains it, these differences are simply there. For example, she feels a touch of pleasure when Rebecca comments on how much she and Jake—who share no genetic link—look alike.

Carrying and Delivering a Baby Forges Strong Bonds

Having just acknowledged that genes are of paramount importance to some people and of relatively less importance to others, we turn to the significance of pregnancy. Even those who would choose a genetic connection over a gestational one if they could make that choice often find that carrying a child for nine months—or sharing a pregnancy with one's partner for nine months—forges powerful bonds. Carla Gordon, who shared a genetic connection with only her first two children, spoke to this bond when she so proudly affirmed, "I grew all of their hearts, I grew all of their brains, and I fed all four of them for nine months and grew them with all the love I could possibly give."

Donated eggs are not for everyone. Some of you will read our first few chapters and decide, for reasons unique to you, that you will take a different path. But for those of you who do choose to attempt pregnancy through egg donation, we hope this observation of pregnancy is encouraging. You may not be able to create your child, but it will be your body that nurtures and cares for your child for nine months, and it will be you who will give birth to him/her.

Couples Can Strengthen Their Relationships as They Journey through Infertility and Gamete Donation

"Whatever doesn't break us, will make us stronger." This certainly applies to infertility, which is, for most couples, a devastating life crisis. Although some relationships may crumble under the stress of infertility, many are strengthened. Surely the process of exploring and possibly attempting an egg donor pregnancy has the potential to strengthen a relationship. The process forces people to take a serious look at why they want to be parents together, how they will share a parenthood that is not genetically equal, how they will respect the importance of privacy while avoiding the hazards of secrecy.

Pregnancy and Parenthood through Egg Donation Are Legitimate and Authentic

If you choose donated ova, you should do so believing that you have a right to this decision and to the child or children it brings into your life. Sadly, we meet women who work so hard to conceive through egg donation and react to a positive pregnancy test by feeling "fake." Although this feeling seems to diminish as a pregnancy unfolds, some feelings of being not-quite-a-real-parent linger, sometimes even after a child is born. We remind you again of Carla Gordon's affirming words, "I grew their hearts, I grew their brains…" If you make this choice and if it works, *you* will grow your baby. More important, still, *you* will raise this child. You'll be the tooth fairy and the car pool pick-up and the one who lies awake at night when your newly minted driver is out on the road. If that isn't real parenthood, we don't know what is!

Consider the Potential for Regret when You Make Decisions

No one has a crystal ball, yet we attempt to predict the future when we make decisions. When faced with difficult life decisions, it often helps to try to imagine yourself in the future, looking back. Deciding to have a child through egg donation may seem like an incredible leap of faith, but that leap may feel less daunting when you consider not having a child at all or choosing adoption and missing out on the pregnancy experience and a genetic link to one parent.

The Meaning of Donor Conception Changes over Time

When they first think about having a baby through egg donation, many people struggle with the concept. Women fear they will not feel like "real" mothers. This is a concern that remains with many, even well into parenthood. However, as time passes, as diapers are changed, these concerns are likely to fade and others arise. Dr. Maggie Kirkman, an Australian psychologist and researcher who has interviewed many women who are mothers through egg donation, confirms, "One of the most notable findings in my research is the way in which the meaning of donor assisted conception, including egg donation, changes over time and according to what else is happening in the family's life." As she picks up toys scattered about, rushes to drive carpool and hurries to get to soccer practice, Carla Gordon will certainly agree that her focus has changed!

The People You Meet along the Way Will Shape Your Journey

As you consider egg donation, you will be talking with physicians, nurses, mental health counselors, parents through donated ova and, possibly, egg donors. The things people say to you and the approaches they take to this decision will influence your decision-making. You will also be influenced by the comments—knowing and unknowing—of friends, family and acquaintances. Ultimately, you will be making your own decision, but it would be foolish for us to suggest that that decision is made in a vacuum. We are introducing you to the Gordons and to others, hoping their experiences will help you navigate your own journey.

Finances and Geography Will Influence Your Decisions

As if infertility wasn't enough, people considering egg donation often face geographical and financial challenges. Depending upon the laws in the state or country where you live, egg donation may be more or less available to you. If you live in Italy, it will be nearly impossible for you to pursue this option. If you live in the U.S., in a state which mandates health insurance coverage for egg donation, the process may be within your reach. Carla and Rob Gordon faced some hurdles in building their family, but they were fortunate, all the while, to live in Massachusetts, where there has been fully mandated coverage for infertility and for oocyte donation since the mid-1980s.

The Blessing and Curse of the Meant to Be

"Oh it was meant to be," well-intentioned people declare upon hearing a couple has had a miscarriage. Or you may say to yourselves, "Maybe we were not meant to be parents?" Both are examples of what we call "the curse of the meant to be." How cruel is it to declare that someone who deeply desires a child is not "meant to be" a parent?

On the other hand, there is a "blessing of the meant to be." The blessing comes when things unfold in an unexpected way and the outcome, although not the one originally intended, is a good one. You have twins through donor eggs. They are wonderful. It was "meant to be." You adopt a little girl from China. She captivates you and you are certain, it was "meant to be."

The Chinese believe that there is a tiny, not quite visible, red thread that connects people who belong together. The blessing of the meant to be and a belief in the red thread offer comfort.

Some Things You Should Know about This Book

Our Readers

Although we would be delighted to hear that this book was helpful to a range of readers, we have written it with certain "populations" in mind. We assume that most of our readers will be women who have learned, for various reasons, that they are unable to become pregnant using their own eggs. We hope that their husbands or partners will also read this book and perhaps, that they will share it will family members, especially if the family is involved in intrafamily donation.

We are both in the U.S. (although in different cities and regions) and hence, much of our reference point is the U.S. However, we have spoken with people around the world for this book and have included their voices and perspectives within it. We hope that our international readers will feel included and forgive us if some of our information, especially the legal pieces, is U.S. specific.

The Book's Organization

When we set out to write this book, we were both overwhelmed by the range of material we wanted and needed to cover. To make the book more manageable for our readers, we decided to divide it into two kinds of material. The first several chapters offer you a "walk through" the decision-making in egg donation. It introduces the topic to readers, lets you know who else considers this option, takes you through decision-making about egg donation in general and then addresses specific questions of donor selection. The section continues with an introduction to the medical process and concludes with chapters on pregnancy and on parenting after egg donation.

In the second several chapters we cover specific topics related to egg donation. In this section, you will be able to read about egg donor programs, where contractual donors are available, and about the ethical issues raised by egg donation. Here we talk also about religion and about the special considerations that arise when gay and lesbian couples explore having a baby through oocyte donation. Finally, we offer a section that contains additional resources.

Repetition

You will find that certain things are repeated in several places in this book. Specifically, we repeat the central themes of the book and we repeat some of the legal and ethical issues in several places. The reason for this repetition is that we do not expect all of our readers to read the entire book. When something needed to be in a particular chapter, we included it, even if we felt it also needed to be included in another chapter.

Some Words about Language

We are aware that some people object to the use of the word *donor* when a woman receives payment, even if it seems clear that the payment is for her time and effort. Some would advise us to say *provider* rather than *donor*. Although we feel that there are instances in which *provider* is the more appropriate term, we like to believe that the majority of women who give their eggs to someone else do see it as a gift. The word *donor* appears to honor that gift more than does the word *provider*.

On the other hand, we will not use the word *disclosure*. This word is often used in reference to truth-telling with children. To us, the word *disclosure* implies a secret. Since we see no secret, we will simply say—again and again—that we feel parents need to be truthful with their children.

Perhaps the biggest semantic challenge we faced in writing this book, was figuring out how to refer to those egg donors who are neither family members nor friends. They have often been called *anonymous donors*, but since we have strong feelings that they should not be anonymous to their recipients and to the offspring, this word did not seem an apt description. Nor did we want to call them *paid donors*, since the fees they receive are considered compensation for time and effort, not payment for ova. Similarly, *commercial donors* did not seem right. Since all donors enter into contracts, the term *contractual donors* didn't work, either. Finally we decided that the clearest term to distinguish between those donors who were friends or family members of their recipients beforehand and those who did not know their ovum recipients beforehand was to refer to the way in which they were located and matched with a recipient—by being recruited by a medical practice or agency program. We will refer to them as *program-recruited donors*.

This book is meant to be both challenging and supportive. We hope you will enjoy it and find it helpful.

Note

[1] ©1987 by Emily Perl Kingsley. All rights reserved. Reprinted by permission of the author. We are proud to be able to properly credit this poignant essay, which is often labeled "author unknown" or adapted without proper credit. Emily Perl Kingsley may be contacted at EPKingsley@aol.com

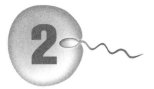

An Overview of Egg Donation

Ovum donation is changing the way we think about family building. Now young women born without ovaries can carry, deliver and parent children conceived with the help of their sisters or friends or strangers. Now women who survive cancer at the expense of their fertility are able to experience pregnancy and the joy of bringing new life into the world. And yes, women can "turn back their biological clocks," extending their fertility past menopause.

Egg donation is still evolving, and should you decide to participate in egg donation, you will be part of its early history. With every new egg donor or egg recipient, all of us learn a little more about the egg donation process—medically, psychologically, ethically and socially. In this chapter, we attempt to provide you with a context in which to view egg donation past, present and future. Although we anticipate that most of our readers will be in the United States, we try here—and throughout the book—to include a worldwide perspective.

Historical Perspective

So how did it all begin? There are published records from as early as the late 1800s of experiments conducted on women who lost their own ovaries at young ages. In the early 1900s doctors began to use intra-uterine insemination with a husband's own sperm. This was followed by the use of artificial insemination with a donor's sperm, which became more and more common. After repeated successes with donor sperm, people began to wonder if it was possible to utilize donated ova as well. A technique called lavage was introduced. This procedure was very complicated and was conducted over a period of several days. As the donor woman ovulated, she was artificially inseminated with the recipient's husband's sperm. After several days, the embryo was "washed" out of the donor's uterus and then implanted into the recipient mother. Unfortunately, sometimes the embryo was not actually "washed out", but instead remained in the donor's uterus, leaving her pregnant. Also, because the "washing" had to occur so early in the pregnancy, sometimes it was done before fertilization had actually occurred. As a result, the chance of becoming pregnant using this early procedure was miniscule (*Getting Pregnant When You Thought You Couldn't* by Helane Rosenberg and Yakov Epstein, Warner Books, 2001).

Then, in the early 1970s, came the development of IVF. IVF involves removing an egg from a woman's ovary and combining it with sperm in a laboratory dish. If fertilization occurs, the embryo is transferred to the woman's uterus. For many years, IVF was in the process of being perfected and was attempted many times by doctors in different countries such as the United States, England and Australia with no success. Finally, in 1978, the first baby conceived via IVF, Louise Brown, was born in England. Soon after Brown's birth, several other IVF babies were born, including Elizabeth Carr, the first IVF baby in the United States, conceived at the Jones Institute in Virginia.

With the worldwide development of successful IVF programs, there was no turning back. Although it had been initially developed to assist women with blocked fallopian tubes, it soon became apparent that IVF had multiple applications: it could be used to assist men with very poor semen analysis, and it opened up the possibility of one woman carrying a baby that was not genetically hers. For women without uterine function, IVF heralded the option of gestational care—the infertile woman and her husband/partner could now undergo IVF and have their resulting embryos transferred to another woman's uterus for her to gestate and deliver. This meant that couples could have their full genetic children even when the woman could not undertake a pregnancy. And more to the point of this book, IVF meant that women without eggs or whose ages were no longer viable could gestate and deliver children conceived with their husband's sperm and eggs donated to them, either from a close family member or friend or from someone who sought to help infertile couples have children. In 1984 the first child conceived through egg donation was born in Australia.

In its early years, ovum donation, though possible, was not readily available. At first, donors were most often infertile women who were undergoing IVF and had produced extra eggs. Since cryopreservation of embryos was not available to all, some of these women could choose only to donate their eggs or to discard them. In addition, some women seeking tubal ligation were encouraged to donate their eggs in exchange for the cost of their procedure. Either way, donated eggs were relatively few and far between, and the process of receiving them was indeed a challenge. One mother of a now 16-year-old through egg donation recalls "constantly cycling and being ready for surgery." What she means by this is that she had to take medications to ensure her uterus was ready to receive an embryo should a donated egg come along. Then, in a time before cell phones, she had to remain "on call" for news that an egg was available. When the call came, there was no asking about who the donor was or what her genetic history revealed. The recipient was to immediately rush to the fertility clinic, where she underwent a full laparatomy (a surgical incision in the abdominal area) and a gamete intrafallopian transfer (GIFT) procedure. The donor's eggs were mixed with the recipient's husband's sperm and placed in her tubes.

Much has changed. Not only has IVF fully replaced GIFT as a vehicle for egg donation, but starting in the late 1980s, fertility clinics began recruiting donors on their own, largely through newspaper and magazine advertisements. It was not uncommon to see a print ad that read,

> "Make a dream come true. Help a childless couple become parents. If you are under 34, healthy, a non-smoker, please consider donating some of your eggs. You will be compensated for your time and effort."

An ad like this one might be placed by a medical program or by an individual couple, who then directed all respondents to a specific egg donor program. This process of locating potential donors turned out to be a challenging one—it was labor intensive, yielded relatively few donors and resulted in long waits for donors and a fair amount of frustration and disappointment for recipients. Medical programs soon began to publicize compensation for egg donation. This increased the population of women willing to donate and provided interested recipients with a list of donors from which to choose.

With widespread advertising for donors, free-standing egg donation programs arrived. These are programs that function much like cryobanks for sperm—they recruit, screen (medically, psychologically and socially) prospective donors, help to match those donors with appropriate recipients, and coordinate everyone's medical care with a fertility center. The arrival of these programs transformed egg donation from something which was difficult to arrange to something that, with financial/health insurance resources and access to medical treatment, could be initiated through a few visits to internet web sites.

Where Are We Today?

Egg donation is still a relatively new procedure, but it is becoming increasingly common. Today there are over 300 fertility clinics in the United States, many of which offer services related to egg donation. Some fertility clinics estimate over ten percent of their patients are pursuing egg donation. Over the past twenty years, over 100,000 babies have been born worldwide as a result of egg donation. This number continues to grow each year, especially as more women are waiting longer to begin their families, as others survive cancer at the cost of their ovarian function, and as still others experience premature ovarian failure, sometimes as early as their late 20s. Similarly, each year, thousands of women choose to donate their eggs to help others achieve pregnancy.

Recently, the media has begun to highlight egg donation, both blatantly and in more subtle ways. A nurse working in reproductive medicine recently commented, "*PEOPLE Magazine* and *US* should be banned from fertility clinic waiting rooms." When asked what she has against two publications which enjoy such widespread popularity, she replied, "They mislead women. The stories of movie stars in their mid-40s give women the mistaken impression they can have babies at any age. The photos of smiling older moms with twins never acknowledge that the children were almost certainly conceived with donated eggs." This critique of the popular press says a lot about ovum donation in the United States, at least in the first decade of the 21st century, by providing readers with false information, for example that egg donation is widespread, that it is often used by women who are beyond menopause, and by not always acknowledging that donated ova have been used. Unfortunately, the feature magazines rarely— if ever—provide any specific information about the trials and tribulations evident in many experiences with the oocyte donation process.

A question that has long been asked is "Can eggs be cryopreserved for future use?" Until recently, the answer to this question was "Not yet." According to Dr. Jeffrey Boldt in *Family Building* (2004), "A key to successful freezing and thawing of any cell is to remove as much water from the cell as possible before it is frozen. If this does not occur, large ice crystals form within the cell during the freeze/thaw process and cause irreversible cell damage." Difficulties in removing water and other challenges thwarted scientists from successfully freezing eggs until the late 1990s. Dr. Boldt reports that his program at Indiana University, one of a number of clinics that successfully perform OCP (oocyte cryopreservation), had a total of twelve pregnancies between 1999 and March, 2004. Of these, four resulted in live births and three other patients were still pregnant when he wrote his article.

So there is hope that OCP will enable some women who might otherwise turn to oocyte donation to be able to preserve their own eggs. However, widespread use of OCP is probably still some time away, and for now, many women are relying on ovum donation, which is also the subject of much study and exploration. With new fertility medications and more sophisticated fertility clinics and laboratories, egg donation is becoming increasingly successful. Every day, advances in oocyte donation continue. Efforts are being made to find ways to administer fertility medications without the use of injections, and to find new treatment methods that make the egg donation experience less time consuming and more comfortable.

Ovum Donation around the World

Although egg donation has enjoyed widespread acceptance and relatively little scrutiny in the United States, this is not the case throughout the world. In Italy, for instance, a law was passed in 2004 completely banning oocyte donation, banning as well use of donor sperm and helping women past childbearing age becoming pregnant via ARTs. The road to this law started in 1994 when Italy made headlines when Dr. Severino Antinori used donor eggs to get 63-year-old Rosana Della Cortes pregnant. Robin Marantz Henig's *New York Times* article (2004) states,

> "We are learning the wrong lessons from our earlier misadventures. Things got a little out of hand, yes, but that is because governments around the world adopted a hands-off policy towards the whole affair. It was too complicated to reach consensus about what steps were too intrusive, about when human life begins, about what risks were worth taking for the sake of having one's own biological child. So governments turned their backs on reproductive technology and allowed the field to be taken over by cowboys."

Still unable to come to a consensus about exactly what should be accepted and what should not, countries like Italy, Austria, Norway, Sweden and Switzerland have nearly eliminated ovum donation. While such strict laws serve to call everyone's attention to the potential for ethical abuses in egg donation, they also create new social problems. There now exists what has been termed "fertility tourism"—people living in countries that ban oocyte donation are traveling to other countries to obtain eggs.

Many countries in which IVF and other ARTs are part of national health care plans, such as France, the Netherlands, Spain, the United Kingdom, Canada and Australia, have legislation in place regulating egg donation. These policies especially place restrictions on anonymous donors. The Human Fertilisation and Embryology Authority (HFEA) is a government body in the UK which regulates and inspects all clinics providing IVF and donor conception. Its governing board, which includes people who have had personal experience of donor conception along with experts in the field of reproductive medicine and bioethics, makes important decisions regarding regulations about the way donor conception is carried out. In January, 2003, the UK announced a registry for donor offspring, which was established in 2004 as a pilot project. This voluntary registry enables donor offspring and donors who participated in gamete donation before 1991, when the HFE Act came into being, to exchange information. Since then, over 18,000 children have been born in the United Kingdom with donated gametes. In 2004, the United Kingdom also announced that after April 2005 anyone looking to donate eggs or sperm would no longer be given anonymity. Similarly, some Scandinavian countries have always had open sperm donor files, and clinics in New Zealand do not accept anonymous donors.

Another worldwide difference of note is the use of IVF patients as a source of egg donation or egg sharing. This is allowed and even promoted in Canada, Denmark, India, Israel, Spain and the United Kingdom, as well as sometimes in the United States. Only in Canada, India, and the United States does the government not pay for IVF procedures. Many European countries, particularly those that support egg sharing, provide government funding to women attempting anywhere between two and five cycles of IVF. Many feel that this method of including egg sharing among government-funded IVF cycles ensures "more bang for the government's buck." On the other hand, New Zealand believes that egg donors are only able to give consent without the pressures of financial incentives; as a result, egg donors are not allowed to be paid in any case.

Perhaps the most controversial issue worldwide involves financial compensation to donors. In Australia and the UK, payment is virtually unheard of (in the UK ovum donors can claim discretionary amounts for expenses). However, on November 11, 2004, the British HFEA announced that it is reviewing the question of payment to donors. It is expected that some payment will be allowed and that it will be more than the approximate $25 currently paid to sperm donors, but less than an amount that could be seen as financial enticement. By contrast, the United States has allowed an industry to develop, in which donors commonly receive $5000, as of this writing, for their "time and effort" in donating eggs, and there are many instances in which higher sums are offered or requested. Arguments for and against payment continue to be made worldwide, with those opposing payment feeling that the money makes eggs—and resultant children—"commodities," and with those supporting payment arguing that a woman must undergo a great deal physically, emotionally and socially to donate eggs and should be paid for her efforts. Those who take this position insist that the payment is for effort and *not* for eggs.

Ethical Concerns

It is obvious that while ovum donation has many benefits, it also raises abundant ethical issues. These issues range from concerns about the offspring, some of whom may be forever separated from their genetic "parents," to concerns for the donors, who some argue are being enticed by the payments to do something about which they may later feel regret, to concerns for the recipients, some of whom may be entering into parenthood at advanced age with inadequate understanding of the challenges involved for themselves or their children. Reproductive technology and egg donation practice are moving at such a rapid pace today that many important social, ethical and legal considerations are lagging behind significantly. Many of us, including leaders in the field of reproductive technology, are unsure what the next steps should be.

The most pressing questions in the field of reproductive technology are about who should regulate oocyte donation and how it should it be regulated. Some in the United States feel that this country should follow in the footsteps of those nations which have implemented governmental regulations and restrictions. Others in the United States prefer to have professional organizations, such as those in the field of reproductive medicine, responsible for making these types of decisions rather than government agencies. Still others argue that since egg donation is a multi-disciplinary field, it should be thoughtfully guided by a panel of experts in medicine, science, genetics, psychology, sociology, theology and law. They feel that these professionals can work together for a common goal: to maintain excellent quality of care while considering the affects on greater society.

Regardless of who regulates ovum donation, the questions around regulation all involve protecting the best interests of all participants. First, the **offspring**—the appreciation for the lifelong impact of donation on all participants has come largely from a worldwide movement of "donor offspring" (although all adult "donor offspring" were conceived through donated sperm, not egg donation, they do not differentiate themselves from anonymous egg donor offspring). Many donor insemination offspring throughout the world have spoken poignantly and powerfully about their experiences.

Christine Whipp wrote an article entitled "Why I Need to Find My Father," (*The Western Daily Press*, UK, January 23, 2004). In it, Whipp writes,

> Luckily through the media and the internet I came into contact with other donor offspring from across the globe…It soon became apparent that we share a commonality in our experiences and have identified many uncomfortable issues with which we must deal as a result of the choices made by our parents. These can include feelings of revulsion at the clinical method by which we were produced; a sense of loss and grief for deliberately severed relationships with unknown biological kinfolk; a fear of accidental incest; anger and frustration at the lack of respect shown for our missing genetic origins and the indescribable emotional burdens which we carry as part of an inherited compromise.
>
> Many donor-conceived adults will freely admit that their sense of identity has been damaged and would concur with Cicero that: "To be ignorant of what occurred before you were born is to remain always a child. For what is the worth of human life, unless it is woven into the life of our ancestors by the records of history?"

Whipp goes on to talk about the anxiety some donor offspring feel about missing medical information and adds, "Our dissatisfaction has also been tempered with the knowledge that adoptees in the UK were given the right to access their birth records as long ago as the mid-1970s, yet no official records concerning donor conceptions have been maintained at all until the setting up of the HFEA in 1991."

Unfortunately, many countries, including the United States, have been slow to react to these concerns. Barbara Sumner Burstyn summarizes these sentiments in her article "The New Underclass," (February 7, 2004 in the *New Zealand Herald*) by stating "allowing technology to willfully create an underclass of people who are unaware of their genetic background and to support parents in denying their children their biological history is to continue the social, medical, and emotional disadvantages that have been suffered for generations by adopted people."

PGD, together with other ARTs, also directly led to the ability to carefully evaluate embryos and eliminate defective ones before they are transferred to the uterus. While this increases the chance that couples will have healthy babies, it has sparked the debate about creating "designer" babies. Just how much say should individuals have about what type of baby should be created or destroyed? A recent article out of Australia illustrates two central ethical dilemmas: should people be allowed/encouraged to create "designer babies" and how can "fertility tourism" be regulated? On September 12, 2004, Infertility Network.org reported about "a scene reminiscent of a science fiction movie plot." The article describes how couples in Australia, desperate for donated eggs, are going to the websites of U.S. programs that allow them to "choose the genetic make-up of their future babies by computer. Features ranging from hair colour to intelligence—all based on the donor mother's genetic make up—can be previewed via a website with the click of a mouse."

Next, the **donors**—Donor offspring are not the only ones speaking out about the consequences of anonymous donation. Men who donated sperm years ago have also stepped forward. In an article, "Sperms of Endearment" published in the *Guardian* (UK), the writer tells of "Charlie," 41, who reportedly made thirty one donations while he was a student at Oxford in 1983-85. Now the father of three children, he says that he spends "considerable time these days fretting about possible extra offspring." He reportedly "worries that children he helped create are out there looking for him, tortured by the fog that blurs their beginnings, when he could make them feel better." Charlie argues that it's the secrecy around what he still considers an altruistic act that has been the killer.

Infertility Network.org, April 26, 2004, tells the story of Alan Sykes, a 75-year-old man who, "having fathered six children from two marriages," is in search of the other half of his brood—six more children, born as a result of his sperm donations in the 1980s. Sykes says, "I'd love to meet them. My kids are so wonderful, these must be too." The article goes on to say that Mr. Sykes is also concerned about what he calls "unconscious incest." "What if one of these children meets another donor offspring and they fall in love and want to get married?"

Although sperm donors and egg donors go through different procedures, including different counseling and preparation, we can only assume that eventually some who donate eggs anonymously will face questions similar to those plaguing some sperm donors.

Finally, the **recipients**—Egg donation has allowed older women, many of whom have entered menopause, to turn back their biological clocks and give birth. There are reports of women in their late 50s, even 60s, having babies While this is still not a common occurrence, ovum donation allows its possibility. This forces us to ask, is this a good thing? Some argue that if a woman in her 50s is married to a man in his 30s, why shouldn't they have a child together? Others support this option for a different reason: they say that age brings a wisdom and maturity that can be as valuable in parenting as "youthfulness" and "energy." Either way, the question must be asked: do women who are contemplating pregnancy after their mid-late 40s *really* know what it will be like to try to raise adolescents when they are in their 60s?

Another ethical concern for recipients involves the promotion of anonymity. Until recently, donors and recipient women were often discouraged, sometimes even prevented, from meeting one another. Fortunately, as a result of increasing work with families doing open adoptions, awareness is growing of the potential benefits to the recipient, as well as to the donor and child, of meeting someone you will, in a sense, be connected to for life. It is increasingly common for donors and recipients to meet and to transform "anonymous" donation into a new form of known donation. These meetings may not include fully identifying information, but both donors and recipients proceed with egg donation aware that in some ways, they will have a life-long connection. In her article "Parents Anonymous," in *New Ways of Making Babies* (Indiana Universuty Press, 1996) Cynthia Cohen, Ph.D. J.D. writes,

> The special nature of this gift—assistance in bringing a child into being—obligates recipients to express their gratitude

by viewing donors as more than anonymous surds. It obliges recipients to view them as actual, characterizable, morally considerable persons who are deserving of respect and appreciation. Donors are individuals whose needs, interests, and rights ought to be taken into account in the process of gamete donation. Givers also incur a moral obligation when they provide a gift—the obligation to give a complete gift and not just part of one. The gift that gamete donors give includes their genetic material. To complete this gift, donors must provide recipients, and ultimately the resulting children, with relevant information that may be carried with the genetic material.

Looking to the Future

As we look to the future, questions abound. One that is on many people's minds is this: will some of the women who are now turning to oocyte donation eventually be able to use their own eggs? We expect that the answer will be yes. There are now several clinics worldwide offering oocyte cryopreservation (OCP). As of this writing, it is estimated that 100-120 children have been born worldwide as a result of oocyte cryopreservation (Boldt, 2004). Efforts continue in many reproductive medical centers to improve methods of freezing eggs and in others, to freeze ovarian tissue. In addition, research will soon be underway to try to identify a marker that will help predict women's future fertility. Each of these investigations involves complex science, but there is another initiative underway which is low tech and potentially very effective: gynecologists are being urged to remind their young patients that fertility declines with age. This effort will not make a difference in the lives of women who encounter premature ovarian failure in their late 20s or early 30s, but it should help many women avoid the anguish that comes when a previously-normally-fertile woman over 40 suddenly realizes that she has moved beyond her fertile years.

Other questions prompt us to turn our attention to the changing nature of families. Egg donation has been but one of the factors in recent years that has altered the definition of family. Stepfamilies, gay and lesbian families and interracial families have all changed the way that families look, at least to outsiders. We wonder, however, if the experience of people living in these families is fundamentally different from that of people in "traditional" families?

Questions abound, and those of you who choose egg donation will help others find answers. You are the pioneers, blazing a trail for those who will follow. We realize that most of you didn't set out to be trailblazers. You never sought to do something different. Rather, you set out for the familiar—you wanted to do something people have been doing since the beginning of time. You set out to have children. To build families. To pass something on to future generations.

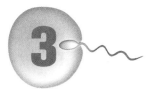

Who Chooses
Egg Donation?

Let's imagine that you are standing in the Departure Lounge for Egg Donation.

It's a large, busy space, and you are, most likely, feeling somewhat bewildered. Whatever it is that brings you to consider egg donation, you are not where you once expected to be in your family building journey. Yes, this departure lounge offers you hope and opportunity, but you are probably feeling a bit dazed. As you look around at others considering ovum donation, you will see a variety of people and a range of expressions on their faces. Some are weary travelers—they have been struggling to become parents for a long time, and their faces reveal the arduousness of their journey. Others look excited and energetic; perhaps this is their first departure lounge. Some women stand alone, some with their husbands or partners, and you may notice a few male couples, as they, too have joined the ranks of those considering and pursuing egg donation.

In the pages that follow, we will introduce the various situations that bring women and men to egg donation—and to some actual people who have chosen parenthood through egg donation. We will also identify some of the specific questions and challenges that face each cohort of prospective egg donor parents. We hope that familiarizing you with fellow travelers will help ease your journey.

Couples in Which the Woman Was Born without Ovaries or without Ovarian Function

There are conditions in which a woman is born without the capacity to produce eggs. The most common of these is Turner's Syndrome, which affects 1 in 2500 female babies. Women with Turner's Syndrome are generally of short stature and have some physical anomalies which include the lack of ovarian function. Most are born with "streaked ovaries"—ovaries that do not contain eggs. Prior to the arrival of ova donation, women with Turner's Syndrome were unable to bear children.

We can easily imagine what the opportunity to carry a baby must mean to someone with Turner's Syndrome. In that regard, they may be "traveling lighter" than others in the egg donation departure lounge. Although some will choose adoption, many will regard oocyte donation as a gift, one which enables them to use that part of their reproductive function that has not been impacted by Turner's Syndrome.

Some Special Issues and Considerations

As we mentioned, couples in which the woman has Turner's Syndrome may face fewer decisions than those with other reasons for considering egg donation. These couples know, usually from the time they first meet, that they will not be creating a full biological child together. The opportunity to share a pregnancy, to have a child connected genetically to one parent and gestationally to the other is inviting. In addition, since women with Turner's Syndrome have a condition that is evident to their family and friends, they are among those most likely to have someone near to them offer to donate.

Unfortunately, it is not so simple. Many women with Turner's Syndrome have a coarctation of the aorta—not enough blood flows to their aorta. This condition makes pregnancy hazardous. In addition, some women with Turners are born with a small uterus, making pregnancy difficult in this regard as well.

....

Meet Tina

When Tina was 16 she received a tentative diagnosis of Turner's Syndrome. She was small for her age and had not begun to menstruate. However, her physician and the specialists she subsequently saw told her that she did not have "classic Turner's." Her heart was normal and she was fortunate that her uterus was of normal size.

"You are a mosaic," they told her.

"I asked what a mosaic was and they told me that I have some of the features of Turner's but not the ones that would make pregnancy inadvisable."

Fourteen years later, Tina became a mother through egg donation. Her first cousin, Rachel, was a few years older, had two children, and knowing Tina's situation, offered to donate ova. "For me it was an incredible gift. I felt that something which had been taken away from me when I was 16 was suddenly returned. I got to have a baby with Dave, my husband, to 'enjoy' all the aches and pains of pregnancy and even to have a child with some of the same family history."

Couples in Which the Woman Has Poor Ovarian Response or Premature Ovarian Failure

Women are born with all the eggs that they will ever have, and, beginning even before their first menstruation, they begin to use up those oocytes very early. Reproductive medicine has long known that female fertility declines from age 20 on, accelerates its decline after age 35 and leaves relatively few women fertile past age 40. Although there are other factors, such as the higher incidence of uterine fibroids in older women, the primary reason for declining fertility is a decline in the quality of the eggs remaining in the ovaries. Surprisingly enough, a woman's uterus may remain quite capable of carrying a baby to term when the mother is well into her 40s and even, 50s, but her supply of ova—and the quality of eggs within that supply—are usually poor by the time she reaches 40.

Because women in their 20s and early 30s are assumed to have "young, healthy eggs," most couples with women in this age group do not anticipate infertility—at least not infertility due to egg quality. Sadly, there are young couples who happily decide to have a baby, expecting that it will happen easily and quickly, who are shocked and surprised to learn that a woman so young can have "old eggs" or even to appear to have entered menopause.

Because there has been no reason to assume "an egg problem," some young women with poor egg quality try for years to conceive (often having early miscarriages) before they learn that their eggs are, most likely, the cause of their infertility. They may learn this when a physician takes—and re-takes—a Day 3 FSH level, or requests that they do a "clomiphene challenge test" or measures certain hormones such as estrogen. Each of these tests can provide some indication of a problem with egg quality.

As if it is not confusing enough, there are some women whose FSH and other levels appear to be fine, but who, nonetheless, are probably infertile due to poor egg quality. These women—and their husbands—are usually considered to have "unexplained infertility" until they undergo a stimulated cycle for an intrauterine insemination (IUI) or in vitro fertilization (IVF). To everyone's surprise, these women are then found to be "poor responders." This unfortunate label refers to those women who, even when prescribed large amounts of potent ovulation-stimulating drugs, "fail" to produce more than a few follicles. Or they may produce follicles that are found to be empty or to contain ova that do not fertilize or that deteriorate soon after fertilization.

However they come upon it, the diagnosis of poor ovum quality or premature ovarian failure (POF) in a young woman is bewildering and often devastating. Women wonder how this could be, what they might have done to harm their eggs, why they had "no warning" of a problem. Indeed, they, like their fellow travelers, will learn, again and again, that reproduction is a mystery. At the time of diagnosis, it is only natural to look for answers, for causes, for blame and responsibility.

Women who learn that they have this problem may focus on what they have heard from popular media. For example, physicians and scientists have speculated that there may be environmental factors, such as exposure to toxic chemicals, which damage both eggs and sperm although there is no clear documentation of this in any scientific studies. On the other hand, they may focus on less "logical" explanations such as fearing that it was anything from ambivalence about motherhood to an earlier abortion that has cursed them with "bad eggs." In fact, other than chemotherapy, radiation and surgery, which we will discuss, there is no explanation for most cases of premature ovarian failure.

Some Special Issues and Considerations

When a young, typically under 35, woman learns that she has "old eggs," she faces several questions. The first is, "Is the condition permanent?" While a 44-year-old woman with high FSH should be pretty certain that her egg supply is not going to be replenished, a young woman may wonder if the condition might reverse itself. Most reproductive endocrinologists have had a patient, here and there, who had elevated FSH, or otherwise documented poor ovarian quality, and who spontaneously became pregnant. Despite high levels of FSH, one egg of decent quality happens to become fertilized. However, we strongly stress that this is not the norm and is most often the result of good fortune.

In addition to the unrealistic hope for a spontaneous reversal and pregnancy, questions inevitably arise about what a woman might do to improve her egg quality. Since it is a mystery how her ova became "old" in the first place, she must also wonder whether there is something she can do to improve her egg quality. Some women have turned to acupuncture, diet or herbal remedies in an effort to reinvigorate or regenerate their eggs. In the book *Inconceivable: A Woman's Triumph over Despair and Statistics* (2001), author Julia Indichova claims to have lowered her FSH through more holistic approaches.

As of this writing, evidence of women improving their egg quality through "alternative" therapies, diet, etc. is anecdotal. Academic research has shown no treatment that is known to create more or better eggs. For the most part, a young woman with premature ovarian failure is left to assume that the eggs she has are the ones she will have.

The young women who come to the departure lounge for egg donation because they have "old eggs," may not be so quick to request egg donation. For one thing, they may need to take some time before they are really convinced that they can't use their own oocytes. For another, they may believe that if they wait long enough, medical science, with its ever unfolding advances, will arrive at a solution. Or they may simply want to wait a bit in the hope that they may be one of the lucky ones who find themselves unexpectedly pregnant.

So one issue for younger women with ovarian failure is the timing of egg donation. Of all the folks in the departure lounge, they will be among the most reluctant to "jump into" egg donation. Hoping that time is on their side, they may choose to delay their efforts.

There are other reasons for waiting. Cost is one. Ovum donation is costly, and young couples are the least likely to have the savings at hand to pursue this option. For them, infertility is all the more devastating because it comes at a time when they are still launching their careers and perhaps saving for a house.

Another reason for waiting is the potential for a sister-to-sister or cousin-to-cousin donation. Of all the prospective egg donor recipients, young women are usually the ones with the greatest likelihood of having a sister or cousin young enough to donate eggs. A young recipient may postpone egg donation efforts because she is hoping a family member will make an offer or because she wants to wait until her sister or cousin has completed her family.

....

Meet Terry

Terry is a woman who exudes vitality. This skin care specialist, athlete, and community volunteer is now 32 years old. Terry and her husband, Dave, have wanted a baby for what seems to be as long as they can remember. They began trying to conceive when Terry was 27, learned when she was 29 that she had "old eggs," and spent the next three years trying to determine what to do.

When Terry first heard about egg donation she was "horrified." A very "traditional" woman and a devout Catholic, she felt it was "weird" and "wrong" for one woman to pay another to donate eggs to her. Terry has a sister who would have donated to her, but Terry felt that that was "even stranger" than anonymous donation. No, it was clear to Terry, at least at the start, that adoption, not egg donation, would be her path to parenthood.

"You will never believe what I am going to say," Terry exclaimed in a counseling session one day last year.

"I've decided to try egg donation."

When asked about her dramatic change of heart, Terry explained, "The past few years have brought Dave and me closer and closer together. Recently, when we were talking about adoption, he said, 'I know you don't want to do egg donation, but I'm curious, because it is half an adoption.' Something clicked with me at that moment. For the first time I thought to myself. 'I'm happy to adopt, but wouldn't it be really amazing to be able to have Dave's child.'"

Couples in Which the Woman Has Lost Ovarian Function Due to Surgery or Illness

With advances in cancer treatment, increasing numbers of people are surviving at the expense of their fertility. A man who is about to undergo chemotherapy or radiation can cryopreserve sperm prior to treatment, but as of this writing (2005), successful pregnancy from thawed frozen eggs is rare enough to still be considered highly experimental. Hence, a woman who is preparing for a cancer treatment that is known to destroy or diminish fertility has to undergo IVF and have her retrieved eggs inseminated with her husband or partner's sperm (or a donor's, in the case of an unmarried woman) and have the resulting embryos frozen for future use. Because this is expensive, because the woman is usually in a crisis and eager to begin her treatment, and because some cancers require immediate treatment, relatively few women undergo IVF with embryo freezing in anticipation of cancer-related infertility.

Infertility after chemotherapy and/or radiation cannot always be accurately predicted. There are women who have aggressive treatment and who are later delighted to find that their menses return. They may go on to conceive and carry without difficulty. By contrast, there are others whose treatment damages their fertility. With chemotherapy, the common observation (a National Cancer Institute Alert, May, 1988) has been that the greater the dose, the longer the duration of chemotherapy and the older the age of the woman at the time of treatment, the more likely the sacrifice of ovarian function.

Cancer is not the only medical problem that causes a woman to lose her ovaries and/or her ovarian function. A woman may have a cyst that ruptures and causes her to lose an ovary. Or a ruptured ectopic pregnancy may result in surgery in which she loses both ovary and fallopian tube. While most women have two ovaries and one may remain after a medical and surgical emergency, there are instances in which a woman loses both ovaries.

Some Special Issues and Considerations

Egg donation after surgery, chemotherapy, or radiation is attractive to some women, but repugnant to others. Those who find it attractive focus on its restorative capacity: here is a woman who has lost half of her reproductive function and who can now use the remaining half—her ability to carry—to bring a new life into the world. For a woman who has been ill, and who probably confronted her own mortality, the opportunity to plant two (or more) new feet on this earth is profoundly moving.

Why, then, would some survivors of illness or surgery feel that ovumdonation is wrong, or at least wron for them? Some say it brings back painful memories of the illness. Until facing their desire to have a family, they had been moving on in their lives, moving away from the cancer. The prospect of being back in a medical setting, of having invasive tests and procedures and of having the constant reminder of their battle with cancer is painful. They may feel that adoption is the right path for them: that cancer forced them to face painful loss and that experience will serve them well in parenting a child who has experienced loss through adoption.

One issue for cancer survivors involves a belief in their future. Some may avoid either egg donation or adoption because they fear the reactions they may see or perceive in others. What if the physician suggests a delay of a year or two or three before pregnancy? A woman could be devastated by this, fearing that her physician is waiting to see if she will have a recurrence. Worse still would be the experience of applying to an adoption agency and being rejected—or (more commonly) delayed—for health reasons. Cancer survivors need to believe in their own futures and, for the most part, to feel confident that others do as well.

If someone is going to think about offering to donate eggs to a family member or friend, she is likely to be prompted by an awareness of some real need in the recipient. What could be a more compelling reason to need ova than cancer survivorship—or some sort of emergency or otherwise serious gynecological surgery? This usually public event often leaves loved ones aware of lost fertility and wanting to help. Ironically, a woman who receives offers from family members and friends to donate may find herself in a bit of a predicament. What if she would prefer the eggs of a stranger? What if she receives more than one offer and has to choose among generous volunteers? Can she feel truly free and clear to decide between egg donation and adoption when she has loved ones eagerly stepping up to the plate?

....

Meet Karen

At 31, Karen appears freshly scrubbed and radiant. Her vibrant dark eyes and warm smile draw people towards her. It is no surprise that she works successfully in human services, navigating her way daily in a large and competitive organization.

These days Karen wears her black hair cropped short—by choice. Seven years ago, that was not the case. At 24, Karen was in the midst of a major battle with Non-Hodgkin's Lymphoma. Although her illness was quite advanced, Karen won the battle. Unfortunately, her survival was not accompanied by a return of her menses.

Karen and her husband, Ted, initially thought they would turn to egg donation. Karen liked the idea of being pregnant and she deeply desired the chance to have Ted's baby. As a couple they were excited about egg donation—until they began exploring the process. Karen doesn't have a sister or other volunteer, and both she and Ted were very troubled by the idea of women being paid to donate eggs. The more they thought about what they describe as "the commercialization of egg donation," the more Karen and Ted were convinced that adoption was right for them.

Karen and Ted are busy these days preparing a nursery, talking with pediatricians, signing up for a baby care class at the local adoption information organization. Their daughter, whom they have already named Lily, awaits them in China. They have sent her photo to their many friends and their eager family and all are enthusiastically awaiting Lily's arrival home. The big question they are asking Karen and Ted is "How many of us can come to the airport when you return from China?"

Couples with Unexplained Infertility

In a time of advances in reproductive technology, unexplained infertility has to be one of the most baffling and provocative of experiences. How is it that a couple can go to a skilled reproductive endocrinologist and be told there is no identifiable fertility problem? Worse still, they can seek a second and even third opinion and hear the same thing again and again, "Something is wrong but we don't know what it is."

In the old days, couples were labeled "normal infertile." How bad was that? Bad enough to prompt people to feel that their problems *must* be psychological. After all, if there was no apparent physical problem, they must be causing their own infertility with ambivalent thoughts, bad behavior, past misdeeds or some other curse.

Couples struggling with unexplained infertility find themselves in the world of trial and error. With little to go by, physicians suggest trying IVF, hoping that the explanation of the couple's infertility rests in the way that the egg is released (or not released) or in difficulties that egg and sperm have when they encounter each other. IVF, especially IVF with ICSI, *should* correct this. ICSI, also called Intracytoplasmic Sperm Injection, is a procedure done under a microscope in which a single sperm is injected into the egg to enable fertilization to occur. This is commonly done in situations of very low sperm counts or nonmotile sperm. And for some folks with unexplained infertility, IVF provides a solution. But what of others? What do you do if your infertility remains all the more unexplained after repeated failed IVF attempts?

Donor ova? Donor sperm? Perhaps a gestational carrier? Maybe it really is the eggs? Or maybe the sperm? Perhaps the problem is one of implantation or some other aspect of early pregnancy? Couples with unexplained infertility ask themselves these questions, consider each of these options and some of them hesitantly make their way to the departure lounge for egg donation.

Some Special Issues and Considerations

Of the three variables—eggs, sperm and uterus—many couples who are considering third party reproduction feel that it makes sense to begin with the eggs. Sperm is easier to obtain but using donor sperm means that the husband has no role in creating his child. Egg donation, by contrast, offers a kind of parity—each member of the couple gets to play a very significant role in bringing their child into the world. However, since egg donation is a far more costly and complicated process than sperm donation, couples with unexplained infertility are unlikely to turn to it unless something points to an egg problem. It goes without saying that the main question for infertile couples with unexplained infertility who seek ovum donation is whether this course of action makes any sense. Trial and error is already a difficult way to undergo medical treatment, but this process becomes all the more perplexing when it advances to the use of donor eggs. If the couple does achieve a successful pregnancy with the help of a donor, they may be able to assume that they made the right decision and indeed, it *was* an egg problem. However, these couples may also wonder whether they would have had the same outcome with donor sperm. Perhaps the problem was not specific to the ova or the sperm, but rather, a kind of reproductive incompatibility? Couples are turning to PGD for answers.

But what of the couple who introduce donor eggs and *still* face un-explained infertility? They are the ones with the more vexing problem. One such couple tried donor sperm and, eventually, a gestational carrier before deciding to adopt. Another tried a second egg donor and lo and behold, just delivered a baby.

So one option for a couple with unexplained infertility is to do trial and error through various third party options (assuming they do not want—or are not ready—to adopt). Another option is to continue trying on their own, knowing that some unexplained infertile couples have spontaneous pregnancies.

. . . .

Meet Cathy

Cathy is now eight months pregnant through the help of an egg donor. This pregnancy, which she has enjoyed immensely, did not come easily. In fact, Cathy and her husband, Don, have been trying to have a baby for five years. They conceived early on in their efforts, had a miscarriage at eight weeks and were then unable to conceive. Cathy, who is now nearly 40, was 35 when they began trying.

As they made their way through infertility diagnosis and various treatments, Cathy and Don's doctor kept saying the same thing to them, "We can't find a problem so you've got un-explained infertility. Your tests look fine but I have a hunch it is an egg problem." As Cathy got older, Dr. S.'s "hunch" became stronger and he became more vocal. When she turned 39, he gave them something of a push to try egg donation. Although this was something Cathy would never have agreed to a year or so earlier, her frustration with the absence of answers and her strong desire to have a baby and move on inspired her to begin looking for an egg donor.

Egg donation provided no "quick fix" for Cathy and Don. They found a donor whom they really liked and were excited about her until they learned that she did not respond to the stimulation protocol. They moved on to another donor, who had five eggs retrieved, two of which fertilized. Yet again, no pregnancy. Cathy and Don felt defeated, but something told them that they should keep on trying. They found another do-nor and decided to move forward with her. Then there was a "glitch"—a glitch that turned into a gift.

"We received a call saying that our donor wanted to meet us. She told the agency that she needed to know she was helping good people whom she respected and whom she felt would be good parents. We were taken aback at first, but felt that we couldn't deny her this opportunity."

Cathy refers to the meeting with Abby, her donor, as being "the best thing we ever did." She describes the meeting as a blind date that went very well. Cathy and Don met Abby, a college student, at a coffee shop near her university. For two hours three people who would be working together to bring a new life into the world talked about their lives, their interests, hopes and plans for the future.

Among the many things Abby told Cathy and Don about herself is that she has a birth half-sister. She explained that her mother placed a child for adoption and in recent years, that child, now a young woman, contacted the family. According to Abby, her birth half-sister is now a valued member of the family. Her search and reunion impressed upon Abby the power of genetic connections and taught her how crucial it is for people to be able to search for those who gave them life.

Abby told Cathy and Don that it was her meeting her birth half-sister, as well as hearing from a close friend about the friend's experience as an egg donor, that prompted her to volunteer her own eggs. However, she added candidly that she was also attracted by the payment.

Cathy and Don appreciated this candor. "I wouldn't be comfortable with someone who was doing it solely for the money, but I believed Abby that there were other motivating forces. And I liked the fact that she felt trusting enough of us that she could speak the truth."

Cathy goes on to say that she and Don left the meeting with Abby confident that they were doing the right thing by pursuing pregnancy through egg donation. Meeting Abby confirmed to them that they could feel really good about a donor. They were pleased that Abby said she would be willing to meet a child who came from her donation and that she would keep in touch with them through the agency, letting them know any important medical information.

Cathy conceived shortly after the visit in the coffee shop. She is currently eight months pregnant and expecting a boy. Reflecting back on the last several months and the last several years, Cathy offers a number of interesting observations.

"I look back at where I was a few years ago and where I am now and am amazed by the differences. Although it was very difficult at the time, I am glad, in some ways, that things didn't work out with the first two donors. At that point we were looking for different things—for someone who looked like me and for someone who would remain entirely anonymous. Now I have a completely different perspective. I thank God we met Abby, because we have that for our son, and I am grateful we picked someone for her character and integrity rather than physical appearance. Abby looks nothing like me, but that doesn't matter. To me, egg donation is like adoption in many ways—the child is coming from another place and the important thing to me is that it is a good place. A very good place."

When asked about her pregnancy, Cathy says that it has been a mixed experience. "For the most part, it has been wonderful. I am so grateful to have had this opportunity to be pregnant. However, there is also a loss. I feel sad sometimes when I think about the fact that I will never have a biological child. That feels like a loss, like someone died."

As she looks forward to parenthood, Cathy also acknowledges some mixed feelings. "I'm excited, very excited, but I'm also nervous. I'll admit that I am worried about the egg donor part. We will tell our son as soon as we can, but we hope we do a good job of it. We want to do what is best for him." She goes on to say that she is already struggling with what to say to other people about her son's origins. "We told both of our families and that felt great. At least at first. Then my mother told my uncle, who told his children, and suddenly it felt very uncomfortable. I am certain our son should know, but I am wondering who else really needs to know."

Cathy says that she worries about what people will think. "I felt uncomfortable calling a pediatrician. I worried about her reaction and was so relieved when she seemed to treat us like any other expectant parents."

And indeed, Cathy and Don are, in many ways, like "any other expectant parents."

Cathy has touched upon several issues that are central to oocyte donation: donor selection, meeting the donor, donor payment, telling others about egg donation, and pregnancy and parenthood. We will be addressing all of these issues in future chapters.

Couples with a Genetic Problem

When a couple is going through infertility, a successful pregnancy often becomes the promised land. It is hard not to imagine that a positive test and evidence of an ongoing pregnancy will not usher in nine months of bliss followed by a lifetime of happiness. Sadly, some couples learn, either through genetic testing before a pregnancy is attempted, or during a pregnancy or after a baby is born that they are carriers of a serious, even lethal, genetic disorder. Some have close family members whom they have watched suffer from a genetic disorder. Some of these families have a baby die in utero. Some choose to terminate pregnancies when such a disorder is diagnosed in utero. Others deliver a child who dies at birth or soon after. Still others parent children with very challenging conditions. Veterans of each of these experiences may turn to egg or sperm donation in an effort to avoid transmitting the genetic abnormality in future pregnancies or they may use PGD.

Genetic disorders may be caused by problems with either genes or chromosomes. They may be inherited—that is, they are passed from parent to child—or they may occur on their own. Some disorders may be caused by a mix of factors (multifactorial). The actual cause of multifactorial disorders is unknown. They can run in families or can occur on their own with no family history. Some disorders can be found by testing, and others cannot. Some disorders can be treated and are not serious.

For dominant disorders, just one gene from either parent can cause a dominant gene disorder. If a parent has the gene, each of his or her children has a 1 in 2 (50 percent) chance of inheriting the disorder. On the other hand, each person carries a few recessive genes. Most of the time, these genes are canceled out by dominant genes. If you have a recessive gene for a certain disorder, this makes you a carrier. Although you may show no signs of the disorder yourself, you still can pass it on to your children.

If both you and your partner are carriers for the same recessive disorder, each of your children has a 1 in 4 (25 percent) chance of having the disorder. If one of you has the disorder and the other doesn't (and isn't a carrier), your children will be carriers.

Genetic disorders also may be caused by problems with the fetus' chromosomes. Most are caused by an error that occurred when the egg and sperm were forming. Extra, missing, or incomplete chromosomes often cause severe health problems. Many children with chromosomal disorders have physical defects and below-average intelligence. The older you are, the greater your risk of having a child with a chromosomal disorder. If you are age 35, for instance, the chance is about 1 in 200. If you are age 40, the risk increases to about 1 in 60. This is another reason that some older women may consider becoming pregnant through egg donation.

Some genetic diseases that are especially concerning to couples trying to become pregnant include congenital heart defects, Tay-Sachs disease, Sickle Cell disease, hemophilia, muscular dystrophy, cystic fibrosis, Huntington's disease, and mental retardation. Many couples who find out they have a high potential of having a child with one of these disorders due to being a carrier or because of advanced maternal age (as with Down's Syndrome) may investigate the option of ova donation so they will not pass the disease or disorder to their children.

Special Issues and Considerations

Couples with genetic issues often face baffling decisions. For one thing, there are a wide range of genetic disorders and these disorders are transmitted with varying levels of probability. For example, if both partners are carriers of the same recessive disorder, each child born to that couple will have a one in four chance of having the disorder. By contrast, if each parent has the gene for a dominant disorder, each child has a one in two chance of inheriting the disorder. Hence, couples who *know* that they are carriers of a particular disorder face two closely related questions. The first is to determine how they feel about transmitting that disorder to a child. For example, parents might be willing to have a child with Marfan's Syndrome, which affects the heart, since people with Marfan's can live reasonably "normal" lives, but that same couple, if carriers of Tay Sachs, which is always fatal within the first few years of life, might do all they could to avoid having an affected child. The second question involves looking at how they *feel* about the odds. For one couple, one in four odds may seem worth playing, while others could easily find such odds unthinkable.

Meet Stephanie and Brad

Stephanie and her husband, Brad, have a 3-year-old daughter, Megan, whom they adore. Megan is the light of their lives, but she is also the reason that life for Stephanie and Brad is extraordinarily stressful. When Megan was six weeks old, she was diagnosed with cystic fibrosis. Her diagnosis was especially upsetting to her parents, since they had been tested for CF during pregnancy and had been told that although Stephanie is a carrier, Brad is not.

Extensive genetic testing has revealed that Brad has some sort of genetic mosaic. Megan's CF is ample evidence that her dad is a carrier, but Brad's CF gene cannot be readily identified. This makes it very difficult for Stephanie and Brad to enter into another pregnancy. They love their daughter dearly but know the resources she needs, as well as the vulnerability of her health. Both are frightened that another CF child would further strain their resources, making it difficult for them to give Megan all that she needs.

Stephanie and Brad discussed both egg and sperm donation and decided on the former because of the "equality" it provides to them—Stephanie will carry the baby and Brad will father him/her. In addition, it is important to the couple, who both enjoyed Stephanie's earlier pregnancy, that they have another opportunity to be "present at the creation" and to care for and love their child pre-birth.

Similarly-Aged Couples in Which the Woman Has Age-Related Declining Fertility

There was a time, not all that long ago, when a woman giving birth after age 30 was labeled a "geriatric mother" or having "advanced maternal age." In fact, there was a documentary in the 1970s called "Joyce at 34" (Joyce Chopra and Claudia Weill, University of Wisconsin, 1973). It was about a couple who decided—at the "old age of 34"—to have a baby. The film shows the couple announcing their "geriatric" pregnancy to Joyce's family, all of whom react with surprise and wonder.

Times have certainly changed! Delayed marriage and parenting and second marriages have brought many women well into their 30s and early 40s before they attempt pregnancy. Although many are able to successfully conceive and carry, female biology has not changed with social norms. The fact remains that women experience declining fertility after age 35 and rapid drop offs after age 40.

The largest group approaching the departure lounge of egg

donation is composed of women in their late 30s and early 40s. They are travelers with worried countenances. Many feel they are racing against a biological clock that is ticking rapidly. Each month that passes weighs heavily upon them. They fear that the last good eggs are slipping away, and they worry that even if they do conceive, they will be prone to miscarriage. FSH numbers loom large, taking on a life and power of their own.

There are some women in this group who are experiencing an early menopause. Because they have higher than "normal" FSH levels (typically above 15) they are given little chance of conceiving with their own eggs. However, many of these women, often still in their 30s or early 40s find themselves in something of a gray zone—they have FSH between 10 and 15, or other indications of diminished but not completely absent fertility.

For some couples in which the woman is over 35, age will be the only cause of infertility. For others, there are additional problems. There may be sperm factors or tubal problems that make assisted reproduction necessary for reasons other than oocyte quality.

Some Special Issues and Considerations

The feeling that time is running out is incredibly stressful for a number of reasons. First, there is regret. Some women look back with profound regret, blaming themselves for not trying to have a child when they were younger (or in many cases, a second or third child.) They may experience anger towards their husbands or partners, if it was their spouse who chose to postpone efforts. Some will regret not having children on their own or in earlier, "bad" marriages. Others blame doctors for not urging them to try sooner, or media coverage of celebrities for promoting the notion that women can have children at any age.

It is, indeed, a very tough place to be. In addition to regret, "older" women face complex decision-making questions. What should they do when their physician tells them, "You probably have about a 3% chance of having a child with your eggs, but you will increase your chances to about 50% if you use donor eggs"? For women intent on having their genetic child, this is a "no brainer"—even 3% is worth trying. For others, whose goal is to be pregnant and preferably sooner, rather than later, a different decision is clear: they should seek donated eggs. Factor in cost and insurance considerations and things become all the more complicated. Some women have coverage for IVF, but not donor egg, some for donor egg but not regular IVF. Some have no coverage and some have insurance that covers all. Except for those with unlimited financial resources, the high costs of IVF, egg donation, and adoption will all enter into their decision making. Fortunately, times are changing. The $10,000 federal tax credit (and for many, adoption benefits of $4-10,000 from their employers) makes adoption a much more affordable.

There is another issue for older women whose only fertility problem is advanced age: "Should we keep trying on our own?" Although many physicians believe that IVF is the optimal treatment for advanced age, since it offers them the opportunity to aggressively attempt to ripen many follicles (and to transfer a limited number of embryos, minimizing the risk of high level multiples, something which would be a problem in a stimulated IUI), there are some couples who "fail" with IVF and then conceive on their own. It seems that, for them, IVF offered no benefit.

Even when continued efforts to try with a woman's own eggs appear fruitless, couples in which the woman is still of childbearing age may be very reluctant to move to donated eggs. After all, one sure way to prevent a spontaneous pregnancy would be to have the woman pregnant with donor eggs. Ironically, donor ova would function here as an inadvertent form of birth control.

Meet Carol

Carol and her husband, Mike, met when both were in their mid 30s. Carol, who had known "my whole life" that she wanted to be a mother, did not delay in telling Mike how much it meant to her to be a mom. She appreciated his ability to listen to her and to understand how important becoming a mother was to her. Without hesitating, the couple began trying to conceive several months before their marriage. Their efforts did not bear fruit, but they did spare Carol the anguish of regret. "We did our best. We couldn't help it that time was no longer on our side."

Time was not on their side, but Carol's close friend, Laura, was. Laura, who had three children of her own, knew of Carol and Mike's efforts, their disappointment, and their deep desire to have a child together. When she heard they were actively exploring adoption, she spoke with her husband, Herb, and together, they made an offer: Laura's eggs. Carol still gets tears in her eyes when she tells the story, "Laura and Herb made it so easy for us to accept their offer. They made it very clear there would be no strings attached. Laura told me that we were already 'practically sisters' and that this would only serve to strengthen the bond between us. It was an offer I couldn't—and wouldn't—turn down."

What Carol left out is the fact that she and Laura look remarkably alike. This was not an important factor in Carol and Mike's decision making, but both considered it a nice "bonus." Prior to attempting pregnancy, the two couples got together several times and spoke extensively of their decision. By the time they moved forward, all felt they had fully explored and addressed what a pregnancy—and child—would mean for them and their families.

Carol and Mike felt strongly that they wanted to give Laura and Herb a gift as a way of thanking them. They knew that nothing could adequately express their gratitude, and, in addition, they didn't want to make Laura and Herb feel like they were being "paid" in any way. After giving the question a great deal of thought, Carol and Mike decided to make donations into each of Laura and Herb's children's college funds. With the donation, they sent a simple note, "You have helped us build our family and, in some small way, we hope this helps your children to grow."

Couples in Which the Woman Is Several Years Older than Her Partner

Once, it was very unusual for a woman to marry a man who was younger than she was, especially if the age difference was more than three or four years. Today, there are many couples in which the woman is five to ten, sometimes even more, years older than her husband. When a woman in her 40s meets and marries a man in his early-mid 30s, the prospect of a pregnancy with donor eggs may be inviting.

Special Issues and Considerations

If a couple is composed of a woman who is 40 and a man who is 30, the "issues" they face in considering egg donation are unlikely to be different from those of a couple in which both members are around 40. However, there are instances in which the woman is over 45, raising questions about the medical and ethical advisability of ovum donation.

From a medical perspective, a woman in her late 40s is at greater risk for complications of pregnancy, including gestational diabetes, pre-eclampsia and pre-term labor. In addition, she is in an age group where her risk of breast cancer is increasing. Hence, it is important that she discuss her medical situation with her primary care physician as well as a high risk obstetrician before embarking upon a pregnancy, Most likely, these doctors will request a mammogram, to confirm there is "nothing suspicious," as well as an electrocardiogram, to rule out cardiac abnormalities that could be affected by pregnancy.

From an ethical perspective, older women and their younger partners should explore what it will mean for a child to have a mother in her 60s when he/she is a teenager. Many argue that there are lots of men who become fathers in their late 40s, 50s—or even older. But "just because we can do something, doesn't mean we *should* do it." Their ethical lens is likely to focus on the age of the male partner. If he is in his early or mid-30s, they may reassure themselves that their child will grow up with one parent of "more normal childrearing age."

....

Meet Donna and Tim

Donna is a warm, outgoing office manager who was swept off her feet by Tim, a client of her office. Although she always wanted to be married and have children, Donna had given up on both goals soon after her 40th birthday, which was a year or so before Tim came along.

"I never saw it coming, but there he was. I knew, from our first date, that this was the man I wanted to spend my life with. He seemed to feel the same way—even when I blurted out my age. Upon hearing it, he replied, 'I don't care.'"

Tim, who was 31 at the time, really didn't care that Donna was older. "What did it matter?" he said to himself, "She's young looking and pretty and full of energy." Tim was not thinking about having a baby, but Donna was. She had wanted a baby for as long as she could remember but had decided against becoming a single mother. Now she had a partner, a possibility—and aging eggs.

Donna and Tim were married less than a year after they met. While they were dating, they spoke often about having children. Tim knew that he would one day want to be a father, but he didn't feel that he was ready and he felt it was too early in their relationship to become parents together. Donna tried to understand how he felt, but she was upset and frustrated. Didn't he understand that time was running out?

Indeed, time did "run out." By the time Tim was ready to attempt pregnancy, Donna was 44. She wasted no time seeking fertility help, but even then, there was not much the doctors could offer. "Egg donation," was all she heard and it was the very thing Donna didn't want to hear. She was determined to keep trying with Tim, even as hope grew dim.

Time passed, things changed and Donna found herself pondering ovum donation. Although she had initially opposed the idea because it seemed "strange" and "weird," Donna's thinking began to shift. She realized that she could see ovum donation as another example of the ways in which women are there for each other in time of need. As this perspective came into focus, Donna spoke about it with her niece, who seemed like she might be willing to donate. Donna found herself fantasizing about being pregnant. Even when her niece decided she wasn't ready to donate, thoughts of pregnancy continued. Then someone told Donna about a program that had a number of donors who were willing, sometimes eager, to meet their recipients. "That turned the corner for me," Donna recalls. "I'm someone who cares a great deal about the bonds that connect women to each other and the idea of meeting and talking with a donor made sense to me. Suddenly egg donation was transformed from some strange, science fiction arrangement to a real life connection between two women."

On a warm, sunny spring day, Donna went to her donor agency to meet Lexi, her donor. She brought with her a big bouquet of flowers from her garden—a fitting gift for the woman who would soon give her precious seeds to grow. Donna had selected Lexi from an on-line profile and had learned a good deal about her from the staff at the agency. But nothing they said could have fully prepared her for the delightful, bubbly, talkative young woman that she met. Lexi, a 27-year-old mother of three, told her that she decided to donate eggs when her sister had a baby through IVF. "I saw what she went through and I looked at my three and felt that no one should be denied having children. I love my children so much and don't know what I would do without them."

Donna floated out of the agency and when she was but steps from it's door, called Tim. "I have been swept off my feet a second time. She's great...and this is all going to be o.k."

Couples in Which the Woman Is over Forty-Five

Before donated ova came along, pregnancy over age 45 was an extremely rare—and usually unexpected—event. Although it remains uncommon, there are some women in their late 40s and early 50s seeking donor eggs. In the departure lounge for egg donation, they are the group whose request for egg donation receives the most scrutiny, both medically and ethically.

Why would a woman in her late 40s or early 50s request donor eggs? After all, this is an age at which women were traditionally enjoying their grandchildren. Or they were appreciating the "freedom" that comes with having raised one's family. The 40s and 50s have been celebrated as a time during which a woman "comes into her own," perhaps launches a career or a new career. Historically, it has not been a time during which women are caring for young children.

Older women seeking egg donation are rarely people who "forgot to have a baby." These are, by and large, not women who woke up one day in mid-life and thought it would be "neat" to become pregnant. Rather, they are most often people who have wanted to have children for many years, but who were not previously in a position in which they believed they should or could become mothers. Some had had children in an earlier marriage, were divorced or widowed and then remarried someone who had not had children of his own.

Some Special Issues and Considerations

Women seeking pregnancy after age 45 face medical, ethical and practical challenges. Confronting these challenges can be draining, especially since there exists little public support for older women seeking motherhood.

From a medical standpoint, physicians will want to feel fairly confident that a pregnancy will not prove harmful to a particular older mother. As we noted in the last section, medical exams will probably include a mammogram and an electrocardiogram. Physicians will also ask prospective older mothers to talk with a high risk obstetrician who will review with them the risks of pregnancy in older women. These include an increased risk of pre-term labor, pregnancy induced high blood pressure and gestational diabetes.

From an ethical perspective, questions will be raised about the best interests of children. Is it in the best interests of a child to intentionally bring him/her into the world knowing that his mother will be in her 60s when at high school graduation? Certainly, there have always been children whose fathers were in their 40s—or even older—when they were born. The argument regarding their well being has been that their mothers were younger. Is it different when it is the Dad who is closer to 30 than 40 when the couple's child is born?

Ethical questions intensify when both partners are over 45. Then the question really arises: "Is this fair to a child?" What would it mean for a child to have two—not one—parents in their 60s at high school graduation? Is this a child who would spend his/her young adult years caring for elderly parents?"

As people examine the ethical questions of older motherhood, it is inevitable that they look beyond the immediate family. What if one or both parents have older children, perhaps now in their late teens or early 20s, who support the idea of another child and who state a preparedness to help raise their half sister or brother? What if there is a large, extended and very supportive family near by? Do these factors mitigate the burden of a child born to older parents?

And then there are the logistical issues. The additional medical tests and consultations may slow down the process of egg donation for older women, usually at a time when they want to accelerate the process. Among their many concerns may be losing out on any opportunity to adopt. Aware that it becomes extremely difficult to adopt a baby after age 45, they recognize that by choosing egg donation, they are effectively "postponing" adoption past a point at which most agencies will place a baby with them. Older child adoption may remain an option for some time.

....

Meet Margie

Margie has wanted to be a mom for as long as she can remember. One by one her single friends married and had children, but Margie found herself past 40 and still alone. Eventually, the long time teacher concluded that she would never find a husband, let alone have the opportunity to be a mom.

Along came Abe. Abe is Margie's husband of three months, the love of her life, the man she longed to meet, but never dreamed would really come along. And there he was, seated next to her at a friend's daughter's wedding.

"We danced and I knew."

Margie is 46. Abe is 44. Margie is giddily happy about her marriage, but also sad that she will never have a biological child. Abe is an agreeable kind of guy and he will do whatever Margie wants—forego having children, adopt or attempt pregnancy with egg donation. At 46 Margie is grappling with what she should do. She is having trouble accepting that she is no longer able to have her "own" baby and hence, neither adoption nor egg donation hold much appeal. At the same time, however, Margie recognizes that she may feel different six months or a year from now, when she has had the opportunity to grieve the loss of biological children and move on. The problem is that at 46, she does not have a lot of time to spare. She knows, also, that her decision is complicated by the fact that neither she nor Abe was able to save much money over the years. With some ingenuity, they believe they will be able to afford either egg donation or adoption—but not both.

Margie would prefer to enjoy her new marriage and put thoughts of egg donation and adoption aside. However, feeling pressured by her age to make a decision, she is pursuing counseling and forcing herself to examine each of her options.

Couples in Which the Man Is Fertile but the Woman Can neither Provide Eggs nor Carry a Baby

Since life is not fair, there are couples who face more than one reproductive challenge. Sometimes it is the woman who is hit with this "double blow"—she can neither produce viable eggs nor carry a successful pregnancy. In some instances, this is something a woman learns early in life and that a couple knows as they enter into marriage and make plans to build a family. In other instances, the "double blow" unfolds sequentially. A woman undergoing a fertility work-up may be advised that she has a uterine abnormality and later learn she has elevated FSH. Or she may have turned to donated eggs because diminished ovarian reserve and had an unsuccessful cycle. Further medical exploration may have discovered uterine abnormalities.

Some Special Issues and Considerations.

The decision to use both donor eggs and a gestational carrier is very different for those who "know from the start" vs. those who "learn along the way." Couples who "know from the start" face one decision: "Do we want to turn to two women to help us bring a child into this world that has a genetic connection to one of us and a parenting bond with both of us or do we want to adopt?" Couples who "learn along the way" face a two part decision. For them, one decision is made. Only after they are comfortable with it and accustomed to it do they face a second decision. As one woman who is now the mother of three children, all through a combination of donated ova and a gestational carrier said, "For us it was a decision made in steps. We ended up doing something we never, ever thought we would do. That is because our reality changed along the way. This experience taught us an important lesson: 'Never say never.' It taught us to be much more open minded."

Couples choosing to have a child through egg donation and gestational care face several issues. One is ethical—is it morally and ethically correct to bring a child into this world when he/she will have neither a genetic nor a gestational connection to his/her mother? A second issue is logistical—it is complicated enough to embark upon either an egg donor or a gestational carrier pregnancy. Combining the two involves a great deal of medical, psychological and legal coordination. Then there are financial challenges—this is undoubtedly a very costly venture, easily upwards of $50,000 simply for the *chance* of conception. Finally, there is the question of what to do if the gestational carrier does not become pregnant. With so many variables, it is difficult to know which one to address. Couples and their physicians wonder if they should try a second time with the same participants and same protocol, change the protocol, change the egg donor or perhaps, the gestational carrier?

Meet Zoë

Zoë is the busy mother of three girls, all under the age of four. Zoë and her husband, Martin, have 3½-year-old twins, Alexa and Emma, conceived with the help of an egg donor and carried by gestational carrier. Last year, they transferred a cryopreserved embryo from the egg donor cycle that created Alexa and Emma and they had Chloe, the twins' full biological sibling, brought into this world by a different gestational carrier.

Zoë smiles when she tells the story of her husband's and children's recent experience in parent-child Sunday school. The teacher was talking about Abraham and Sarah and the difficulties they had having children. Alexa turned to her dad and said, "Well our family certainly didn't have that problem." Martin didn't say anything at that moment, but later in the day, he and Zoë sat down with the girls and began to tell them the remarkable story of how their family came to be.

Zoë and Martin had begun trying to have a child when they were both 30. Zoë had endometriosis, but did not anticipate this preventing pregnancy. However, when initial efforts did not succeed, the couple moved quickly on to IVF. To their surprise and profound disappointment, Zoë did not produce any eggs. Stunned and in disbelief, the couple was told to consider donor eggs.

"We didn't know what to think, but we decided to put one foot in front of the other and to learn about egg donation and adoption. We went to a number of meetings at adoption agencies and then one at a reproductive center where there were couples talking about egg donation. I have to say that it was what we heard at those meetings that shaped our decision. The adoption agencies scared us away and the donor parents encouraged us. We came away from the adoption meetings feeling that we had heard, 'You have no control in adoption and it is fraught with risk.' With egg donation, you are not being rejected and you feel like you have some control."

And so Zoë and Martin moved on to egg donation, assuming it would work. Zoë notes that doctors neglect to remind people that egg donation is only a chance, and often, it does not work. Indeed, Zoë and Martin ended up disappointed after working with their first and second donors.

After the second egg donor attempt met with disappointment, Zoë's physician encouraged her to think about a gestational carrier. "He called it a 'gestational uterus' and I was horrified. I was so upset that I changed doctors. But it didn't take very long for me to realize that he had been right."

So there they were, a couple who had worked hard to decide between egg donation and adoption, confronting a new question: Do we adopt or do egg donation with a gestational carrier. "We were already there at the egg donor decision but now we had to look at gestational care." Zoë remembers taking many of the same steps she and Martin took when they first looked at egg donation and adoption. They attended adoption agency meetings and they went to a seminar where people who were parents through gestational care told their stories.

Once again, adoption came up short for them. Zoë notes that if she had heard different things, she might have a different family now. No better, no worse, but different. Yet once again, Zoë and Martin heard many cautionary stories about adoption and a host of enthusiastic ones about gestational care. They left the meetings clear what their next steps would be. They would find yet a third egg donor and they would seek a gestational carrier.

"Along the way, we had to change our priorities. We had wanted a donor who was willing to meet us and who had never donated before. We had to abandon the first goal early on since at that time, 'semi-anonymous' donation was not available. Then, when two donors failed to produce viable eggs, we decided we needed someone who had donated before. In fact, we ended up with a woman who had donated many times. At that point, we wanted it to work."

Indeed, Zoë and Martin's story is one of evolving priorities. Both look at their children with a sense of wonder and with a bit of amusement. Surely when they married, twelve years ago, neither could have anticipated the path they would travel to build the family they longed for.

Do they have any regrets?

"Just one," Zoë replies. "And it is not one we can do anything about. I wish I had met or at least been in contact with our donor. I wish I had that for our children, but it wasn't possible at the time. I am hoping something will make it possible for them to find out about her in the future."

Single Women

There was a time, not *that* long ago, when becoming pregnant "out of wedlock" was a shameful thing. So shameful, in fact, that it was the reason why many women placed children for adoption. But as we know, times have changed and perhaps in few areas more dramatically than attitudes towards single motherhood. No longer shameful, out of wedlock pregnancies are often pursued with a vengeance.

Look around any fertility center waiting room and there are single women who have decided to try to have a baby "before it is too late." Most started with simple donor inseminations, but as they work their way up the fertility center food chain, they often find themselves all the way at IVF. And if that doesn't work, then what?

We think that it is safe to say that many people would feel it is unfair to a child to create him or her through anonymous donor eggs and donor sperm. However, there are women who have an identified sperm donor. He may be a friend who offered to donate sperm when he learned she wanted a baby.

Some Special Issues and Considerations

If we assume that it is unfair to a child to be the product of two anonymous donations, a single woman seeking egg donation will have either a known egg donor or a known sperm donor. Either way, the relationship between the two participants will need to explored, with both encouraged to talk extensively about what this will mean for them. In the instance of sperm donation, these conversations will be all the more significant since the participants will need to agree on what role, if any, the donor will have in the child's life.

An additional ethical issue arises with single women: Is it fair to intentionally create a child who will have only one parent? This question becomes all the more poignant when the intended parent is older. Add to that the fact that the one parent is not the child's genetic mother. Going through this list, it becomes easy to see why many would say, "Stop. This is too much. Reproductive medicine has gone too far when it creates a child who will not be parented by either of his/her genetic parents, will have only one parent and that parent will be of advanced age." Everything seems clear in the abstract, but not always so much when there are real people. Like Jenny...

Meet Jenny

Jenny is a 47-year-old physician and the over-the-top-in-love mother of Olivia, now nearly two. Like so many women who eventually turn to egg donation, Jenny wanted to be a mom for most of her life. However, medical school and the demands of her training, plus a dose of bad luck, brought her into her early 40s without marriage. A "very traditional person"—or so she thought—Jenny could not seriously entertain the idea of having a child on her own.

Then came Pierre. Pierre, three years her junior, was the love of Jenny's life. She met him through friends and they were engaged within a few weeks and married in six months. Jenny and Pierre began trying to conceive before their marriage and went right to treatment after a few months of trying. Even with the invasive tests and procedures, they were blissfully happy and totally delighting in finally having lasting love.

But it was not meant to be. Pierre was not feeling well, lost some weight inexplicably and complained of a strange itching feeling. Jenny pushed him to see his doctor, who was initially reassuring but who soon suspected that Pierre had a malignancy. Indeed, he was diagnosed with leukemia, and although aggressive chemotherapy seemed to be working, Pierre succumbed to the disease barely two years after he and Jenny were married. He left Jenny with several vials of frozen semen which he had cryopreserved upon diagnosis.

Jenny was 44 when Pierre died. She allowed herself several months to grieve but then began thinking, perhaps more intensely than ever, about pregnancy. Jenny questioned whether it was wise for her to embark upon single motherhood in her mid-40s but felt more optimistic when her younger brother and his wife, parents of three children themselves, were supportive of the idea. Their offer to be guardians of a child further bolstered Jenny's confidence. She consulted her doctor about using Pierre's frozen semen and was told, "Your eggs are old now. It's a real long shot, but you have nothing to lose by trying."

Jenny saw it differently. She *did* have something to lose. Something big—Pierre's sperm. For her it was more important for her to have Pierre's baby than one conceived with her eggs. Although her doctor and others offered little support for the idea, Jenny began looking for an anonymous donor. When she found her, their collaborative efforts brought Olivia into the world.

At 47, Jenny is filled with energy and vitality. She acknowledges that she is fortunate in this regard. She is able to work full time, spend considerable time with Olivia and, amazing as it is, still get to Yoga twice weekly and to dinners with friends. She acknowledges wishing that Jenny had two parents but says that wish is far overshadowed by the joy she feels in seeing her daughter grow and flourish and in remembering Pierre.

Until now we have talked about those couples and individuals who come to the departure lounge of egg donation with some form of infertility. But there are others in the throng—people who are considering egg donation for different reasons. Let's introduce them, acknowledging that they come to this option having traveled other journeys.

Male Couples

It is no longer unusual to find two men sitting together in the waiting room of a reproductive medicine clinic. Eager to have children together and often discouraged from adoption, a number of pioneering gay couples have turned to egg donation with a gestational carrier. Theirs is a very complicated and costly path to parenthood, but one that affords them the opportunity to share in a pregnancy, to lovingly create a child and to have a child with a biological connection to one of them.

Since two men intending to have a child together know for certain that they need ova, they confront none of the "what if" questions that many heterosexual couples face. There is simply no question of trying another medication protocol or seeing another physician as a means of attaining better egg quality. Hence, gay couples, for all the challenges they face, are at least spared the question: "Do we really need an egg donor?" They do.

Some Special Issues and Considerations

Needless to say, there are many special issues and considerations for gay couples. Some remain societal—although their families are increasingly accepted, there remain many who are against same sex unions and are even more opposed to gay couples having children. Gay couples who seek contractual egg donors and gestational carriers inevitably begin with the question, "Will this woman be o.k. donating to/carrying for a gay couple?"

Gay couples must decide who will provide the "genetic material." "Do we want to have one of us be the biological father and have the other partner's sister donate eggs?" If so, then there does, of course, need to be a sister who is ready, willing and able to donate. What if there are two sisters? What if both offer to donate? What if neither offers? Do we ask? What if each man has a sister and both are willing to donate? In order to maximize their chances of having a baby, a gay couple might find themselves trying to figure out which one of the partners and which one of the sisters is likely to be most fertile. It's easy to see how this could all become very complicated, very fast!

Some gay men do not have sisters willing to donate or they may simply prefer to go with anonymous donation. If so, other questions arise about genetic connections, since presumably only one of them can father a child at a time. We say "presumably" because we have known gay couples who have chosen to have embryos inseminated with sperm from each of them and to have one embryo transferred from each batch, hoping to have twins.

Gay couples must also figure out how to put all the pieces of their parenting project together. What do they do first? Find a gestational carrier? An egg donor? Do they seek both simultaneously? And what of all the medical and legal procedures?

A major consideration for many gay couples is cost. Unless they have family members or close friends volunteering to donate eggs and to carry the pregnancy, costs will be high, probably around $50,000. Since gay couples are likely to be younger than heterosexual couples seeking egg donation, the enormous cost of becoming a parent comes at a time in their lives when they are just launching their careers, perhaps saving for a home or paying student loans.

Meet Joe and Justin

Joe and Justin were college sweethearts. They met twelve years ago at an Ivy League School and have been together ever since. After college, Joe followed Justin to Philadelphia, where he earned his MBA, and then Justin came to Boston with Joe so that Joe could attend law school. Now both are well established in their careers. They own a four bedroom home in the suburbs and are quite ready to become parents together.

At first Joe and Justin felt totally overwhelmed by the prospect of trying to create a child together. They looked into adoption, but learned that it, too, would be difficult to accomplish. Besides, they realized that they would love to raise a child with whom they had a genetic connection. As Joe put it, "I would love to father a child but I would be equally thrilled to parent the child of the man I love."

Joe and Justin have a friend—Joe's former colleague—who offered to carry a child for them. That was great, but the offer did not last. Once Ginger really thought about carrying a baby and separating from it at birth, she changed her mind. Joe and Justin were left to confront the costs and complex process of finding a contractual carrier.

To make a long and often difficult story short, Joe and Justin are now awaiting a pregnancy test. Their determination eventually led them to Sara, their gestational carrier, and then on to Lynn, an egg donor. They are hoping that Sara is pregnant. Both are jittery and eager about the pregnancy test, but say that whatever happens from this point forth, they feel they have gained a great deal from this process. They've learned a lot about themselves and their relationship as they have made their way through interviews with two very different and very interesting groups of women.

Female Couples

Perhaps it seems odd to think that couples consisting of two women might find themselves in the departure lounge of egg donation. After all, with both partners capable—we would assume—of producing eggs, we would expect that one, if not both of them, would be able to be the genetic mother of their child. Indeed, there are lesbian couples who have viable eggs *and* who undergo egg donation.

For legal reasons and for parity, some lesbian couples decide that one will donate the eggs and the other will carry their baby. Hence, each becomes an equal player—legally and emotionally—in creating their child. In some instances, there may be medical reasons for the donation: the partner desirous of pregnancy may not be the one with "good eggs."

Lesbian couples occasionally have other reasons for seeking egg donation. Perhaps they have asked one of their brothers to donate sperm. If so—and if the unrelated partner is unable to produce eggs—the couple will need to seek an egg donor in order avoid having a child created by a union of siblings.

Finally, there will be lesbian couples who wish to share a pregnancy, but neither of whom has viable eggs. When this occurs, they may turn to a family member for either oocyte or sperm donor, trying to ensure that the child has a genetic connection to at least one of his/her parents.

Some Special Issues and Considerations

To state the obvious, lesbian couples require sperm donors. Hence, those who are also pursuing egg donation intend to create a child who is not the genetic offspring of either parent. As we noted above, some couples deal with this by making sure that at least one of their donors is a biological relative. Still, more ethical questions arise when parents use both egg donation and donor sperm than when one of them uses her own gametes.

Lesbian couples choosing donated ova face countless challenges that extend far beyond their donor cycle. At a time when single sex marriage and parenthood are still highly controversial, these pioneering couples face a multitude of questions as they create their families. These questions center largely on whether they, as partners and parents, will have the rights and privileges of marriage.

As we have seen throughout this chapter, people enter the departure lounge of egg donation for a variety of reasons. Many of our travelers carry a heavy load—they may be parenting a child with a significant genetic disorder or they have endured a number of pregnancy losses or perhaps they are in a marriage that feels like it will crumble if this next effort to have a child does not work out. Other travelers arrive feeling less burdened. Women with Turner's Syndrome and their husbands may have been looking forward to egg donation for several years. Male couples probably feel overwhelmed by costs and the complexity of the process, but appreciate finally having a place in any departure lounge for parenthood.

Some of our travelers will spend some time in the departure lounge of egg donation, but ultimately decide to take a different course to parenthood. Others will acquaint themselves with egg donation and feel fortified to pursue it. In the next chapter we will take a look at the ways in which people approach egg donation, at the questions you are likely to ask yourselves, at some of the answers you may find.

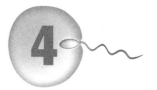

Deciding Whether to Pursue Egg Donation

"Two roads diverged in a yellow wood…"
—Robert Frost

Here you are at a crossroads in your journey toward parenthood. You can either travel down the road of oocyte donation or you can choose another path. Before you focus intently on whether or not to use donated ova, we encourage you to pause for a time and consider all of the possible choices that lie before you. Since most of you will be traveling as part of a couple, we encourage each of you to turn to your companion in this journey and to remind yourselves that you must come to decisions that will work for both of you and for your relationship as a family.

Elements and Influences, Some Reminders

Like all travelers, you should plan well for the journey. We'd like to begin by reminding you of some of the elements of and influences on decision making that we addressed in Chapter 1 and then offer additional suggestions

Decisions Are Made Sequentially

If you have been struggling with infertility, you have probably already figured out that as your reality changes, so do your perceptions of your options. How many of you once thought, "I'll *never* do IVF?" By now many of you are veterans of IVF cycles many times over. As you traveled down one path, you discovered that options which once seemed daunting or disturbing could actually have become attractive.

Never Say Never

You have probably figured this out as well. It is easy to say you will *never* do this, or *never* do that, but as we said before, as your reality changes, so do your decisions. Remember also, that *not yet* does not mean *never*. For instance, your partner may say "Not yet" to something that you think you want to do. Listen carefully to your partner, talk openly about your concerns, and repeat after us, "*Not yet* is not *never*."

Husbands and Wives Move at Different Paces and This Is Not Necessarily a Bad Thing

Remember that we said, "*Not yet* is not *never*." We remind you of this so soon because if you are like most couples facing decisions about using donated ova, one of you will be ready to consider this alternative path to parenthood before the other. When this happens, the person who wants to move forward is often upset and angry with the one who says, "I'm not ready" or "We need to try…again."

You are perhaps puzzled by our saying that this is not necessarily a bad thing. In fact we have found that couples have a way of balancing each other. One of you can sound—and feel—eager to explore options beyond conventional treatment in part because you know that your partner will slow you down and help insure that you make wise, informed decisions. Similarly, you who are trailing at the rear can afford to take it slowly because you know from past experience that your spouse is well prepared to take the lead.

Your History Will Inform Your Decision Making

Remember that you and your partner have different histories as well as a shared one. Inevitably, decisions about using donated ova, adoption and other options will be shaped by your past experiences. If your favorite cousins were adopted, you will have one set of associations about adoption. If the worst trouble maker in your elementary school was adopted, you will have different notions about people who joined their family through adoption. If you were a birthmother and placed a child in adoption, your feelings about adoption will be influenced by this experience, and if your cousin's daughter was a program-recruited oocyte donor, you will have her as a reference point for egg donation.

Be prepared for significant losses to help shape your perceptions of each of these options. This leads us to...

Loss and Grief Are Part of the Journey

Surely you will feel loss and grief along the way. After all, things are not working out the way you had hoped or expected. However, if you may still succeed in having a biological child (or another biological child), you may not face the full loss and grief encountered by those who learn or realize that they will never fulfill their dream. Nonetheless, you are experiencing loss—loss of the hoped for spontaneous conception, loss of feeling that you can plan your time (let alone your family!), loss of money, loss of a great deal of emotional and physical energy already invested, loss of the perception that hard work always pays off. Be prepared for a journey—or the continuation of a journey—that involves loss and grief and ever unfolding new realities. We hope that you, like others who have traveled before you, will discover the unanticipated rewards that come from being able to accept loss, to grieve, and then to celebrate your new realities.

Infertility researcher Dr. Stacy Ellender captures this in an essay she wrote about her own infertility experience and her daughter's arrival from China in *Experiencing Infertility* (Josey Bass, 1998)

> Ellender writes, "Someday, my daughter will learn that she was 'forsaken on the street,' abandoned under unknown circumstances, and waves of pain may send her reeling. But I like to think that I will steady her, that we will share our stories of loss and redefinition. I can hold her hand in mine and show her how to face pain with honesty, integrity and a deep wonder at its unexpected potential to shape our lives."

Don't Punish Yourselves

Remember that you have made the best decisions you could along the way. Regret is a painful, poisonous feeling, and infertile people are often the maestros of regret. It is so tempting to look back and second guess yourself. "I should have been less focused on my career and we should have tried earlier." "I shouldn't have had an abortion when I was 22. It might have been my only chance to have a baby." "I should have pushed my husband when he said we had time to wait." "I should have met him earlier." "I should have tried to marry a younger woman."

Although none of us make decisions expecting to regret them, sometimes the choices we make turn out to be the wrong ones. We wish we could tell you that you can be fully spared regret about future decisions, but you cannot be. It is almost inevitable that you will look back and contemplate how things could have been different if only you had made a different choice. All we can ask is that you try to be gentler with yourselves and each other and remind yourselves that in most instances, you did the best you could with the information you had at hand. As we know, hindsight is twenty/twenty, but in looking forward, all we can do is to try to see things as clearly as we can. Now is the time to look forward with hope rather than back with regret.

The People You Meet along the Way Will Shape Your Journey

Be prepared to meet some wonderful people, perhaps people who will change your lives.

People struggling with infertility find one another in doctors' waiting rooms, on line through sites like INCIID.org and fertilethoughts.com, through infertility support groups like RESOLVE and the American Fertility Association, the Infertility Network, and the Infertility Awareness Association of Canada. People considering using donated ova and adoption turn for guidance to others who have traveled these paths before them. How reassuring it is to attend an adoption agency meeting and see a couple smiling happily as they dote over their newly adopted baby. And you say to yourself, "They look just like regular parents!" How comforting it is to see a woman pregnant through egg donation, glowing and very much "with child." You feel tickled as again you say to yourself, "She looks no different than any other pregnant woman."

The people you meet along your journey will have a lot to do with the choices you make. This is, for the most part, a good thing. We expect that you will find mentors and friends. But take caution as well. You are vulnerable. You will be listening carefully and with emotion to everything you hear about the options that lie before you. If someone has had a bad story using an option that you are considering, that doesn't mean that everyone's experience is bad or that yours will be.

You will meet people along the way who will become friends for the journey. You may also meet people who will become friends for life.

You Have the Right to Make Your Own Decisions and to Feel That You Are Doing So Free and Clear of the Influence of Others

As you travel this journey, you will surely find that others will offer advice. First of all, you will receive a tremendous amount of medical information and advice, requested and unrequested, from physicians, nurses and other caregivers. Medical and program staff's information is given so that they can be sure that your decision is made autonomously and that your consents are fully informed. You should take all of this information in and consider it carefully before making your own unique decision. Advice about non-medical options in family building or the non-medical aspects of gamete-donation, on the other hand, is unauthorative when coming from medical personnel, and should be thought of as such.

You will receive additional advice from what we call "the self-appointed experts"—the family members, friends and complete strangers who want to give you such sage advice as "Relax and you will get pregnant" or "Parenthood is not so great anyhow" or "Why don't you just adopt?" You will need to remain strong and sure-footed as this advice comes your way, often when you feel least equipped to cope with it.

Speak from a Position of Strength

Do not tempt advice givers! If you let people know only the basic facts about your situation—that you want to have a baby and that you are doing your best to make that happen—you are less likely to invite unsolicited advice. And this is really all that anyone needs to know. They don't need to know that you are contemplating using a donor's egg or adoption or another IVF cycle.

When you do have some news that you want to share, speak from a position of strength. If you say, "We're thinking about using a donor ovum" or "We are looking into adoption," you may get upsetting responses such as, "Oh we're so sorry IVF didn't work for you," or "Are you sure you've seen a good doctor? We know someone who had 25 miscarriages and then saw Dr. So-and-So in North Rural, South Dakota and..." or "Whatever you do, stay away from adopting from That Country. We know people who..."

What you need to say—if and when you say anything at all—is "We have *great* news. We've decided to ..." or better yet, "We have great news, we're expecting a child through...."

Realistically Assessing Whether You Can Use Your Own Eggs

As we saw in Chapter 3, some couples turn to oocyte donation because of a genetic problem rather than because of egg quality. However, most exploring ovum donation has reason to believe that they are unlikely to succeed in having a child with the woman's oocytes. Short of a genetic disorder or the absence of ovaries, what "proof" does a couple have that donor eggs are needed?

Unfortunately, there is no test that can perfectly predict a woman's ability to become pregnant with her own ova, so we will discuss some of the tools that physicians and nurses use to assess what is known as "ovarian reserve," but first, it is important to acknowledge the role that natural aging plays in diminishing fertility.

Nurse practitioner Carol Lesser of Boston IVF in Brookline, Massachusetts, works with many women in their early 40s who are seeking pregnancy. She notes that they are, for the most part, a youthful, energetic, optimistic group who had looked forward for many years to having children. Sadly, many are now filled with regret and anger when they learn that their chances for having children using their own eggs are slim. "They are angry at themselves for delaying parenting, and they are angry at physicians for never warning them of the natural hazards of aging."

Lesser has found that before she can offer medical guidance, she must help her patients with their feelings of anger and regret. She begins by assuring them that they have not done something "wrong" and reminds them that they are experiencing a normal aging process. She explains that the ovary ages more rapidly than any other organ in the human body and that by the time a woman reaches age 43, approximately 85% of her eggs are abnormal, regardless of her FSH (Seifer, Grifo and Battaglia, 2000.)

With over twenty years of experience in the field of reproductive medicine, Lesser acknowledges that it was not until recently that obstetricians and gynecologists fully appreciated the impact of age on reproductive ability. "Society has changed, but biology has not. In the past, when people did not live as long, a woman who completed her childbearing by age 30 or so was able to raise her children to adulthood. It made sense from an evolutionary standpoint. Today people are living longer and often preferring to have children later in life, but our ovaries are aging just as rapidly as they did a century ago. It is often very hard for women to have to accept this, but they should understand that they are not the cause of their problems—they are simply experiencing an aspect of normal aging."

IVF arrived 24 years ago and in the excitement about rapidly progressing advances in reproductive medicine which offers cures for reproductive problems that had been intractable for generations, an important message was not sent to the women of the first two birth control generations—medicine can't stop the effects that normal aging has on women's ovaries—at least not yet.

With no perfect, predictive test of ovarian function, how can a woman assess her chances of pregnancy with her own eggs? In addition to paying attention to chronological age, she can turn to the Day 3 FSH test, the most common measure of ovarian reserve (FSH is follicle stimulating hormone). Typically, on the second, third or fourth day of a woman's menstrual cycle, blood is drawn to measure FSH. Because testing for FSH varies from state to state, clinic to clinic and lab to lab, we cannot offer a universal guide for FSH results. However, a relatively low number is desired and a high number suggests decreased ovarian reserve, with sustained high levels seen in menopause. For example, many clinics hope that their patients will have Day 3 FSH numbers under ten, will interpret numbers between ten and fifteen as "borderline," and will see numbers over fifteen as worrisome. So, you might conclude, "If my FSH is low, my eggs should be fine."

If only it were that simple! FSH, as we said, measures "ovarian reserve," or the number of eggs that a woman has left. For some women, quantity is related to quality, but for others, it is not. Hence, it is possible for a woman to have a higher FSH, indicating fewer eggs, but still have some very good quality eggs remaining. We'll talk about assessment of ovum quality after this discussion of measurement of quantity.

There are other tests of ovarian reserve. Some physicians focus on Inhibin-B levels or on MIS levels. In their paper "Early follicular serum mullerian-inhibiting substance levels are associated with ovarian reserve during assisted reproductive technology cycles," (Fertility and Sterility, 2002) researcher David B. Seifer and colleagues demonstrated an association between early follicular phase serum Mullerian inhibiting substance (MIS) levels and the number of oocytes retrieved. Seifer et al found that higher serum MIS levels were associated with greater numbers of retrieved oocytes.

Antral follicle assessment of a woman's ovaries provides yet another measure of ovarian reserve. This test, an ultrasound, is performed on day two, three or four of a woman's cycle. Antral follicles are small potential egg sacs. Ovaries that have no antral follicles at the start of a woman's cycle are likely to be difficult to stimulate. By contrast, those with five or more antral follicles are likely to be easy to stimulate.

Some physicians employ the clomiphene citrate challenge test, a test considered by some to be more precise than the simpler Day 3 FSH test. With the clomiphene citrate challenge test, 100 mg. of clomiphene citrate is taken for five days (usually days 5 through 9) early in a woman's cycle. Her FSH is measured on Day 3 and then again on Day 10. Optimal results show FSH dropping on Day 10. Conversely, if it rises at that point, it is thought to indicate diminished ovarian reserve. Estradiol is also measured on Day 3.

In addition to a decline in quantity, most women also experience a decline in the quality of their eggs as part of the normal aging process. This too can be examined. Lesser recommends looking at FSH alongside levels of Estradiol. Estradiol is the most powerful form of estrogen produced by the ovary and is responsible for the uterine lining and estrogen released by each follicle. The more follicles a woman has, the higher her E2 or estradiol should be. Lesser notes that a higher than normal E2 (estradiol) can artificially lower a woman's FSH. Lesser explains that some older women have high levels of estrogen inappropriately early in their cycle that serve to lower FSH. Hence, when women have E2 levels over 75 or 80, they may actually have artificially lowered FSH.

Lesser reminds women that chronological age is as—or more—important as ovarian age. She notes that women with advanced ovarian and chronological age generally have a lower chance of a successful pregnancy using their own ova than either younger women or women with "younger" ovarian age. But again, she emphasizes that there is no absolute way of predicting fertility. She is thankful to have seen women with elevated FSH or E2 occasionally conceive and carry healthy babies to term, either on their own or with treatment.

It is also possible for a woman to have eggs that are plentiful, look good and fertilize well, but which, when fertilized, still do not create a healthy embryo. The most likely reason for this is again maternal age. As we mentioned earlier, a substantial percentage of the eggs of women in their 40s are genetically defective. In recent years pre-implantation genetic diagnosis (PGD), a procedure originally developed to assist carriers of genetic disorders to have healthy babies, has become a tool in assessing ova/embryo quality. PGD is not a simple procedure, and it is not inexpensive. It involves removing one cell from an eight cell embryo produced in vitro and looking for certain chromosomal abnormalities. Physicians are now introducing PGD as a diagnostic tool for those couples who create a number of healthy looking embryos but who fail to conceive after transfer or who frequently miscarry. In some instances, a number of these embryos are found to contain a chromosomal abnormality not compatible with full term pregnancy. It is thought that most of these abnormalities originate in the egg, not sperm. In addition, with knowledge gained from the Human Genome Project, physicians and scientists are just beginning to identify and learn about genes which cause countless defects, including oocyte defects.

So what does all of this have to do with the fork in the road? A lot. Inevitably there are some women who have elevated FSH who will conceive. Similarly, there are women 43 and 44 who will succeed in becoming pregnant and who will give birth at an age at which some women are already grandmothers. How then do those of you who are at the fork in the road decide between IVF and egg donation or between trying on your own and using donor eggs? A first step is to be absolutely certain about your feelings about the importance of genetic connection. If you find that this still feels of great importance to you, then you will probably want to have most of the above tests run to get a clear sense of your odds for successful conception and delivery using your own eggs.

Some women attempt to lower their FSH level. There are many anecdotal stories of success with acupuncture, as well as with herbal supplements or special diets, including one that recommends eating large amounts of wheat grass, weekly acupuncture and meditation. It is difficult to assess whether or not any of these approaches actually make a difference, since there are natural fluctuations in FSH and since pregnancies can occur in a few instances with elevated FSH levels. Lesser has found that when someone has a "miracle" pregnancy, she is likely to credit the success to whatever she was doing and to want to share her recipe for cure with others. This exuberance comes from a good place, but it can be misleading to others, especially since women undergoing infertility treatment are often eager and willing to try new approaches.

Instead of looking at "curative potential," many clinicians focus on how people feel—emotionally and physically—when they are utilizing "alternative" approaches. Many women find that they feel better in a number of ways. Some report more energy or increased calm. Many report a generalized sense of improved well-being. And perhaps most important, in the face of a dreadful sense of helplessness, many women are grateful to be able to do something that feels pro-active. As many have reported, "Even if I don't become pregnant, I feel better after my acupuncture sessions, and I feel they are helping me to lead a healthier life." It has long been widely accepted in the scientific community that women have a finite number of eggs that dwindle throughout one's earlier years and diminish exponentially in the latter reproductive years. This is in dramatic contrast to men, who have a steady, replenishable supply of sperm.

And, for those for whom using their own genetic material remains a high priority, before looking further at using donated ova and comparing that to other alternatives, we want to offer some brief discussion of two treatment options that could result in the birth of a couple's full biological child.

Continuing to Try on Your Own (without IVF)

Some women are not ready to give up on the possibility of having a child with their own eggs, but they choose to try on their own rather than with IVF. What distinguishes this group from those who try IVF—or more IVF—before taking the ovum donation fork in the road? Financial cost is a significant factor for many, but there are other issues as well. The most important involves determining whether IVF offers any benefit over "trying naturally." Surely it does when a woman has blocked tubes or there is a severe male factor, but what of the couple that is considering egg donation only because of oocyte quality?

Carol Lesser observes that the higher the FSH, the less treatment matters. She explains that if a woman has a low FSH, she is likely to have many eggs. Even if most of the eggs are flawed, some good ones should remain. IVF, with its controlled hyperstimulation and retrieval of eggs, enables the physician to go after a large group of eggs all at once. Hopefully that large group will contain at least one egg of good quality. Perhaps two or three will fertilize, and if all are transferred, the result may be an on-going pregnancy. Lesser's point is that by doing IVF, someone with a large number of eggs, but declining fertility, is able to condense several natural cycles into one month. Unfortunately, this is not a guarantee of success. If most eggs are of poor quality, more is not necessarily better.

Without adequate ovarian reserve, women are less likely to benefit from IVF. There aren't as many eggs and so an IVF cycle is unlikely to yield the quantity of oocytes that would enable someone to condense several months of retrievals into one. Lesser and many others have observed that women with high FSH who become pregnant often do so on their own spontaneously, unless, of course, blocked tubes or severe male factor renders this impossible.

Trying on your own, without IVF, before choosing egg donation, offers a number of benefits, assuming a couple can afford for time to pass. For one thing, there is that matter of "the lucky egg." If a "lucky egg" is going to come along, you can't be pregnant with a donated egg. So those who hold out some hope that they will conceive on their own benefit from delaying an egg donation pregnancy.

Another reason for trying on one's own comes back to that thorny issue of regret. Over and over and over again, moms through donated ova who came to the decision slowly and after years of infertility credit their readiness for their happiness. As one woman, now pregnant with her second baby through oocyte donation, put it, "I remember not liking the idea of egg donation at all when it was first mentioned to me. But by the time we got to deciding to do it, I really felt we had exhausted all fertility options. At that juncture, it seemed like the natural next step."

Finally, trying on one's own buys time. It buys time to save money for egg donation or for adoption. It buys time possibly to benefit from medical advances. It buys time for a woman to grieve not being able to pass on some special part of herself and time for her partner to grieve this loss as well. It allows a couple to grieve the fact that fertility treatments did not work for them, to re-group and replenish their relationship, to feel that when they get to the next fork in the road, they will be all the better prepared to make the best decision for themselves.

Continuing to Try on Your Own with IVF

And for those still hopeful of using their own eggs there also remains the option of moving to IVF (or, for many reading this book continuing with IVF treatments for a while more.)

In vitro fertilization refers to fertilization outside the human body. In "regular IVF" a woman takes medication that causes her to produce several ovarian follicles. Follicular growth is carefully monitored by ultrasound, as well as by blood tests. When a number of follicles have grown beyond 15 centimeters, eggs are retrieved in what is a minor surgical procedure. They are then mixed with the intended father's sperm, placed in a special culture medium for two to five days, and transferred back to the intended mother's uterus via a catheter. "Regular IVF" differs from an egg donation cycle in that the fertilized eggs returned are those of the genetic mother rather than those of a donor.

The Costs of IVF

Costs of IVF are real and they are steep. Because the laws governing health insurance companies vary from state to state, where you reside will determine many of your costs. If you are fortunate to live in one of the sixteen states (as of this writing) that have either "mandate to cover" laws (which require that health insurance companies provide coverage of infertility treatment as a benefit included in every policy) or "mandate to offer" laws (which require that health insurance companies have policies available for purchase that offer infertility treatment coverage) your treatment may be covered or partially covered. In considering your options, it is important to talk with a financial specialist at a reproductive medicine center, as well as with a representative of your insurance company, to determine what treatment is covered, how much coverage is offered (some policies limit the number of treatment cycles) and under what circumstances coverage may be denied. For example, even the most generous of mandates may deny coverage to someone who has had "voluntary sterilization"—tubal ligation or vasectomy.

Depending upon whether you live in a state with an insurance mandate or in one that has none, and depending upon your personal finances, the decision to try—or continue to try—"regular IVF" or to turn to donated ova may be driven by the costs involved.

Let's look for a moment, then, at some of the cost variables.

IVF in a Mandated State

Assuming that you have medical insurance, there is virtually no financial cost involved in trying IVF. (There are other costs, in terms of time and energy, but we will get to those).

IVF in a Non-Mandated State

IVF is expensive (anywhere from $10,000 to $20,000 per cycle) and even if you can afford it, you may feel that you would be "throwing money away" if you or your physician considers your odds of success is considered a "long shot." Some programs offer money-back guarantees to excellent-prognosis patients or may offer various payment plans. We will talk about those later.

What Now?

If you have reached this point having determined that you cannot use your own eggs to achieve a pregnancy and parenthood, you have reached another fork in the road. Available to you now are the following options:

- Donor oocytes
- Other collaborative (third-party assisted) options
- Adoption
- Accepting life as it is and moving forward positively

We believe that the best way to proceed from this point is to at least cursorily consider all of the options open to you. Since the focus of this book is deciding whether or not to use the option of using donor eggs to achieve pregnancy and parenthood, we have chosen to frame the discussion of the other three options as they *compare* to using donated eggs.

We believe that making any of these choices, however, requires beginning at the beginning—looking carefully at your motivations for parenthood.

Exploring Your Motivations for Parenthood

How and why does anyone decide to become a parent? If we were to pose that question to one of your fertile friends, she might respond, "I didn't think about it very much—I just knew I wanted to be a mom" or "It was just the natural order of things—you get married, buy a house, have a kid...." or "I love little babies and couldn't wait to have one to take care of."

We could add to the list, but, instead, we hope that you see our point: people who don't face difficulties conceiving don't always give a whole lot of thought to what it means to be a parent. In addition, they are never called upon to consider the relative significance of different aspects of parenthood—how important it is to them to share a pregnancy experience, to have a genetic connection with their child or with one another, or to continue a bloodline. They don't have to consider the impact of having their bodies and their sex lives invaded by a team of "helpers" in order to become parents. They don't have to ask themselves what it would mean to parent a child of another race or a child who was half genetically theirs or, perhaps, was their full genetic child gestated by another woman.

The decisions that may lie before you are very complicated ones that you may not feel qualified to make. "How," you might ask yourself, "can I know how it would feel being the Caucasian mom of a little Chinese girl?" or "If I've never been pregnant and certainly never been a mom, how can I possibly know how I will react to having a baby through egg donation?"

Although there are no easy answers to these and the multitude of other questions you will ask yourself, there are many things that you can begin to do that can help you to obtain plenty of information and to see things more clearly. We propose that you begin by asking yourselves the following questions and writing down your responses. If you have a partner, we suggest that you do this homework separately and then come together to share with each other your responses.

1. Why do you want to be a parent? How many of your responses have to do with having a physical connection to the child—genetic or gestational? How many have to do with your expectations and dreams about the parenting role and experience? If you have a parenting partner, how many have to do with the notion of blending your genes with your beloved's in creating a child to parent together? Together you may discuss your thoughts and feelings about the relative importance of each of these.

2. What kind of parent do you want to be? Again, infertility has probably forced you to avoid this question, but now, with decisions and options before you, it is something to think about. Do you envision yourself as "strict" or "lenient," "pushy" or "laid back," "playful," "instructive," a "role model," a "mentor?"?

3. What are the values and the traditions in your family, your culture, and your faith that you wish to pass on to a child? Consider what it means to be a member of your family. Is your family one in which there has been inter-marriage—religious or racial? Is your family one with a strong ethnic or cultural identity? Is it one that celebrates diversity? Do you have nieces and nephews who are of a different race than you are, either because of adoption or transracial marriage? Have there been divorces, remarriages, step-families within your clan? How do you see your becoming a parent as altering your relationship with your extended family?

4. What do you see when you see parents and children? What is it about parenthood that you look forward to?

5. Look around you at pregnant women and at parents. This is probably something you have been avoiding if you have been

struggling with infertility. Now you need to start looking and taking notice. When you see pregnant women, remind yourself that they may be pregnant with a donor oocyte or donor embryo or donor sperm. Can you tell? Do the parents through donors look different to you in any way?

In thinking through these questions openly and honestly by yourself and in discussing them just as honestly with your partner (if you have one) you will have gained a great deal of information that will help you to make choices. For example, if genetic connection ranks high with you, adoption may move lower on your list of options—at least for now. The importance of genetic connection to a wife without "good eggs" can produce the need for some real soul searching before she considers using the genetic material of a donor to achieve a pregnancy. If the actual experience of being a parent is the most important thing to the two of you, you may be willing to forgo the physical, emotional and financial risks of pursuing any more options that involve treatment and plunge straight into adoption.

Comparing Other Options to the Option of Egg Donation

So here you are at a fork in the road. One path leads towards using donated ova. The other fork sends you down a different path—at least for the time being. As you face this next decision, remember that your perspective may change as your reality changes. You may travel down one path only to reach another fork in the road and the need for a different decision. But here you are at this fork. So let's take a look at the decisions you face and at the choices you see before you.

Egg Donation and Other Collaborative (Third-Party) Options

One set of options you might want to consider involve collaborative or third-party options. Of course egg donation is one of these, but it is not the only collaborative reproductive option. Donor sperm, surrogacy, gestational care and embryo adoption are collaborative reproductive options which can be attractive to those who are also considering egg donation, though of course not all of them would "work", depending on your medical issues. As we said before, because this is a book centered on oocyte donation, our format will be to compare each alternative to the option of using donated ova to create a pregnancy.

Embryo Adoption vs. Ovum Donation

In the earliest years of the 21st century, a new path to parenthood became available: embryo adoption. This is the pre-pregnancy "adoption" of an existing embryo. Embryo adoption became an option because there are couples who go through IVF, cryopreserve embryos for possible future use and then, for a variety reasons, do not seek pregnancy with their frozen embryos. This may happen when embryos remain after the couple has twins or triplets on the first IVF cycle, or has a second or third successful pregnancy using some frozen embryos or decides, for other reasons, including divorce and death, not to use the remaining embryos.

For some parents who were assisted by IVF, having "extra" embryos does not pose a problem, either emotionally or ethically. They see their embryos as having "potential" for life and feel they are fundamentally different from fetuses. Such couples generally feel comfortable either discarding "extra" embryos or donating them to science

Unfortunately, there are some couples who go through IVF and end up with embryos that they are prepared neither to parent, to discard nor donate to science. Included in this group are those who believe that life begins with an embryo and who are aware, as they enter into an IVF cycle, that the process may put them in the unenviable position of being "high tech birthparents."

There are others who enter a cycle with no particular concerns about their embryos, but who later find themselves in a very painful predicament. This happens to some who feel so barren that they cannot imagine having more embryos than they are prepared to parent, as well as to those who discover, in the course of the IVF process or after having children, that their feelings about the origins of life have changed.

Psychologist Maggie Kirkman, PhD, of the Key Centre for Women's Health in Society at the University of Melbourne interviewed women who decided for and against embryo donation. She notes that it is the maternal feelings that some mothers feel towards their embryos that prompts them to donate them to another couple. Kirkman quotes Wilma, who considered reasons for and against donating and concluded, "One embryo became our second child, who is absolutely wonderful. Who were the others? Just as wonderful? They at least deserved a chance at life." Kirkman also writes of Yolanda, who became a mother after an egg donation from her sister. She decided against donating remaining embryos because "a baby is not an empty vessel; it is born with an inheritance and a corresponding right to know its origins." Kirkman goes on to say, "This sense of 'child of ours' was marked in embryo donors and others who had contemplated embryo donation. It could be explained in terms of pre-implantation parental feelings known to be experienced by people undergoing IVF who look through a microscope at the dividing cells of their potential children.

Kirkman tells of Samantha and her husband, an Australian couple who had two children from donated embryos. They had planned to have only one child "and would have happily carried out that plan had no embryos been left over; but the three remaining embryos were related to Stephanie and "if those embryos had gone to another couple and a child was conceived from them, we would have been devastated."

However they get there, couples who have extra embryos and who believe that life begins with an embryo, not with a beating heart, are in a very difficult predicament: they feel they must find parents for their embryos. Until a few years ago, they were left to try to resolve this dilemma on their own. Ironically, some felt they had to attempt a pregnancy they didn't want or they found themselves as unwitting and unassisted birthparents, trying to "make an adoption plan" for their embryo. With little, if any help, from reproductive medicine centers and with none from adoption agencies, these high tech birthparents were left with a very private sorrow. ("Grief reactions following an invitro fertilization treatment" by Greenfeld, Diamond and DeCherney in *Journal of Psychosomatic Ob and Gyn* [pp. 8, 169-174]).

As adoption agencies became aware of the dilemma of embryo birthparents, some stepped in and began to formalize and facilitate the process of embryo adoption. While their efforts undoubtedly provide some relief to embryo birthparents, embryo adoption raises profound moral and ethical questions. Since this book is for individuals and couples considering egg donation, we will focus here on how you might compare egg donation with embryo adoption. However, it is our hope that physicians and mental health counselors working with pre-IVF couples will counsel them, as best they can, to help avoid the creation of extra embryos. This can be accomplished, at least in part, by encouraging those who believe that life begins with an embryo to inseminate only the number of eggs they feel they can transfer. In addition, all pre-IVF couples should be alerted to the possibility that their feelings about the origins of life may change in the course of their treatment.

They should pay particular attention to a shift in their feelings and do what they can to avoid having extra embryos (e.g. A couple who might have wanted to avoid a multiple gestation and transfer only one embryo could elect to transfer two or three in order to reduce or eliminate the risk of having extra embryos).

As you explore your options for family building, should you consider helping these unwitting birthparents by adopting their embryos? For some of you, this option offers two substantial benefits: it can feel like the "right" thing to do and it can be more cost effective than egg donation since intended parents (or their insurance) will have covered IVF costs. However, there are some important issues to consider:

The Child's Story

As you begin to think about embryo adoption, remember that children who enter their families through this process will have birth families with full biological siblings being raised by the people who originally created them. Embryo adoptees will grow up knowing that their full biological siblings were given the opportunity to be raised by their genetic parents but that they—because of a decision made by their parents, their parents physicians and embryologists—must grow up without a genetic connection to their parents. As they mature, they will grapple with the knowledge that it probably took a split second for the embryologist to decide which embryos to transfer to the genetic parents and which to cryopreserve for some other future.

We see the story of a child created through embryo donation as similar to, and yet fundamentally different from, the story of the traditional adoptee. The traditional adoptee may also have full siblings being raised by his birthparents, but what he knows, painful as it may be to accept, is that at the time of his birth, his parents were not prepared to parent another child. By contrast, the embryo adoptee grapples with a very different story: at the time of his conception, his parents deeply longed for a child or twins to parent. Because of medical and lab decisions, he was not included in the pair of embryos offered that opportunity. It seems to us that this knowledge is likely to prompt an embryo adoptee to feel a profound sense of displacement. And since all of us sometimes wonder how we landed in our families, we imagine he may face a lifetime of recurring feelings that he is the wrong person, in the wrong family. Knowing his birth siblings and birthfamily may help answer some of his questions but could further intensify his sense of disconnect. We worry about how embryo adoptees will accept their adoptive families, and whether they will have feelings of anger, loss, confusion and resentment towards the medical caregivers and their birthparents. We are concerned that they may resent their adoptive parents, their birth siblings and others who have rendered them this unique status of embryo adoptees.

The story of a child created through egg donation is fundamentally different from that of an embryo adoptee in several respects. First, in terms of genetic ties, the child created by egg donation does not have full siblings being raised by their genetic parents. In addition, this child has a genetic link to his/her father and to the father's entire family, past, present and future. And perhaps most significant, for the child created through egg donation, there never were other intended parents. He/she has the opportunity to be raised by the people who sought to be his/her parents from the start.

Birth Family Concerns

Embryo adoption raises profound questions not only for the offspring for whom an adoption was planned, but also, for the entire birth family. Even embryo adoptive parents who do not plan to maintain contact with their child's birth family will recognize the birth family played—and continues to play—an important role in their child's life. How can embryo adoptive parents escape from the somber awareness that the birthparents—people who believe that life begins with an embryo—have to live with a feeling of estrangement from their biological offspring? Imagine, also, what the siblings, who were transferred to their intended mom as embryos, will feel knowing that others were adopted rather than transferred.

Because of these issues and others, many choosing embryo adoption will choose an open arrangement. While this arrangement may spare the offspring—both adopted and raised by the genetic parents—some bewilderment, it does not necessarily make things easy for both sets of parents. How can birthparents really anticipate how they will feel in the future as they watch others raise children they desperately wanted and worked so very hard to create? What might happen if one or more of the birthparents' children become ill or have a disability, while the adopted-out children thrive? Or what of the reverse? Will the birthparents be plagued with guilt and will the "adoptive" parents feel they are being judged for the way they handle these challenges?

Unfortunately, the list of potential questions and anxieties for the birth family is extensive. We have raised but a few of the most likely sources of loss and regret.

Comparing "Traditional" Birthparents and Embryo Birthparents

As you consider embryo adoption as a path to parenthood, we encourage you to think about the experience of "embryo birthparents." All of us have learned, from "traditional adoption," that birthparents do not forget the children they placed for adoption and that many go on in their lives with a profound sense of loss. Since all members of the adoption triad—adoptees, adoptive parents and birthparents—are in many ways, connected for life, the losses experienced by birthparents touch the hearts and minds of adoptees and adoptive parents.

Because embryo adoption began only a few years before this writing, we do not have the experiences of many embryo birthparents to draw upon. However, we can imagine that they will experience some feelings of loss similar to those of "traditional" birthparents. In addition, the way in which they become birthparents is likely to further impact their feelings. It seems, in some ways, like the ultimate irony that they, who struggled so much to have their children, should find themselves feeling the need to find parents for one or more of their offspring.

Unlike "traditional" birthparents, embryo birthparents do not experience pregnancy and labor and delivery. They do not feel a baby move inside them, nor hear his cries at birth, nor hold him moments after he enters this world. From this perspective, embryo birthparents seem to have an "easier separation"—they say good-bye to an embryo that is usually lodged in an embryology lab rather than to a baby in a hospital nursery or adoption agency office.

Although the parting may be simpler and "easier," we wonder if the long term impact of placing an embryo for adoption will be any less painful than it is in traditional adoption. Although embryo birthparents do not experience saying good-bye to a real live baby, they are raising a child or children conceived at the same time as the embryo(s) they placed for adoption. What will it be like for these parents when they watch their child or children grow and know that there could be a third or a fourth child in the family? We expect that those who have open adoptions will wonder what it would be like if that child had been part of their family. And for those with closed adoptions, there will inevitably be feelings about the child who is "out there in the world. The feelings of separation and loss in both open and closed adoptions may seem similar between traditional and embryo birthparents, but we fear that with embryo adoption there will be added feelings of guilt and responsibility. Traditional adoption is a solution to a problem: a child needs a home. Embryo adoption grows out of a different problem: people have turned to science in an effort to become parents and the science has yielded more offspring than the parents feel prepared to raise. For a group that believes that life begins with an embryo (otherwise, they would probably discard the embryo or donate to science rather than choose adoption), this may be profoundly troubling. "Did we violate the natural order of things?" they may wonder. "Was it wrong for us to pursue assisted reproduction when this was the outcome?" "Have our lives become a science fiction story?" they may ask.

It is too soon to know how this will all play out. Having experienced the pain of infertility, embryo birthparents may feel grateful to be able to help others become parents. They may go on in their lives feeling content that their efforts to build a family brought additional new lives into the world. Or they may be burdened with feelings of loss and confusion, wondering if what happened was really meant to be.

As we said at the start of this book, assisted reproduction, egg donation and here, embryo adoption highlight the blessings and the curses of the "meant to be."

Risks

In a sense, embryo adoption is a step closer to pregnancy than egg donation and might therefore *seem* to have fewer risks. After all, the embryo already exists and simply needs to be transferred to a womb. By contrast, egg donation requires several preliminary steps—medical and psychological screening of the donor, stimulation, egg retrieval and finally, fertilization. Nonetheless, embryo adoption seems to us to carry with it many more risks than egg donation—most of them the mental health risk to embryo adoptees and to their birthparents described above.

We caution people considering this option now to think about what it will mean for them and their children to be pioneers in this new and uncharted form of family building.

Truth Telling

Although families built through gamete donation (sperm donation has been practiced for over 100 years) were historically encouraged to make their choices a secret, most have learned, from the experiences of others, that secrets can be lethal and that the happy story of how they became a family should be proudly shared with children. Parents and children can sort out, in an on-going and ever unfolding way, what they want to keep within the boundaries of their home and which parts of their story they will choose to share with others.

For families created through embryo adoption it is much more complicated. For one thing, how do parents share this difficult story with their children? How do they explain that the birthparents *really, really,* wanted them but that the embryologist chose someone else for transfer? How do the children process this story and can they tell others the truth about their origins without feeling lonely, isolated, different and perhaps, even teased or ridiculed? And do both sets of parents—birth and adoptive—have a responsibility to bring the children together, at least on occasion, so they can know their full biological siblings?

....

Meet Angie and Gino...

"Because that's the way it is." Gino, a 35-year-old electrician, hears these words a lot these days. His wife, Angie, also 35 and pregnant for the first time through embryo adoption, invokes them a lot. When her parents ask her to explain why she and Gino chose to become parents through embryo adoption, she responds, "Because that's the way it is." When friends ask her how she will explain things to her child, she says "Because that's the way it is." When she anticipates talking with a pe-diatrician about the fact that the donor couple—Gino's former colleagues—used a donor egg, Angie says, "I'll tell her 'that's the way it is.'"

That's the way it is. Angie and Gino, both first generation Italian Americans, never anticipated being trailblazers. When they set out to become parents five years ago, they assumed it would all happen "the old fashioned way." Indeed, Angie did conceive easily, but that pregnancy ended in miscarriage. Another treatment ended in miscarriage, followed by a third pregnancy which proved ectopic. Along the way, the couple learned that Gino had serious defects in his sperm that Angie's tubes were blocked, and, while the physicians were at it, her eggs were "just so-so." The couple was exploring adoption when they received a call from Maria, an acquaintance. "I hear that the two of you are going through infertility. Remember Pat and Ryan? They went through infertility, had a little boy and decided not to have more children. They've been looking everywhere for a couple to adopt their frozen embryos. There are three of them."

"For a few seconds, I didn't know what to do. I had never really heard of embryo adoption, let alone think of doing it ourselves. I assumed, once we heard that Gino's sperm was bad, that we'd use donor sperm. But when we tried it for one cycle, Gino became depressed. He said he'd feel left out if it worked. We were glad when it didn't."

Once Angie and Gino decided they needed to be "on equal footing with a child" they knew that neither egg donation nor donor sperm would work for them. Adoption was attractive but the costs were discouraging, especially for Angie and Gino who had full insurance coverage for all forms of treatment, including gamete and embryo donation. Then came Maria's call and it set a whole new process in motion.

Angie and Gino did not enter into embryo adoption lightly. They talked a lot together and then talked with Pat and Ryan. The two couples agreed that they would be fully open about how their families were formed. The children would grow up knowing each other and would share important occasions. Both couples met with lawyers and with mental health counselors. Angie says that each step along the way confirmed to her that this was the right thing to do.

"I'm not an overly religious person, but I do have faith. I decided that God had things happen for a reason and then brought Pat and Ryan back into our lives for a reason. It feels like fate or destiny. And that's the way it is."

Donor Sperm vs. Egg Donation

Sounds like an odd choice, doesn't it—for a couple reading a book about egg donation because they "need" oocytes to also consider using donated sperm? Since an egg and a sperm are each essential ingredients in pregnancy, why would anyone be choosing between them? In fact, there are two groups of couples who could find themselves in the position of choosing between donor eggs and donor sperm.

Couples with Genetic Problems

Couples in which both partners are carriers of a serious genetic condition have two options if they want to avoid transmitting that condition to their child: they can do IVF with PGD, something which is very complicated and expensive or they can eliminate one of them as a carrier.

Take Alice and Larry, for example, both are cystic fibrosis carriers and the parents of two sons, Matt and Alex. Matt has CF, Alex does not. Alice and Larry want another child, but are afraid to roll the dice again. They can try IVF with PGD or they can decide to go with donor oocytes or donor sperm. The obvious advantage of donor sperm is that it is much less costly and does not require assisted reproductive technology. However, with donor sperm, Larry is very much out of the pregnancy loop—Alice has both a genetic and a gestational tie to their next child and he has neither. If they choose egg donation, it will be more costly, but it will offer the couple "parity"—each will play a crucial role in bringing their child into this world.

Couples with Unexplained Infertility

Although many with unexplained infertility do learn more when they try IVF, there remain couples whose infertility continues to be entirely unexplained even after IVF. They could try PGD or they can introduce either donor sperm or donor ova to see if that makes a difference. Their decisions will be influenced by whether either or both partners have children and by costs, since donor sperm is much less expensive than oocyte donation.

Surrogacy vs. Egg Donation

In the early years after the development of IVF, when the procedure was experimental and not very successful, couples with female infertility problems had limited treatment options. Commercial surrogacy arrived to fill a service gap. Those who wanted to have a biological connection to one parent sometimes turned to surrogacy as an alternative to adoption. With surrogacy, a woman willing to bear a child for another couple enters into a pre-conception adoption agreement with a couple. She agrees to become pregnant by being inseminated with the male partner's sperm and to place the children with the couple following birth in a legal process very akin to a step-parent adoption. This option was pursued by a number of infertile couples in the 1970s, but ceased to be widely sought once IVF was improved. For one thing, women who were unable to conceive because of blocked or absent fallopian tubes now had a greater chance to become pregnant. For another, IVF soon made egg donation possible, enabling a woman with a functioning uterus to carry and deliver her baby.

Finally, IVF made it possible for couples to create their own embryos and have them transferred to another woman if the intended mother was unable to gestate them. This woman became known as a gestational carrier and we will refer to the experience she undertakes as gestational care, though you may also hear it referred to as gestational surrogacy.

So what became of "traditional" surrogacy? It continues to have a place for some couples. They include couples in which the woman can neither produce viable eggs nor carry a pregnancy. Such couples can combine egg donation and gestational care, but may choose not to do so either for financial reasons and logistical reasons (surrogacy can be a very simple, low tech process) or perhaps, because a special person in their lives has volunteered to be their surrogate.

Surrogacy occasionally has a place for gay couples. After all, they need an egg and a uterus and there are women willing to provide both. For those couples who do choose surrogacy, the process can be less costly and less medically invasive. The surrogate can simply be inseminated by the sperm of one of the intended fathers (men are advised not to try to mix their sperm in one attempt, but can do so in alternating inseminations). However, although this may appear attractive for its relatively simplicity and its cost effectiveness, many gay couples are reluctant to turn to traditional surrogacy. They worry that the surrogate, who is truly the child's birthmother, may change her mind and may then have parenting rights. Many also feel that they are looking for different qualities in an egg donor than in a surrogate and prefer to seek those qualities in two different women. Finally, they look at surrogacy through the child's lens and wonder how a child will comprehend that his/her birthmother entered into a preconception adoption arrangement.

Gestational Care with Egg Donation

We turn now to an option that has become more common in recent years: Gestational care with egg donation. This is an option rarely decided upon all at once, but rather, it is one that people come to *after* they have decided on egg donation or *after* they have chosen gestational care. Having reached a fork in the road and traveled down one path, they now find themselves at a second fork.

Gestational care is the process by which a woman carries a child to whom she has no genetic connection, gives birth to that child and transfers his/her care to the couple who created him. It can be combined with egg donation either for a gay couple or for heterosexual couples who prefer this option to adoption. Often these are couples who have made sequential decisions. First they were told that the woman had either a uterine problem or an egg problem and, depending on which problem it was, they were advised to consider gestational care or egg donor. As a couple they decided to move forward with the option offered, only to later learn that there was an additional problem that was preventing pregnancy. When a couple learns they need more help than they anticipated, they find themselves at a second fork in the road facing yet another major decision.

Recall Zoë and Carl...

Zoë and Carl never expected that they would be one of those "very fertile looking couples" with three children under the age of two. But here they are—the parents of three young daughters, born to them through the help of an egg donor and two gestational carriers. Zoë and Carl's older two daughters are two year old twins, Emily and Angela and their younger daughter, Hayley, is 6 months old.

Zoë and Carl's story began like many other infertility sagas, They were in their early 30s, tried to become pregnant and learned that Zoë had a fibroid that needed to be surgically removed. She underwent surgery, the couple resumed their efforts to conceive only to learn that at age 34, Zoë had elevated FSH indicating she had a decreased number of eggs. "Egg donation" their physician said. "Not so easy," responded Zoë and Carl, who were quite interested in adoption.

"We visited a few adoption agencies and had really disappointing experiences. Each place we went to seemed to go out of their way to let us know how difficult adoption was. No one seemed to want to present a positive, optimistic picture. We began to feel pretty deflated and then we heard about an egg donation workshop. To our relief, it was completely different! We heard from several couples and a few physicians about how 'easy' and 'wonderful' egg donation was. After that meeting, we knew what our decision would be."

Unfortunately, Zoë did not become pregnant through egg donation. One donor, then another. After efforts failed with a second donor, the couple received more bad news. "We think your fibroid is growing back." Still undaunted, the couple decided to try with yet a third donor. Two embryos were transferred to Zoë, who ended up in the hospital for pain control because of endometriosis. When a social worker came in and said to Carl, "You can't do this to her anymore," he responded, "You're right." That was when the couple realized they were at the next fork in the road—once again they were ready to compare two options: egg donation with gestational care or adoption. Once again, adoption came up short—they went to adoption agencies that told horror stories and to a gestational carrier seminar where they heard more good news. "What we were hearing about adoption was making us feel it was not a good decision for us. What we were hearing about gestational care was reassuring—we would be there from the moment of conception to birth…we would be in the delivery room and no one was going to change their mind. And having decided on egg donation, we knew now we would have the same child we would have had had I not had the hysterectomy."

Zoë goes on to say, "I completely believe that being able to listen to the people and to hear them juxtaposed to each other was incredibly helpful. Earlier I had been totally offended when a doctor suggested I get 'a gestational uterus.' I never would have done something as totally weird as this in my entire life— there is what you think and all the steps you go through and that changes your reality."

Additional Resources

If, in light of what you've read above and your discussions with your partner, you believe that you owe it to yourselves to consider more seriously any of the other third-party reproductive options, we offer you the following carefully selected list of resources, each of which has a different purpose, and each of which can lead you to additional resources as needed for your decision making.

Helping the Stork : The Choices and Challenges of Donor Insemination by Carol Frost Vercollone Heidi Moss, Robert Moss (Wiley, 1997)—a thoughtful exploration of the practicalities and the ethics of choosing to parent by donor insemination with helpful discussions applicable to those who choose any third party option.

Experiences of Donor Conception: Parents, Offspring and Donors Through the Years Caroline Lorbach (Jessica Kingsley, 2003) by—a thoughtful discussion of donor conception enlightened by anecdotal material from those living the experience.

Experiencing Infertility: Stories to Inform and Inspire by Ellen Glazer (Jossey Bass, 1998)—moving essays by parents who choose egg donation, known gestational care, sperm donation, international and domestic adoption.

New Ways of Making Babies: The Case of Egg Donation, edited by Cynthia Cohen (Indiana University Press, 1996)—a series of wise, thoughtful and provocative essays about egg donation.

Adoption vs. Donated Oocytes

Adoption, like egg ovum donation, comes in various shapes and sizes. Domestic adoption, international adoption, same race adoption, transracial adoption, infant adoption and older child adoption, the adoption of children who are healthy or who have various levels of health issues are all questions one must consider in making a decision to adopt. And for ovum donation carries its own set of choices to make. There is sister-to-sister donation, other intrafamily donation, friend-to-friend, contractual program-recruited anonymous donors and contractual program-recruited known donors. Surely, there are some people who will make decisions between using donor oocytes and adopting based on the availability of particular kinds of adoption or egg donation. For example, a sister's offer to donate might prompt someone otherwise intending to adopt to seek egg donation. Or, the offer of a healthy newborn baby, born to friends of friends of friends, might sway a couple off the donor course.

The decision to choose adoption over egg donation or vice versa is ultimately, like most other important decisions in life, a matter of the heart. People can (and should) go to great lengths to analyze the pros and cons of their decision, but ultimately, they are guided by what *feels* right. Nonetheless, they do take the following into account as they examine their feelings.

Importance of Pregnancy

People's sentiments about pregnancy play a big role in determining how they feel about egg donation vs. adoption. If there is one single factor that clearly distinguishes the two paths to parenthood—especially for women—it is pregnancy. With egg donation you have it, and with adoption, you don't.

For some, pregnancy is an essential ingredient in a parent-child relationship. They feel that bonds between mother and child begin in utero and that a child benefits from hearing both of his parent's voices in the months before birth. They also value pregnancy because they know that what a woman eats and does not eat, drinks and does not drink during pregnancy can play a role in a newborn's health. In addition, some would-be parents look forward to pregnancy as a "countdown to parenthood," anticipating nine months of preparation for a child's arrival.

Not everyone feels such awe about pregnancy. Couples who have suffered devastating pregnancy losses cannot help but feel that pregnancy brings enormous pain and suffering. Those who have difficult pregnancies, marred by severe nausea, depression or physical illness, have similarly lost their respect for this supposedly "perfect state of the unions." For those who have had negative experiences with pregnancy, it becomes, at best, a means to an end—their goal of parenthood.

Feelings about pregnancy often change in the course of infertility diagnosis and treatment. Some who may have had little interest in pregnancy find themselves longing for it. Others may find themselves moving in the reverse direction, seeing pregnancy as an experience that lasts nine months and parenthood as one that lasts a lifetime and is available without pregnancy.

Relationship with the Child

Everyone who sets out to be a parent wants to have a child they will love and cherish and who will feel authentically their child. For many, adoption feels like an incredible leap of faith. In signing on to adopt, they feel they are making a lifelong commitment to a total stranger. This is daunting. A common concern voiced by prospective adoptive parents is "I fear I will be living with a stranger."

Of course, some of this fear is based on a misunderstanding of how bonding and attaching works between human beings, Some assume that "real bonding" is a result of a nine month gestation, and they wonder if they could ever attach to a child not genetically related to them. The truth is that bonding is an emotional connection between human beings that is based on a growing sense of the ability to trust one another. Those of us who will be parenting in pairs have already proven to ourselves that we can attach to someone genetically unrelated to us: we share an attachment with our partner.

Still, for some would-be parents, oocyte donation feels like less of an emotional stretch than does adoption. They are reassured by the fact that the child will have a genetic connection to the father and with intra-family egg donation, to both parents. They are reassured, also, by the fact that the mother will have a gestational connection to the child. Although no one knows for sure what an unborn child feels and experiences, many assume that a child that was intentionally created by his/her parents and is eagerly awaited will somehow know this in utero and will enter the world with the beginnings of a strong connection to his family.

Others see bonding and attachment through a different lens. Some couples feel it will be much easier for the two of them to connect with a child that is adopted into the family with no genetic connection to either parent, than it will would be to face what for them is the more complicated task of raising a child with a genetic connection to just one of them.

Egg donation is also attractive because it offers couples the opportunity to "be present at the creation." Yes, they are assisted by another person, but the child conceived is *intended to be their child.* Despite the questions some have about whether children conceived with donated gametes will have a difficult time understanding their donor parent's motivation, these would-be parents are reassured to know that the child is unlikely to experience the feelings of rejection and loss that are so often troubling to adoptees. In addition, they are comforted to know that there are no "other parents" out there.

Health of the Child

Almost everyone wants a healthy child. Certainly, there are people who seek to adopt a child with a special need, but for the most part, intended parents hope that the child that enters their family will be healthy, physically and emotionally. So what is the more likely way to have a healthy child: egg donation or adoption?

Some say adoption. When you adopt a newborn child domestically, the child has been born and assessed by a hospital pediatrician, who will be discharging a healthy baby to your care unless you voluntarily accept a child with a medical problem. With international adoption there is a similar added benefit. The children are usually at least several months old. Adoptive parents of internationally-born children are now encouraged to share the medical profile they receive of a child referred to them with a growing number of pediatricians across the U.S. who are especially trained in issues of international adoption medicine. These clinics should be able to confirm a strong likelihood that the referred children will walk, talk, hear, see and most likely, be free of major cognitive impairments.

Egg donation offers no such sureties. With ovum donation, you have a pregnancy and you "get what you get," just as you would in using your own eggs to conceive. Offspring born as a result of oocyte donation, like any other baby, can be born with any number of anomalies (1-4% of all babies are born with some genetic anomaly). "On the other hand," would-be parents say, "we can pick the genes, do our best to 'control' the prenatal care, and we don't have to worry about our child being harmed by poor foster or institutional care." Both views are accurate. With adoption, you get a healthy baby or toddler or young child, but you have little if any say in selecting his birthparents and you have no say in where he/she was before coming to you. Egg donation offers the father's genes on one side and the opportunity to select a donor—whether known or anonymous—for her genetic makeup. And it offers the intended parents the opportunity to control—as best anyone can—the prenatal environment and to make obstetrical choices.

Feelings of Family Continuity

What does it mean to carry on a family line? In some families any child who enters a family is a full fledged member of the family tree, regardless of whether they were adopted or conceived with donor assistance. However, others view family continuity through a different lens. For them, it is difficult to "graft someone onto the family tree."

For those who subscribe to the "any child of ours is part of the lineage of our family" perspective, it doesn't much matter whether they choose egg donation or adoption, at least with regards to family continuity. However, those who regard genetic and/or gestational ties as very significant are likely to see egg donation as less of a stretch than adoption. Surely that will be the case on the father's side of the family, but perhaps also for the mother, since this child, although not her genetic offspring, was born to her.

Then comes the question of how important it is to feel a family tie to generations past and future. Although this is a compelling need for some, it is relatively unimportant for others. In the course of doing adoption home studies, I (Ellen) have met several couples who chose to adopt without ever trying to have a biological child. Some had something in their genetic heritage that they preferred not to pass on, but others did not. In both instances they seemed somewhat puzzled that people would feel a desire to carry on a bloodline.

Efficacy

Will it work? Most people who are comparing using a donor's oocytes and adoption have met with disappointments and frustrations along their path to parenthood. They want to find a light at the end of the tunnel and to head for it. How do egg donation and adoption compare?

Adoption is a sure bet. It *will* work. That doesn't mean that it will be easy or that it will necessarily work on the first try. Some would-be parents from non-traditional situations (age, sexual orientation, single status, etc.) may need to be more flexible when it comes to age of the child and/or country of origin. Since more and more domestic adoptions of babies today involve matching with an expectant mother weeks or months before her delivery date, adoption can include "fall throughs" when a new mother decides to parent her baby herself. Some agencies, some countries, some case workers and it can be create situations fraught with frustration, but in the end, for those who persevere there is a child to parent. It will work.

Using donated eggs is not a sure bet. It has a good success rate, especially for those who are able to try more than once or twice. However, there are those who try egg ovum donation and do not achieve successful pregnancies. When this occurs, some move on to adoption, having lost time and money along the way. Lost time may not be of particular concern for younger couples, but for those who first try egg donation in their mid-late 40s, the delay in time may significantly reduce their adoption options. It is important for women in this group to discuss success rates for older women as some clinics report a lower on-going pregnancy rate in women over 45.

For couples who hope to have more than one child, egg donation offers a potential bonus: twins. Although many egg ovum donation pregnancies are singletons, twins come along often, especially if two or more embryos are transferred. The arrival of twins, while challenging physically and in other ways, may provide parents with the "instant family" they longed for. Fertility centers, recognizing the increased risks associated with multiples, remind patients that it is important to transfer as few embryos as possible in order to minimize the chance of twins multiples. Unfortunately, many couples have struggled so long and want children so desperately that it is hard not to think "the more the merrier" —not "the more the scarier"—when warned of multiples.

Financial Costs

Both egg donation and adoption involve substantial costs, and with each option, there are a range of costs. Adoption of older and special needs children through state social service agencies can involve very little, if any out of pocket expenses. However, for private (non-profit) domestic or international adoption, fees range from about $15,000 to $40,000. Fortunately, the federal government softens the sting of these high fees by providing families with a $10,000 tax credit, if their incomes are under $150,000, and reduced credit for incomes between $150,000 and $190,000. In addition, many U.S. employers, including major companies, universities, and medical institutions, offer employees an adoption benefit, often in the $5000 range. So a couple with a combined income of under $150,000, who have adoption benefits from each of their employers, could begin the adoption process with a $20,000 reduction in their out of pocket costs.

Oocyte donation comes with no neither tax credits nor employee benefits. However, in mandated states, the medical costs are covered, assuming the egg problem is not age related. If a woman has a sister willing to donate and medical coverage for treatment, her out of pocket costs will be limited to medical co-payments and legal fees. On the other hand, if prospective recipients do not have medical coverage for egg donation *and* have to pay fees to a contractual donor program-recruited donor and agency, the costs—per try—for using donor ova could approach $25,000.

If a successful pregnancy is achieved, the costs of egg donation are likely to be similar to the costs of adoption. However, if egg donation does not work and a couple moves on to adoption—or to trying with other donors—costs mount.

Ethical Considerations

Dr. Aaron Lazare, Chancellor of the University of Massachusetts Medical School and founder of Center for Adoption Research at U/Mass said the following of adoption, "What other institution is socially correct, morally correct, politically correct, economically correct?" Indeed, adoption, which finds homes for children who need them, is "ethically correct." Yes, there have been "black market" adoptions and other deplorable practices, but here, at the start of the 21st century, adoption is governed by state, national and with the passing of the Hague Convention, international regulations. These laws strive to eliminate any risk of "baby selling," or of birthparents or entrepreneurs profiting in other ways from adoption.

In the United States, egg donation is essentially an unregulated industry. The American Society for Reproductive Medicine offers guidelines for practice, but there are no enforceable rules and regulations. At this point in time, virtually anyone can call themselves "an egg donor agency" and recruit young women as donors. Similarly, nearly everyone can present at a medical clinic and pretty much demand medical assistance with egg oocyte donation. No laws or guidelines exist to say "this woman should not donate her eggs" or "this couple should not be permitted to create a child through egg donation."

In the absence of regulations, egg donor programs and fertility clinics are left to regulate themselves. This is extraordinarily difficult, since even those who feel strongly about working in what they see as an ethically sound way are met with challenges. Take the egg donor agency that feels there should be a cut off at age 45 for recipients. What do they do when one of their donors goes to a program that permits a 48-year-old woman to attempt pregnancy with egg donations? Similarly, what does a medical program do when a determined patient brings in a donor who is charging them a $10,000 fee "because she has high SAT scores?"?

Another ethical concern raised by egg donation is whether it is ethically correct to intentionally create a child who will not be raised by both of his/her biological parents.? Some say, "Of course, the child will be created in love and will be deeply wanted." However, others will argue that donor offspring enter life facing an avoidable loss—the loss of genetic connection to one parents."

Humanitarian Considerations

No one should ever feel that a history of infertility instructs them to be humanitarians. However, for some, the opportunity to "do good," to "make a difference in a child's life," to "offer a home to someone who would otherwise not have one" is inviting. We spoke before about the "blessing and the curse of the meant to be." This is an example of the blessing—sometimes it feels that things "happen for a reason."

Egg donation offers no humanitarian opportunities, but no one ever said that someone need do a good deed because they were infertile.

Accurate Information

In order to decide between egg donation and adoption, people need to have accurate information about each. Unfortunately, this is not always the easy to obtain. There exist many misperceptions about adoption and some about egg donation as well.

Five Common Myths about Adoption

The child will want to leave you and seek his "real parents."

Those who familiarize themselves with adoption learn that adoptees who search do so to find information about themselves, not to find new parents.

The birthparents will come back and take the child.

Changes of heart in adoption almost always occur during pregnancy or just after birth and before placement. The few frightening and highly publicized court cases which have promulgated this myth involved cases where birthparents' rights were not legally terminated appropriately. Those who have accurate and ethical legal advice would not find themselves in a situation of being asked to return a child who had already been placed in their home.

Furthermore, just as adoptees don't leave their parents to find "real parents," birthparents don't come looking for the children they placed for adoption. More and more adoptions today involve ongoing contact between birth and adoptive families. This openness does not in any way involve co-parenting, but the communication does help everyone involved by-pass the predictable "fear of the unknown" that was part of adoption generations ago. Yes, it could happen, but so could many, many more frightening things.

There are no white babies available for adoption.

In fact, couples and singles seeking to adopt a white newborn infant in this country can do so generally within a year or so with ease. It may be more difficult if you already have a child or if you are in your late 40s, or for non-traditional families, but they, too, can do this, with accurate information and good professional support..

Children placed for adoption are born to drug addicts and others who don't take care of themselves during pregnancy.

All sorts of people find themselves expecting a child that they are unable to parent. Yes, a drug abuser could seek adoption, but so could a recent college graduate headed for more schooling or a married couple with three children who have decided to divorce. Interestingly, recent statistics show that about 65% of women planning an adoption for a newborn today are already parenting one child with success by themselves but believe that they do not have the resources needed to parent two children..

Adoption takes "forever."

No again. Most domestic adoptions and many international adoptions are completed in one to two years for families working in major metropolitan areas,International adoptions are taking only a little longer. Of course factors such as whether you already have a child, marital status, age, sexual orientation may lengthen the wait for some, but those who have good information and are working with ethical and experienced professionals do not experience delays of multiple years.

Four Common Myths about Oocyte Donation

You have to wait a long time for an egg donor.

The arrival, in recent years, of programs that recruit and match egg donors, has greatly reduced the time that people wait for a donor. You can go to a number of programs and have a donor within days of application.

Egg donation is for "women who forgot to have a baby."

While there are some women in their mid and late 40s pursuing egg donation (and most of them did not "forget" to have a baby), this option serves women of all ages. It is not unusual for a woman in her mid-late 30s to learn that her eggs are of poor quality.

Ovum donors are "just doing it for the money."

Although there are some women who become oocyte donors because they need money, they do not represent the majority of donors. Many egg donors have had a family member or friend suffer with infertility. Moved by this person's experience and the desire to help others, women offer to donate eggs.

Egg donation is really no different from adoption—you are "just adopting an egg."

Egg donation differs from adoption in a fundamental way: you get to intentionally bring a new life into the world and you have the opportunity to have a partial genetic connection to that child.

Accessibility

Decisions regarding egg donation and or adoption will be influenced by how accessible each option is to a particular family. Factors that make one option more or less available and accessible include: finances, geography and the "eligibility" of the intended parents. We'll say a bit about each...

Finances—If you live in a mandated state, have a volunteer donor and cannot afford many out-of-pocket expenses, egg donation will be more available to you than adoption. If you have no coverage for egg donation, no volunteer donor, income under $150,000 and benefits from two employers, adoption will be more accessible to you than donated eggs.

Geography—Egg donation relies on reproductive technology. If you live in a rural area, far from medical services, adoption will probably be more accessible to you than egg donation. You will need a home study and an adoption agency, but they can be accessed long distance.

Eligibility— Not everyone can adopt a baby and not everyone can undergo egg donation. The main reason that an individual or couple would be turned away from either option would be age. For example, a couple seeking to adopt a baby from Korea would be turned away if either partner is over 45. Similarly, we like to think that responsible medical programs will deny egg donation to couples due to advanced age. Definitions of "how old is too old" will vary (see Ethics chapter).

Since egg donation is unregulated, very few would-be parents are turned away from this option for reasons other than age or other medical issues which would make pregnancy unlikely or unwise. Adoption, by contrast, does adhere to rules and regulations. Prospective parents with serious criminal histories, couples with obvious marital issues and people with grave, life threatening illnesses will be denied—or postponed—access to adoption.

Legal Considerations

When people have struggled long and hard to bring a child into their families, the last thing they want is to fear losing that child. While neither adoption nor egg donation nor anything else can fully protect people from accidents, illness and other tragic losses, there are legal safeguards that protect adoptive and egg donation parents from loss due to others claiming parental rights.

Egg donation works fairly simply. A legal contract is generally signed at the time eggs are donated. This contract clearly establishes the fact that the donor does not have and will never have parental rights. For an expanded discussion of this, see Chapter 6.

Adoption is more complicated legally. In nearly every state there is a window of time (sometimes a matter of hours, most often a matter of days, occasionally a matter of weeks or months) during which a woman can change her mind about whether to place her child. Good adoption professionals educate would-be parents about these waiver periods when a placement is at legal risk and may even suggest that the child go to foster care during that window of opportunity. Once finalized, depending upon the state and the country a child is born in, an adoption may be more or less legally secure. Adoptions which follow the laws of the state in which they occur are absolutely safe. When the participants live in more than one state, the laws of both states must be followed. International adoption includes the laws of another country. Working with professionals who are knowledgeable about the laws and are committed to following them ethically is the most important guarantee that a finalized adoption is completely safe. What is important for people to know when they are deciding between egg donation and adoption is that there are many adoptions that are entirely secure from the time of placement. These include adoptions in states that have no revocation period, meaning that if a child's birthparents surrender their parental rights according to pre-determined state protocol, they cannot change their minds and return seeking custody of the child. Legally secure adoptions also occur in foreign countries, such as China, where children available for adoption have often been abandoned and where adoptions are almost always finalized at the time of placement.

Social Norms

Adoption has existed throughout history and has long been accepted as a means of family building. Ovum donation arrived only in the 1980s and, hence, is less familiar to most people. For many, egg donation still feels "weird," "unnatural," "like science fiction." People who react this way *and* who are comfortable with adoption are likely to choose the path that is familiar.

Some are drawn to egg donation because it is "invisible." With adoption—especially transracial adoption—"everyone knows." For those who want to be sure they "fit in" and "look like everyone else," egg donation is attractive. Many feel that their child is the only one who really needs to know how their family was built.

Talking with Children about Their Origins

Although we like to think that everyone who adopts a child or has one with a donated ovum will feel comfortable and confident talking with their child about how they entered the family, many intended parents are understandably uneasy. Thankfully, their discomfort tends to diminish once there are real, live children in their homes, but in advance, the anxiety can be daunting. "How will we talk with our child without upsetting him and without feeling rejected ourselves?"

In thinking about talking with children, some prefer the simplicity of an adoption story to the "new fangled" oocyte donation tale. Yes, adoption involves loss and possibly feelings of rejection, but it feels simple and uncomplicated because adoption is public, it is widely accepted and respected. Parents can talk with their children, confident that the children will know others who joined their families through adoption. In addition, in recent years adoption has become very fashionable, so much so that there are adoption "specials" on TV, feature stories of celebrity adoptions etc.

For an expanded discussion about talking with children, please see Chapter 10. However, we want to take a moment here to remind readers that although ovum donation is "newer" and provides fewer models to follow, families can learn from both adoption and from donor sperm offspring and they can have wonderful conversations within the privacy of their own homes. Remember that children are very self centered and they love to hear stories about themselves. Instead of approaching disclosure from a self-conscious, "What will I do wrong" perspective, we encourage parents to think about the positive conversations they can look forward to having with their children. How wonderful it can be to tell a child how much he was wanted, how thrilled you were to know he was coming, how much joy he brought when he *finally* arrived.

Sadly, some parents considering using donated eggs don't see it this way. When they think about talking with their future children, they are filled with a kind of irrational fear and anxiety. Some comfort themselves by saying, "We don't really have to tell if we decide not to." Others acknowledge the need to tell, but anticipate that when the time comes, they will want to avoid or postpone conversations. Again, we remind readers that this is a happy a story: "We wanted you, someone helped us make you, we loved seeing you grow in Mommy's tummy and we were over the top with happiness when you were born. The donor doesn't see the egg as a potential child—she sees it as an ingredient to help another family create a child." The adoption story includes some of this joy, but there is also the other side of things—there *were* other potential parents and for whatever reason, they were unable to parent at this time.

Existing Family Composition

People will look at the family they have when it comes time to consider ovum donation or adoption. Some, who have a biological child, choose egg donation because they look forward to another pregnancy and want a child who will be half genetically connected to his/her sibling. They may look at egg donation and observe how similar it is to "regular" biological parenting—the couple plans for the child, the mother carries him/her, the dad is the genetic father and the couple gets to share pregnancy, labor and delivery. It all seems remarkably familiar.

Others see things through another lens. Adoption offers an opportunity to expand the family in a different way. Parents always worry about "comparing" their children and about whether having a second child will live up to their experience with a first. Adoption—especially international adoption—invites parents to depart from comparisons and to celebrate differences.

Since more and more people are marrying for a second time after divorce or the death of a spouse, there are many couples considering egg donation or adoption when they are older and when one or both has other children. These experiences, also, will influence their decision. When a man who has never had a child marries a woman who is the biological mother of her child, egg donation can be especially attractive. When both partners have had children, adoption, especially international adoption, offers them the opportunity to share a new experience together.

Your Child's Story

Everyone has a personal narrative about how they entered their family. "I was planned," "I was named after my grandfather," "I was an accident," "My parents were still trying for a girl" etc. Joining one's family through adoption or egg donation surely adds a dimension to the story. We think it safe to say that egg donation is never a first choice and that adoption is usually not a first choice. One of the reasons why it is so important for parents to really come to terms with the "second choices" they make along the way is that we don't want to have children whose personal narrative includes "second choice."

Loving parents will do what they can to convey to their children that they were very much wanted and are deeply loved regardless of how the parents *originally* felt about a second choice path to parenthood. For some parents this is easier to do with adoption: they feel that the child can develop a positive personal narrative based on the story that he was born to parents who loved him, but could not parent him, and that his "now and forever" parents were thrilled to have him. For these parents, egg donation provides more challenges. They wonder how a child forms a secure personal narrative based on the knowledge that she came from two women.

Others disagree. "How hard is it," they ask, "for a child to see one woman as offering important baby making ingredients to two eager parents in need of them?" What a happy, positive personal story these children will form, one built on the solid foundation of knowing their parents intentionally created them to be part of the family they live with and belong in.

The Family Story

And finally, we come to the family story. Anyone who considers using a donor's eggs and most people who consider adoption have to relinquish their original vision of what their family would look like. Indeed, most parents are forced to abandon this fantasy somewhere in their lives, although for many, it comes when they are raising children, not bringing them into the family.

So what, then, does your second choice family story look like? Again, how you look at this may be determined by whether you have children already and whether this is a first marriage for each of you. For some, egg donation feels like less of a "second choice" because it feels "closer to what we originally wanted—to be pregnant, to share child-birth, to have at least some genetic connection."

Faced with loss and disappointment, others take a different approach to creating a "second choice family story." They think, *If it has to be a different family than the one we imagined, then let it really look and feel and be a different family.* Some who choose adoption, especially an international and transracial adoption, discover that family building can truly be an unexpected adventure, filled with travel and cultural rewards they never anticipated.

....

Meet Terry and Mark...

Terry and Mark were "on the fence" for a long time. When they married, at 45 and 35, both knew it was unlikely that Terry would be able to become pregnant with her own eggs. Since she had been thinking about adopting as a single woman for several years, Terry simply assumed that Mark would be happy to join her in an adoption. Mark has a cousin who recently adopted from China, and perhaps more to the point, Mark joined his own family through adoption. And so it came as a surprise to Terry when Mark said, "I'd rather do egg donation."

There they were—Terry preferred adoption and Mark preferred egg donation. Each voiced very compelling reasons for their choice. For Terry, pregnancy at 45 or 46 seemed scary and she felt, "unnatural." She described egg donation as "sci-fi" and embraced adoption as "a good thing for everyone concerned." She pointed to Mark and his family as "great proof that adoption works" and wondered why people would want to create a child through eggs donated from a stranger. In addition, she reminded Mark that his birth sister is schizophrenic and questioned whether they should be worried about "passing on mental illness genes."

Mark, by contrast, advocated for egg donation. He spoke poignantly to Terry of his desire to have a biological offspring and also, of his wish to share a pregnancy with her. He spoke with some skepticism about adoption "these days," contrasting current practice with the "good matching" that he felt went on at the time his parents adopted. However, he added that he would be willing to adopt if they had a child through egg donation first or if they tried egg donor and it didn't work.

This was not an easy situation. Terry and Mark had each waited a long time to find the right life partner and each agreed they were lucky to have found each other. But how were they to resolve what felt like an impasse. Many discussions ensued, including several with a counselor, who helped them to listen carefully to the other's concerns and desires. Ultimately, it was Terry who decided she could make a shift in her thinking.

These were Terry's words, "I grew up knowing my biological family so I can't say, first hand, what it feels like to not know people to whom you are connected genetically. Yes, Mark was lucky enough to find his birth family as an adult, but when I thought about it, I realized that did not erase the impact of the years of not knowing. When I thought about it that way, I decided that Mark deserved to enjoy a parent-child relationship that included a genetic connection, not only because it was important for him as a father, but also because he felt so strongly about it for his child."

Cost

Sadly, there will be people who will turn away from adoption, egg donation and other options because of the costs involved. Although saving for the costs can easily postpone treatment or an adoption, we like to think that people will not turn away from parenthood entirely, solely because of the costs. Though financial assistance with the most complex of and expensive of treatment options can be difficult to find, especially in adoption there are opportunities for parenthood that are affordable to almost anyone whose goal is parenthood, period.

Additional Resources

If, in light of what you've read above and your discussions with your partner, you believe that you owe it to yourselves to consider adoption more seriously, we offer you the following carefully selected list of resources, each of which has a different purpose, and each of which can lead you to additional resources as needed for your decision making.

Adopting after Infertility (Perspectives Press, Inc. 1992 to be revised in 2005) by Patricia Irwin Johnston—a step-by-step guide to adoption-related decision making: first, is adoption for you? And, if so, whether to adopt infant, toddler or older child, domestically or internationally, through an agency or independently.

The Adoption Resource Book (HarperResource, 1998, 4th edition) by Lois Gilman—a guide to finding and evaluating the professionals and resources to assist you on your journey to adoption

www.adoptivefamilies.com—the website of the oldest, broadest and most authoritative periodical on adoption, providing links to hundreds of articles, book reviews, and many additional helpful websites.

Life without Children or, in the Case of Secondary Infertility, a One Child Family

There are individuals and couples who travel a long, arduous road through infertility and, after examining many options decide not to pursue parenthood through adoption, or any of the third party collaborative options. Some of you already have a child or children and decide to stay with the family you have rather than to try to add to it via an alternative route. Others do not have children but realize that alternative paths to parenthood are not right for them. There are several factors that may prompt each of these decisions.

Age

Although adoption is sometimes available to couples in their early 50s and egg donation is often accessible to women in their late 40s, there are many people whose careful thinking tells them that, for themselves, they have "aged out" of parenthood. Many think about the ages of their parents when they were born, look around at parents they see on the local playground or in the supermarket and conclude that it is "simply not fair to a child to have parents this old." Some may have considered older child adoption, in an effort to "reduce the difference in our ages," but may have concluded that this path to parenthood is just not for them. Although deeply saddened, people who make the decision to stop pursuing parenthood because of their ages often feel some sense of relief.

Satisfaction and Priorities

There are couples who start down the road of infertility diagnosis or who travel a long way through treatment or who carefully examine alternative paths to parenthood and ultimately conclude that their lives are full and satisfying without children. Many are couples who met later in life and who rushed into infertility treatment because they knew that time was running out. Some find as they look at their options that their glass is mostly full. For some who have begun to feel this way, it may come as a big relief to step back, celebrate the relationship you have and enjoy some of the fruits of your labors. Parenthood can be satisfying, gratifying and pleasurable, but it is also frustrating, stressful and sadly, for some, it brings sorrow.

Those who already have a child may find that after exploring other options and finding them wanting, for you, you can live happily and feel fulfilled with one child. There was once a stigma about only children, but thankfully, that stigma has vanished. Today, people are creating all kinds of families, making one child families more common and less isolated. If you have a healthy child, who is thriving, you may feel it is time to "count blessings," rather than to seek new ones.

Additional Resources

If, in light of what you've read above and your discussions with your partner, you believe that you owe it to yourselves to consider more carefully living childfree or accepting your family as complete with the number of children already there, we offer you the following carefully selected list of resources, each of which has a different purpose, and each of which can lead you to additional resources as needed for your decision making.

Sweet Grapes: How to Stop Being Infertile and Start Living Again (Perspectives Press, Inc., rev. 1998) by Jean W. Carter and Michael Carter—a guide to deciding on and embracing a childfree lifestyle after infertility by a couple who have been there and done that!

"Married No Kids" *http://www.bellaonline.com/subjects/3180.asp*— Bella Online's guide to childfree living after infertility.

You and Your Only Child: The Joys, Myths, and Challenges of Raising an Only Child (Perennial, 1998) by Patricia Nachman and Andrea Thompson—a guide to deciding on an only and then raising him well, this book is commended by its reviewers for being inclusive of families who didn't start out to raise an only child.

Parenting an Only Child: The Joys and Challenges of Raising Your One and Only (Broadway Books, 2001) by Susan Newman, Ph.D.—an advocacy guide for the one child family.

http://www.onlychild.com—an online community for the families of single children.

But What if the Goal Remains a Full Biological Child?

As you have gone through infertility diagnosis and treatment, you have found yourself thinking about why you want to have a child (or another child, in instances of secondary infertility). IVF, with its ability to separate the genetic, gestational and rearing mothers, forces people to examine the relative importance of pregnancy, genetic connections, genealogy and day-to-day parenting. Some conclude that pregnancy, when all is said and done, is really not essential. Others conclude that genetic ties can be relinquished. Some conclude that being a parent doesn't really depend upon who carried the child or who created the child, but is grounded, almost entirely, in who rears the child. And some feel otherwise.

There are people who know, either at the start of treatment or somewhere along the way, that they seek "the whole package"—pregnancy, genetic and generational ties, labor, delivery, If you are one of these people, you may already be parents or you may be childless. Either way, you feel that for you, parenthood is tied to biology and genetics. You may conclude that there will be other satisfying ways to have children—or more children— in your lives, but these ways will not be defined as parenthood.

When you feel this way, but the medical issues that prevent you from becoming pregnant and delivering a child genetically related to both of his parents and the alternative to parenthood are unacceptable, you are stalemated. We're sorry, but you've reached the end of the road.

What to do? Infertile people in this position will grieve deeply. That's normal and predictable, but the danger is that they can become stuck in this grief and unable to move forward. To simply exist in a life that feels ruined by disappointment in family building colors ever other aspect of our lives—our relationships, our jobs, our faith. If this is where you are, give yourself six months to go through the natural process of grief. If you remain stuck at time, we urge you to find an infertility-experienced therapist who can help you accept what is and move on in a more positive way.

Additional Resources

If, in light of what you've read above and your discussions with your partner, you believe that you owe it to yourselves to consider more seriously stopping your efforts at building or expanding your family, we offer you the following carefully selected list of resources, each of which has a different purpose, and each of which can lead you to additional resources as needed for your thinking about embracing the life you have.

Shoulda, Woulda Coulda: Overcoming Regrets, Mistakes and Missed Opportunities (Perennial, 1990) by Arthur Freeman and Rose DeWolf— demonstrates how cognitive therapy can help to overcome the crippling effects of regret.

Ambiguous Loss: Learning to Live with Unresolved Grief (Harvard University Press, 2003) by Pauline Boss—a practical discussion about moving beyond grief from difficult to acknowledge losses

Full Circle—Coming Back to the Option of Using Donated Ova

If you have taken the time—most likely days or weeks or in some cases even months—to carefully consider the possible options we've mentioned above (other collaborative reproductive options, adoption, accepting your life as full just as is), if your infertility issues make you a candidate to try using oocyte donation, and if you just don't feel ready to make any of those leaps, you've come full circle from the beginning of this chapter. Using a donated egg remains an option you need and want to explore more fully.

We may be leaving some of our readers here. There are those of you who will decide not to pursue egg donation, perhaps because of something we have said in this chapter or in a previous one. But many of you will move on. We hope the chapters that follow will provide you with practical information and emotional support as you need to make a good decision about and/or pursue egg donation.

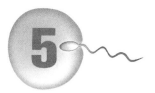

Choosing Your Donor

Here you are at another fork in the road. You've explored other options and you've pretty much decided to move forward with egg donation. One big decision has been made, but another sits before you: finding an egg donor. For some of you, the decision may seem simple and straightforward: you have a sister or a cousin or a friend who has volunteered her eggs and you are delighted by her offer. However, for most people, deciding on the *type* of donor they desire and then, on the *specific* donor are formidable decisions.

In this chapter, we will look at how people identify their donors. In keeping with central themes of this book, we encourage you to look at each of your options through the "bi-focal" lens of the best interests of the child and of parental pride, satisfaction and security. Which egg donor decision—if any—will you be able to look back ten years from now and be able to say, "It was absolutely the right choice"? It provided us with a child whom we love and cherish and with whom we can speak securely and openly about the wonderful way that he/she joined our family. It left us with gratitude to our donor, whom we feel gave us a gift that enriched not only our lives and those of our families now and for future generations. It is our belief, also, that by giving to us, the donor enriched her own life as well ours."

There are three categories of donors:

- Family members— including sisters, cousins and in some instances, nieces, or possibly daughters.

- Friends and acquaintances—including close friends, casual acquaintances or even people one meets solely for the purpose of voluntary donation.

- Program-recruited donors, including women who receive financial compensation to provide eggs whether on an anonymous, semi-closed or fully open basis. These women might more accurately be termed *providers* than *donors* because of the payment involved.

Obviously, a wide range of women participate as egg donors for a wide range of reasons. How can recipients sort through their options and look through the bi-focal lens with clarity? We suggest that you consider each type of donor along the following parameters, and we have constructed this chapter in a way to encourage you to do this

Availability and Accessibility

Is this type of donor available and accessible to you? For example, not everyone has a sister or a friend who is willing and able to donate them.

Costs

Is this type of donation affordable to you? The costs with donation vary, with some intended parents paying more for medical costs and less for donor fees (e.g. a couple living in a state without an insurance mandate but working with a volunteer donor) and others paying less in medical costs and more towards a donor (e.g. a couple in a mandated state paying fees to both a donor program and a donor).

Fertility

Is this donor likely to help you achieve pregnancy? Some very willing donors may have diminished fertility.

The Child's Story

Will working with this type of donor provide you with a story that you will feel comfortable sharing with your child? Included in this will be considerations about to whom else your child is related.

Ethical Considerations

Will you feel that your donor is donating for reasons that are "right" for her and which you can confidently share with your child?

Our Family

Will this type of donor help you to create a child that you will feel "fits" in your family—racially, ethnically, in terms of intelligence and appearance?

With each of these parameters in mind, we turn now to the three categories of donors. As you review them, we encourage you to remember some of the messages we conveyed in Chapter 4. Again we remind you…

Never Say Never

As your reality changes, so may your ideas of what is right for you. You may begin this process, saying, "I'd never do this with a stranger," but come to find that program-recruited donation turns out to be the right option for you. Perhaps, for example, a sister who offered will end up changing her mind.

You Have the Right to Make Decisions for Yourselves and to Feel That You Are Free and Clear of the Influences of Others

You will find that people have some strong opinions about ovum donation. Some will say, "How can you do it with a sister? Won't the child be confused about who his real mother is?" While others will counter, "How could you accept eggs from a total stranger? Isn't that weird?"

As with all other aspects of infertility, you will find that egg donation is filled with "self-appointed experts." These people, sometimes well intentioned, seem to think that they know what is best for you. Needless to say, they are wrong—only you can determine what will be right for you and your family. You may choose a path that is unpopular or that others do not understand, but what matters is that you and the other participants have a clear sense of what you are doing and why.

Loss and Grief Are Part of the Journey

Oocyte donation has a good success rate, meaning that many who choose this path to parenthood succeed in achieving and carrying a pregnancy. What you must remember is that among those who have children through donated eggs are many who had to change donors, many who experienced failed cycles, and worse still, many who suffered pregnancy losses, including some late losses. Sadly, a history of loss does not protect you from additional losses when you venture into egg donation.

The People You Meet along the Way Will Shape Your Journey

You could never imagine having your sister donate to you, and then a neighbor tells you that a "wonderful thing" has happened in her family: one of her sisters has donated eggs to her other sister. You hear the news, look at your neighbor's smiling face and think, *Maybe? Maybe I could do that? Maybe I could ask my sister?* Or you attend a support group for women considering donor egg. The group leader has invited a panel of parents to speak about their experiences. You listen keenly as one woman, holding adorable one year old twins, talks about the donor she found through a program. They met prior to the cycle, talked by phone during it and now stay in touch every several months or so by card or email. Suddenly it all sounds so natural, so easy, such an obvious and workable way to build a family.

Counseling Can Assist You in Your Decision Making

One of the people you will probably meet along the way is a mental health counselor—a psychologist, social worker, nurse clinician, licensed marriage and family therapist or perhaps, a psychiatrist. We want to say a few things about counseling here, since it is likely that a counselor will be an important companion in your decision making process.

A counselor who is well versed in reproductive medicine will help you sort through questions of which type of donor—if any—is right for you. The counselor can also assist you with such additional questions as "What do I do if my sister offers to donate and I prefer to have a friend?" "What if my sister and I want to do this but my parents object to the idea?" "My sister/cousin/friend and I have been competitive with each other in the past—is this likely to get in our way in ovum donation? I don't want to have her donate and then 'hold it over me?'" and "What if my sister offers but I really feel she was 'pushed' into this by our mother?"

You will notice we use the word *counseling* and not *psychotherapy*. This is because *counseling* is the appropriate word in this regard. The mental health professional you meet with will not be "shrinking" you. Rather, she/he will provide you with informed guidance. Having explored these issues with countless others, your counselor should be an able guide, helping you take the next steps in your journey.

So let's take a look at the different types of donors.

Intrafamily Donation

For a number of reasons, intrafamily egg donation makes a lot of sense. It offers recipients the opportunity to create a child with genetic connections to both of his/her parents. It provides the child with a personal story that makes sense (e.g. "Mommy and Daddy needed help making a baby and so they asked Aunt Cathy or Cousin Sally or ...to help them"). It avoids ethical concerns about payment for eggs, since family members are rarely, if ever, compensated for their donation. And it is more affordable, since there are no fees to agencies.

If only it were that simple. Intrafamily oocyte donation can be immensely attractive, but it can also be filled with frustration and tension. As all of us know, families are very complicated entities, often filled with rivalries, resentments, favoritism and allegiances. One sister's offer to donate to another may sound wonderful at first but be undermined if a third sister feels left out, if a mother or father feels this is "too weird," if the sisters' husbands don't like each other, or if the recipient talks with her physician and concludes she would have a better chance of success with a program-recruited donor.

In considering intrafamily egg donation, recipients need to know which family members might be considered appropriate. In general, sister-to-sister and cousin-to-cousin donation is considered ethically sound and is often medically and psychologically appropriate. From a medical perspective, physicians look for donors who are under 35 and who have had children (most physicians will not turn away a sister who is over 35 or who has not had a child, but will advise recipients that the viability of this donor's eggs is questionable).

From a psychological perspective, mental health clinicians will be looking for a donor who does not feel coerced into donating, either overtly or covertly, and who has, if possible, completed her own family. The psychologist will want to confirm that the donor has carefully considered how she will feel seeing the child at family events, how she will feel about that child in relation to her own children, how she will deal with differences in child rearing philosophy between herself and the recipient of her eggs, and how she will feel if she decides to have more children and is unable to do so.

Some prospective recipients look beyond sisters and cousins for potential intrafamily donors. Nieces and daughters are other potential sources of donation, but both groups are considered ethically problematic by most mental health professionals and physicians, since there is more likelihood that the younger woman will feel pressured –either directly or subconsciously— by the older one.

In November, 2003, The American Society for Reproductive Medicine published guidelines for intrafamily donation. They conclude that familial donation is acceptable and note that intergenerational donation is more challenging because it is unlikely that a mother will be young enough to donate to her daughter. Marshall ("Intergenerational Gamete Donation: Ethical and Societal Implications" *American Journal of Obstetrics and Gynecology*, 1998) talks about the "complex web" of family relationships arising from inter-generational gamete donation.

Occasionally, there will be requests for a daughter to donate to her mother, if the mother is now married to someone other than the daughter's father. Dr. Elaine Gordon, author of *Mommy, Did I Grow in Your Tummy* and a respected expert in egg donation, cautions families making this request. "I worry that daughter-to-mother donation is inherently coercive. It may prove very difficult for a daughter to refuse her mother's request. In addition, it can feel strange, particularly if the mother's new husband is close to the daughter's age. In these cases it is important to assess the potential for sexual innuendo. Also, daughter-to-mother donation turns the convention of mothers taking care of their daughters on its head, asking daughters to take care of their mothers"

Many programs will accept a niece donating to her aunt, as long as the relationships between the two women and between them and the donor's mother (recipient's sister) are discussed and explored. Dr. Gordon encourages these donor-recipient pairs to carefully consider the feelings of the donor's and recipient's existing children, as well as those of hoped for future children. Gordon emphasizes that this decision will re-shape a family in significant ways, and it is helpful for people to clearly define their roles. "Everyone needs to be clear who is 'aunt' and who is 'mother.'"

Psychiatric Clinical Nurse Specialist Sharon Steinberg of Harvard Vanguard Medical Associates in Boston informs participants, "If a mother divorces and remarries and asks her daughter from her first marriage to donate to her, this decision has an impact on more than the two women and the potential offspring. I remind the would-be mother that it is her ex-husband who will be contributing to the baby's genes. How will her current husband react to a baby who is one quarter the genetic offspring of his wife's ex? Will the ex-husband want a relationship with his genetic grandchild? This is but one of the ways in which daughter-to-mother donation can be a lot more complicated than it initially appears."

We turn now to the seven parameters we noted earlier, looking at how each might apply to intrafamily donation.

Availability and Accessibility

Not all recipients have sisters or cousins who are "suitable" egg donors. A woman may be an only child, or have only brothers and no female cousins or, more likely, have sisters and cousins who are too old to donate. Sisters and cousins may be unable to donate for other reasons—their own infertility, their youth (a sister or cousin could be too young to really give informed consent), or she may have physical or mental health problems with a strong genetic component.

Some women have sisters or cousins who could donate, but don't feel comfortable doing so. Many sisters or cousins would love to be helpful, but regard their eggs as their "potential children" and don't feel that they can donate them. In some instances, a sister or cousin may want to donate, but her husband raises objections, including the possibility that her health may be adversely impacted by the donation. There are also instances in which family members do not offer because they don't approve of ovum donation in general or because they oppose the prospective recipient (for example a single or older woman) participating in egg donation.

When a woman needs eggs and has a sister or cousin who would be a suitable donor, she may find herself waiting and hoping for an offer. Indeed, some prospective donors do come forward offering to help, but others do not. Recipients are left wondering, "Does she know she could donate to me and has decided not to, or might she be unaware of this option or perhaps, be reluctant to offer?"

It is our impression that family members are more likely to offer in some instances than in others. When a young woman loses her ovaries to cancer, family members are so moved by her loss that they start thinking about how they can help. However, in other instances of infertility, family members may not understand what is needed and how they might help.

If you are in need of eggs, you have one or more family members who are potential donors and you have not received an offer, you will need to find a way to ask for help. That might seem like an impossible task.We have some suggestions...

> You might send a "general" letter to "family and friends," in which you introduce your desire for donated eggs. In the letter you can explain what is involved and you can outline the characteristics of an appropriate donor (age, fertility etc). The letter, which may really be targeted for one or possibly two people, can be mailed out to several people (or can *appear* to be going to several). At the end of the letter, you can ask that "anyone who might be interested," contact you. By doing it this way, with the "general mailing," you don't have to worry about putting an individual "on the spot." You can simply send the letter and hope.

> A second approach is to be more direct. You may want simply to ask the prospective donor, prefacing your request with several reassurances that you will fully understand if she is not comfortable with what you are about to say. You can ask her in person or by letter. The advantage to the letter is that it gives you the opportunity to carefully choose your words and it gives your reader a chance to sort out her feelings on her own, without feeling any pressure to respond to you immediately.

There is a significant downside to the direct approach: once the question is asked it cannot be taken back. One woman who agreed to donate for her sister acknowledged feeling very uncomfortable with the request. However, she felt obliged to consider it carefully and so spent several weeks talking with friends, family members, clergy and a counselor about her decision. Ultimately she decided to donate, not so much because she truly wanted to donate, but rather because she found herself anticipating regret. "I am afraid," she said, "that if I don't do this, I will always look back and regret my decision. I pride myself in being a good and giving person and I am afraid that if I don't do this, I will never again feel like such a good person." The counselor explained that she saw it as part of her job to help prospective donors get out of difficult situations, rejecting them "for undisclosed medical or psychological reasons." But the woman held fast to this position even when her counselor offered to help her out of the situation.

Another version of an "accessibility problem" arises when two people offer to donate. While this is a problem that many people would like to have, it poses a real challenge to those who find themselves in this situation. How do you tell one sister that you would rather have another sister donate? The answer to this is relatively easy if the sisters' suitability can be differentiated by age or fertility history. But what if they appear "equally fertile," "equally appropriate?" And what if there is an apparent difference, but you prefer the sister who is the less apparent choice?

We suggest that you talk with both sisters together and that the three of you try to sort things out. You may find that one of the volunteers would feel relieved if she knew the other sister was donating. Take the burden off yourself by asking them for their advice and get them to help figure out what makes sense for all of you. By bringing all of you together, you avoid having "factions" and causing family hurt when one sister feels left out. Whether they are donating or not, both sisters can be active participants in this experience.

Clinical Nurse Specialist Sharon Steinberg encourages sisters to talk in terms of donating one time. If the first donation doesn't work, this decision can always be revisited. However, Steinberg feels it is important that an offer to donate not be open ended. "The donors need to see how they feel about the process and the donation before committing to do it a second time."

Costs

Intrafamily oocyte donation appears to be cost effective since sisters or cousins are unlikely to expect or seek payment as part of their donation. However, since family donors may not be as fertile as program-recruited donors, it is possible that intrafamily donation will not always be less costly than cycles that involve payment to donors. If a couple lives in a state without a mandate and ends up paying for repeated donor cycles with a sister or cousin, the process could become quite costly. On the other hand, if all goes well and the first or second donor cycle work, intrafamily donation will save the recipient couple upwards of $10,000.

Fertility

In considering a family member as a donor, it is crucial that you not ignore fertility. It is tempting to focus solely on the advantages of the genetic connections, especially for a child who will have a clear sense of where he/she came from. However, all advantages vanish if your donor isn't fertile. Before you and your sister/cousin become too involved in this endeavor, it is important that you listen closely to her fertility history (how old is she, has she had a baby in recent years and does she have a history of miscarriages?). It is also important that you consider her general physical and emotional health, since they may influence her ability to donate and they will be factors in what is passed on to a child.

The Child's Story

If there is a compelling reason to have a family member as your donor, it is for the child's story. Throughout history, there have been sisters who raised their sisters' children, grandparents who raised the child of their child. In many cultures, children belong to an extended family and grow up feeling close ties to cousins, grandparents, aunts and uncles. In this sense, egg donation is simply an extension of time-honored tradition.

Some see this through a different lens. They argue that sister-to-sister donation is confusing since a child "could be confused about whether his aunt was his aunt or his mother." We don't see it this way, but we recognize that there are some potential sister-to-sister donations that would not work. Indeed it would be extraordinarily difficult for a child if the donating sister somehow felt she had some parental authority over the child.

Ethical Considerations

From an ethical perspective, intrafamily donation has much to recommend it. For one thing, it does not involve financial compensation, and hence, escapes any implication that it is a business transaction. For another, the child will have a genetic connection to both parents, and hence, is likely to face fewer "Who am I?" questions than someone conceived through program-recruited donation. Finally, there are the benefits of altruism—the donor has the opportunity to make a real difference in the lives of people she loves as well as in her own life (since she is helping to create a niece or nephew for herself and a cousin for her child or children.)

It is not always so simple, and unfortunately, there are instances in which sister-to-sister or cousin-to-cousin egg donation raises ethical questions. Most of these involve the question of coercion—either overt or covert. The following are some examples of problematic situations:

Donation Following Illness

When a sister loses her ovaries to cancer or other serious illness, there may be pressure in the family for a sister to donate. But what if the "designated" donor does not feel comfortable with this, either because she sees her eggs as *her* potential children, or because she has not yet had children of her own, or, perhaps, because she doesn't like her brother-in-law or she feels they have a poor marriage or because she feels they won't be good parents?

Donation When the Relationship Involves Competition

Sibling rivalry is certainly not a new or unfamiliar concept. Two sisters may be very close and may love each other immensely; however, their relationship may also be competitive, perhaps judgmental or critical. Relationships in which these are prominent features may not be good candidates for sister-to-sister donation. I (Ellen) am reminded of one client who was all set to accept her younger sister's offer to donate until she visited her sister for vacation. Spending several days with her sister reminded her of how competitive her sister is and how much stress there can be in their relationship. Although she much preferred the *idea* of donation within the family, the potential recipient returned home knowing that she would choose anonymous donation.

Donation When One Sister Feels that the Other "Owes It to Her"

Chicago social worker Judy Calica has come across an occasional sister pair in which one sister seems to feel that her sister "owes her an egg." Calica notes that this can arise after illness or other hardship in the recipient's life, but that this experience does not provide a mandate for her sister to donate to her. Ironically, this expectation of entitlement usually advises against sister-to-sister donation despite the fact that the recipient may have endured great hardship.

The emotional challenges of sister-to-sister donation have been explored in "All in the Family: Social Processes in Ovarian Egg Donation between Sisters" (1993). Lessor et al. discuss the "intricate psychological ramifications in the sibling relationship of sister-to-sister donation.

And of course, those who challenge all of ovum donation will include intrafamily donation in their scrutiny, wondering whether it is ever ethically sound for one woman to take potent drugs and undergo a surgical procedure all to help another create a child that is not biologically hers.

Our Family

"What will our family look like?" This is a question that couples ask themselves while they are in the throes of infertility treatment and when they are pursuing alternative paths to parenthood. For many, the prospect of a family member as donor is very inviting, as the hoped for offspring is likely to "fit in," to bear some physical resemblance to both his/her parents, to feel familiar. However, there are others who feel that these likenesses will feel odd or awkward as they will serve as a constant reminder that baby Sara or Alex was born from an egg from Aunt Cathy or Cousin Meg.

Meet Andrea and Margaret and Their Families...

Andrea and Margaret are the first- and second-born in a family of four girls. Like their two younger sisters, Andrea and Margaret each have two children, coincidentally, a son and daughter, three years apart. Although they are already very busy people, whose lives are full to overflowing, Margaret and her husband, Tom, are very excited to be adding a baby girl from China to their family. Her older sister, Andrea, marvels, "Margaret can do more in one day than many of us can do in a week."

Indeed Margaret learned at an early age that time is precious. When she was 22, she was diagnosed with lymphoma and underwent treatment, which rendered her infertile. At the time she was single and far away from being prepared to be a mother. However, Margaret remembers thinking that she would not let her illness prevent her from becoming a parent.

Margaret and Tom met in their late 20s, married, and decided to become parents through oocyte donation. Living in Australia at the time, they sought treatment with an anonymous donor and conceived their son, Ricky, who is now 8 years old. After enjoying an easy and uneventful pregnancy and the arrival of a healthy baby, Margaret and Tom decided to wait a short time and then seek another donor. They knew they were moving back to the U.S. and would need to begin their second round of treatment at a new clinic.

Margaret and Tom found a clinic they liked in Pennsylvania, where they are now living, and they found a donor. The first cycle *appeared* to go well, but Margaret did not conceive. It was the same with the second and third cycles. After the third disappointment, the couple spoke with their physician, who told them they could try another donor, consider adoption or content themselves with their one child. When Margaret asked the doctor whether she might ask one of her sisters to donate, he advised against it. "Your older sister is definitely too old. She is practically 40. Your younger sister, 36, is also a bit old for donating. And this isn't a good time for your youngest sister, 33, who is in the middle of planning her wedding. You should just move on to another anonymous donor."

Margaret, who tends to think "out of the box," heard this advice and decided to dismiss it. She knew that Andrea was "too old," but she also knew that she loved the idea of having Andrea donate. The two sisters had always been close, and Margaret admired Andrea for her calm, even tempered, gentle approach to life. She convinced Tom that it would be worth a try with Andrea, assuming, of course, that Andrea would say yes.

"I didn't know how to react when she asked me," remembers Andrea. "I wanted very much to help her, but I didn't know what the process involved, and I didn't like the idea of taking a lot of heavy duty medications. I was happy to give her my eggs, but I wanted to be sure I could deal with the way that the doctors would get them."

Andrea did some reading, talked with her husband and some friends, and said yes. From there, the two sisters and their husbands were sent to a psychologist for counseling and then on to the medical clinic where Andrea would be tested. "They were incredibly pessimistic," remembers Margaret. "They said we were all silly to be trying with 40-year-old eggs."

Never inclined to take no for an answer, Margaret told Andrea she wanted to forge ahead. Even if there was only a small chance of success, she wanted to try. Although initially worried about the medications and the procedure, Andrea was now fully on board with her plans to donate to her sister and agreed that they should do it.

As predicted, Margaret did not become pregnant with Andrea's eggs—at least not the first, "fresh" batch. Although the physician declared that the egg quality was "poor as expected," there were three embryos that might be suitable for cryopreservation. Ever the optimist, Margaret insisted the embryologist attempt to freeze them and when this proved successful, she followed it with a request for transfer two months later. And that is when her daughter, Sara, was conceived.

Sara is now 5, two years younger than her Aunt Andrea's daughter, Melissa. The two cousins live four hours apart but see each other several times a year because their parents make an effort to get together. They are very different children, but like their mothers, their relationship seems to thrive on differences. Sara is loud and boisterous, while her cousin, Melissa, is much more mellow.

When asked what it is like for her when she sees Sara, Andrea says, "It's great, but no different than when I see Ricky or any of my other nieces or nephews. I wonder if I will feel different when she is older, especially if she reminds me more of one of my children, but for now, she is no different than any of my sisters' other children."

Three months ago, Margaret and Tom traveled to China to bring home 1-year-old Lily, their youngest child. Her infectious smile and spunky personality has captivated all of the older children, who wasted no time in making her an integral part of both families.

When asked who knows about how Margaret and Tom's family was built, Andrea and Margaret say that they are, for the most part, private about it. "Needless to say, everyone knows how Lily came! But as far as Ricky and Sara, we're more private. Our family knows, a few close friends, but mostly we don't talk about it." The sisters explain that some of this is privacy and some of it has to do with the differences that Ricky and Sara will have to deal with. They feel that Ricky, who knows how he was conceived and has some understanding of it, will have some feelings when he puts it together that Sara shares a bloodline with their mom.

Andrea has not told her children the story, because she is waiting until Margaret and Tom talk more fully with Sara. However, when asked about it, Andrea responds with optimism and confidence, "I've had some great conversations with both my children about how babies are born. We've been talking about gay marriage and they've been asking me lots of questions. I'm convinced that children are accepting, and that they take all sorts of family situations in stride. The key is to talk with them early. When they are young they accept things that might be harder to grasp when they are older."

Meet Carolyn and Arthur and Carolyn's "Half-niece" Rebecca

Carolyn and Rebecca are part of a large, complicated extended family that has grown exponentially in recent years. The women are connected through Carolyn's half brother, Neal, who is Rebecca's biological father. We say "biological," because Rebecca has never had much contact with Neal, who was divorced from her mother when Rebecca was 2 years old. Instead, it has been Peter, her mother's second husband, that Rebecca has called "Dad."

Carolyn and Rebecca have been in touch over the years, but have never been especially close. There are ten years between them in age, and most often they were separated by many miles. However, the two women did become closer two years ago when both were pregnant: Carolyn with her second child and Rebecca with her first. Rebecca went on to have a healthy baby girl, but, tragically, Carolyn, who has a daughter, gave birth to a baby boy who lived only a day. Carolyn was 43 years old at the time.

When Carolyn and Arthur felt ready to resume their efforts to expand their family, they consulted a fertility doctor. She advised them to consider donated eggs since Carolyn was now nearly 45 years old. Although initially put off by the idea, both Carolyn and Arthur were eventually able to embrace it. They began doing a "mental inventory" of the extended family and landed, before long, on Rebecca. After much discussion and several rehearsals, Carolyn phoned Rebecca and asked.

Rebecca remembers having a wild mixture of feelings about Carolyn's request. She ranged from feeling "special" and "honored" to feeling "worried" and "burdened." She moved quickly from thinking, "Of course I could do that," to feeling doubtful, wondering how she would react to the child. Since her own family is not yet complete, her thoughts went, also, to her own fertility. She also found herself thinking about her place in the family and her perceptions of Carolyn's place. From Rebecca's vantage point, she has always been something of an "outsider" and Carolyn is in the "in crowd." Rebecca wondered if donating would enable her to feel more included, more valued by the family.

Rebecca spent several weeks soul searching before ultimately deciding to donate. When asked about her decision, she indicated that she had tried to predict how she would feel in the future if she donated and if she decided against it. Her conclusion was that she would regret not donating, but she could imagine few reasons why she would regret the decision to donate. In Rebecca's words, "When Carolyn first asked me, I thought, 'Of course I could do that—that's no big deal.' Then I began to think about it and it seemed like a very big deal. Now I have come full circle—I've thought and thought and thought about it and concluded it is really not so big after all."

Hearing this story and listening to Rebecca speak about her decision to donate, it is difficult for us not to see her as pressured in some ways. The loss of Carolyn and Arthur's second child, followed by a direct request for donation and Rebecca's initially positive response, seems to have put her in a position where she felt she really could not say no.

Friend-to-Friend, Acquaintance-to-Acquaintance Donation

Many people seeking egg donation would like the donor to be someone they know, but they either don't have a family member who can or will donate or they prefer to have the donation occur outside the family. Some of these couples turn to friends or acquaintances for ovum donation, either because the friends or acquaintances make an offer or because the prospective recipient feels comfortable enough asking someone to donate.

Friend-to-friend donation offers many benefits. It enables people to bring a child into the world who will know the woman who provided half of his/her genes. It gives the recipients the reassurance that the egg comes from a good person and is being offered for altruistic reasons. Less likely to be burdened by family issues of coercion and competition, friend-to-friend donation may feel more free and clear with "no strings attached."

So is there a down side to friend-to-friend donation? Of course there is, since no option is perfect. Friend-to-friend donation can be less than ideal if the friend is not fertile or if the friend's husband or others in her life are less than enthusiastic about this decision. Clinical nurse specialist Sharon Steinberg cautions friends about entering into a donor pregnancy without careful exploration of their relationship with the prospective recipient—past, present and future. Although friend-to-friend donation can be a wonderful option for couples who seek the benefits of a known donor who will remain part of their lives, it is not without its potential complications and challenges.

We turn now to the seven parameters, making note of how each applies to friend-to-friend or acquaintance-to-acquaintance donation.

Availability and Accessibility

Depending upon your age, the age of your friends, the breadth of your social circle, and your openness about your situation, you may or may not have several people in your life who are available to donate eggs to you. Friend-to-friend donation is probably best suited to women in their early to mid-30s. Hopefully, many of your friends will have completed their families by this point and still have eggs that are "young enough" and healthy enough to be suitable for donation.

Older or younger recipients may have a harder time identifying someone in their social network who could donate to them. For older recipients whose friends are approximately the same age, the issue is older eggs. For younger recipients, the problem is that friends and acquaintances are less likely to have completed their families.

Anyone seeking a known donor from among friends and acquaintances faces the question of how to "access" that donor. Some people are lucky enough to receive an offer, but this does not often happen. Remember that in many instances, friends would love to help, but they don't know that someone close to them is hoping to be offered an egg. In the absence of an offer, how do you ask?

Asking a friend or acquaintance to donate should be easier than asking a sister or a cousin. In the latter instances, there is always the risk that the person asked will feel pushed to donate. Our hope is that with friends and acquaintances there will not be this inherent pressure, and that people will feel free to either offer or decline. Part of the reason for this is that if a friend declines, there are usually many other people in the recipient's life who are "eligible" to donate. This is in contrast to what may be one sister or one cousin who has the potential to help the recipient pass on family genes.

Our recommendations for asking friends are very similar to our recommendations for asking sisters or cousins. You can ask someone directly, or you can take the more indirect route of sending a general letter. In many ways, we prefer the letter, especially when it comes to friends and acquaintances. After all, you really have no way of knowing who will want to donate and by sending a letter out to several people, you "can cast a wide net and see who swims in."

The down side to sending a letter is that it diminishes your privacy. Once a letter goes out, many people in your life will know that you are considering or pursuing oocyte donation. This doesn't mean that they have to know if and when you decide on a donor, but if the letter states unequivocally that you need eggs in order to conceive, people will assume that any subsequent pregnancy involved donor eggs, which invites speculation about who the donor was.

Costs

As with intrafamily donation, friend-to-friend donation may be very cost effective. It is unlikely to involve substantial payment to the donor, and in a mandated state, there will be few medical costs. However, as we noted earlier, egg donation in a non-mandated state can be very costly, especially if the donor is not very fertile and requires more than one stimulated cycle and retrieval.

You will notice that we said "unlikely to involve substantial payment to the donor, " rather than, "it doesn't involve payment." The reason we phrased it this way is that there will surely be instances in which the recipient wants to give the donor a gift as a way of saying thank you. While this is unlikely to be a large sum of money, some recipients will make a donation to the donors' child's (rens) college fund, indicating that just as the donor helped them form their family, so, too, do they want to help the donor better launch her own children.

So what does this mean in terms of dollars and cents? If the recipient couple gives the donor a gift of say, $2000, "for college," and all medical costs are paid for, there will remain only legal and counseling fees. These are unlikely to exceed $2500, making the entire cost of the donor cycle under $5000. However, if anything fails to go smoothly—the donor doesn't stimulate well, the recipient conceives and miscarries, the insurance doesn't pay—then costs mount. It is not difficult to imagine a friend-to-friend egg donation costing upwards of $10,000.

Fertility

In general and as a group, volunteer donors—whether family members or friends—are assumed to be less fertile than program-recruited donors. The reason for this is that program-recruited donors are selected, in part, for their known or presumed fertility. Volunteer donors, by contrast, are usually asked—or offer—for other reasons. In addition, volunteer donors are often older than program-recruited donors and hence assumed to be less fertile.

A volunteer donor who is under 35 and has had a successful pregnancy within the last year or so is likely to be a fertile donor. A volunteer who is younger and has recently had a baby is an even stronger bet. While most programs will not accept a program-recruited donor who is over age 32 or so, many will work with older family members and friends, recognizing that the advantages of a known donor may make the diminished chance of success "worth it" to some people.

The Child's Story

From the child's perspective, friend-to-friend donation is inviting. Many see it as the best of both worlds. The child has all the benefits of knowing and feeling close to his/her donor, but none of the drawbacks that could come from intrafamily donation. The child grows up knowing where he/she came from, has an up-to-date medical history, knows other genetic relatives, including the donor's children, and appreciates, first hand, the importance of having friends who will help you when you need them.

Ethical Considerations

From an ethical perspective, friend-to-friend donation raises fewer issues than does intrafamily donation. Friend-to-friend donation probably won't feel coercive, and unlike program-recruited donation, payment is not involved. Those who challenge all of ovum donation will include friend-to-friend donation in their scrutiny, wondering whether it is ethically sound for one woman to take potent drugs and undergo a surgical procedure all to help another create a child that is not biologically hers.

Our Family

"You can pick your friends but you can't pick your family"—or so they say. With egg donation, friends sometimes become "family." You will need to be comfortable with this—with having your child have genetic ties to your friend and to your friend's family. For some people, this can feel like a natural extension of their friendship—one which feels entirely comfortable. For others, it may feel like the boundaries of their family would become porous—that it would simply feel "too weird" for them to create a baby with their friend. "Will our donor's mother think she is our child's grandmother?" "Will our child and her children be confused by this, wondering if they are 'really' sisters?" "And what about the husbands—will it be strange for them as well to have the two of us sharing such a unique and intimate bond?"

....

Remember Carol...

We met Carol and her husband, Mike, in Chapter 3. They are the couple who became parents through the help of Carol's close friend, Laura. They had pretty much given up on pregnancy and were pursuing adoption when Laura approached them with "the offer we couldn't—and wouldn't—turn down."

Things have gone remarkably well for Carol and Mike, as well as for Laura and her husband, Herb. Carol became pregnant on the first donor egg cycle and gave birth to a healthy baby boy. When he was only a few months old, his parents, who were now in their mid-40s, wanted to transfer their cryopreserved embryos "rather than let ourselves get any older." They were advised to wait six months before embarking on another pregnancy. When the requisite six months had passed, two embryos were transferred. The result: Carol is pregnant a second time.

When asked how the pregnancies have affected their relationship, Carol and Laura look at each other, smile, and say, "We're closer than ever." Laura went with Carol for the initial ultrasounds, and each time she was introduced to the technician as "my egg donor." Both women say that they were pleased when the ultrasound technician acknowledged Laura's contribution but readily focused her attentions on Carol, her patient.

Although Carol and Laura are very open about their experience with medical people and with their immediate families, they say that most people do not know about the oocyte donation. The women feel that it is private and that only their children, their close families, and Carol's pediatrician need to know.

Carol remembers a time when her infertility weighed heavily on her and she felt pretty overcome with grief. Those feelings are now long since gone, and when asked if she continues to feel loss, Carol says no. Instead, she replies, "I feel that Laura has given us an incredible gift. Our child is a miracle baby who came to us from God. Laura transformed our lives, and for that we will always be grateful."

"And do you have any regrets?" Carol is asked.

"Only one," she replies. I wish I were younger. I am 44 now, and I feel that this is the maximum age that someone should have a baby." Then she smiles and points to her son, "But he is doing his best to keep me young."

Program-Recruited Donors

We are identifying women who receive some payment for their efforts to donate as *program-recruited donors*. Although sisters and friends also enter into contracts with the recipients, *program-recruited donor* seemed to be the best umbrella term to use to refer to women who are recruited by agencies or clinics, who are almost always previously unknown to the recipient, and who often remain anonymous during and even after the donation process.

This group is made up of women who decide to become egg donors and then apply to commercial egg donor agencies or to medical practices seeking donors. This includes women who respond to an advertisement for an egg donor in a magazine, newspaper or on a public bulletin board or who go to internet websites investigating egg donation. Regardless of how they get there, these women have fundamentally made the same decision: they wish to voluntarily donate eggs to strangers.

"Why," you might ask, "would a woman want to give her eggs to a stranger in order to help establish a pregnancy? Why would a woman want someone else to conceive, carry, deliver and parent a child who came from her?" The answer to this is complex and will be addressed in greater depth later. But to begin…

Remember, first, that most women do not choose to make their eggs available to strangers. This cohort of women who become involved in egg donation is relatively limited and seems to consist of women who are motivated first by an appreciation of motherhood. Chicago social worker, Judy Calica, has interviewed hundreds of such donors and observes that many already have children and want other women to experience the joy of motherhood. Her findings have been confirmed by researchers Lessor, Balmaceda, Cervantes, Asch and O'Connor in "An Analysis of Social and Psychological Characteristics of Women Volunteering to Become Oocyte Donors" (*Fertility and Sterility*. Vol. 59. No. 1, Jan. 1993) and by Australian psychologist Maggie Kirkman (*Social Science and Medicine*, 2003). Lessor et al. found that most of the women they interviewed "expressed generally altruistic ideas about the value of their contribution," while Kirkman writes about the women who have the belief that "someone needs to be a mother."

Another primary motivation for program-recruited ovum donation is what Calica calls "volunteerism." She has found that these women make altruism a central tenet of their lives, feeling good about being able to help others. Kirkman supports this and quotes a donor, "I donated eggs because I wanted to do something special. I will die knowing I have made a difference to someone else's life." Others who have found altruism to be an important motivation for egg donors are Klock, Braverman and Rausch (1998) and Maggs-Rapport (1999).

Questions inevitably arise about payment: how much is it a motivating force for program-recruited egg donors? Nurse Katrina Twomey, Director of Dream Donations in Newton, Massachusetts, notes that while some women are initially attracted by the offer of payment, the applicants to her program who go on to donate appear to be more motivated by factors other than money. In their 2001 article, "Anonymous Oocyte Donation: A Follow-up Questionnaire" (*Fertility and Sterility*. Vol. 75. No. 5) researchers Patrick, Smith, Meyer and Bashford found that donors who have children were less likely to be motivated by money. These authors note that this finding was consistent with the findings of Raoul-Duval; Letur-Konirsch; and Frydman in France, (*Fertility and Sterility* 1992) which found that the "gratification of maternity desires may be a motivation for these women." In addition, they found that those donors who acknowledged being motivated by financial reward had less satisfaction than those with other motivations.

Finally, there are women who have had close friends or family members struggle with infertility. They have wanted to help their loved ones, but, for a variety of reasons (including infertility factors other than egg quality), donating eggs to them has not been an option. Sometimes these women seek program-recruited donation as a way of fulfilling their need to give to someone who longs to have a baby.

Another group of program-recruited donors is made up of women who are undergoing IVF and who are offered a discount for the treatment in exchange for some of their eggs. In 1997, as many as 23% of the medical programs offering donated eggs (ASRM/SART registry 1997) included egg sharing as an option. We worry about these donors. We see them as fundamentally different from other program-recruited donors, in that their donation is not really voluntary. Their willingness to donate eggs in exchange for medical treatment seems more likely to be the result of their deep desire to become parents—whatever the cost—than to want to help another infertile couple. We worry that this system is coercive and has the potential to render lifelong pain to these "involuntary volunteers." However, we acknowledge that researcher Maggs-Rapport presents a different perspective in her 1999 article "Egg Donation: A Gift of Love (*Nursing Standard* 13 [27]). In interviewing women who participated in what Maggs-Rapport calls "egg sharing schemes," she found that infertile women who donated did so with pride and a great sense of satisfaction and of the rightness of their decision.

Program-recruited oocyte donation is an evolving field. We can easily remember a time when the only way to obtain a donor who wasn't a friend or family member was to advertise on your own either in a magazine or paper or on the internet or to wait endlessly on a waiting list through a medical program. It was not until well into the 1990s that programs which are not part of medical practices which recruited, screened and matched egg donors became prevalent. It has been much more recent that programs have offered donors and recipients the opportunity to participate in open—or semi-open—egg donation.

We turn now to the six parameters that we used in discussing intrafamily and friend-to-friend donation to discuss program-recruited donation, whether it been conducted in an open, closed or semi-open format. However, since we see some degree of openness as a positive ingredient in egg donation, we will address this issue in all parameters to which it applies (all but cost and fertility).

Availability and Accessibility

Program-recruited donors are readily available, especially if prospective recipients seek a Caucasian donor. Donor programs report fewer Asian, Latino, and African American donors, although these groups, also, are represented in the donor population. According to Shelley Smith, Director of the Egg Donor Program, a large program in Los Angeles, 25% of her donors are women of color.

After checking for reputability and ethics, prospective recipients can go to the websites of any of these donor egg programs and find a substantial number of women who are currently available to donate. When recipients have selected a donor, or are seriously considering her, her profile will identified as "on hold," or there will be some other way of letting prospective recipients know that she is currently unavailable to donate. We will discuss repeat donations in the ethics chapter, as this practice does raise some ethical questions, but it is important to note here that many women do donate more than once. Hence, recipients who locate a donor they like, but who is currently unavailable, may choose to wait a few months until after her current donor contract ends.

One of the reasons given by some programs for making program-recruited donation anonymous has been that they "are concerned for the donors." Practitioners have worried that women might not choose to participate in ovum donation if they were required to meet the recipients or "worse still," if their identity were to be revealed to these recipients. However, there appears little evidence to justify this fear. In their 1990 study "A Comparison of the Attitudes of Volunteer Donors and Infertile Patient Donors on an Ovum Donation Program" (*Human Reproduction* Vol. 5), Power, Baber, Abdalla, Kirklund, Leonard and Studd found that more than 80% of anonymous egg donors in the U.K. would still choose to donate even if records were open. Similarly, researchers Lessor, Cervantes, O'Connor, Balmaceda and Asch (1993), who did a follow-up study of 95 program-recruited donors, found "an overwhelming majority who indicated their comfort at meeting the recipient if she so desires." They go on to say, "Recipients and donors have reported that these meetings have gone well, an observation confirmed by treatment team observers."

Shelley Smith, Director of the Egg Donor Program in Los Angeles, further confirms this anecdotally. Smith, who routinely asks the young women she is interviewing for her program whether they would be willing to meet recipients, reports that many of her donors say "Sure." Smith adds that these young women have been open to meeting recipient couples before commencing a cycle as well as after pregnancy has been confirmed. After participating in many of these meetings, Smith and her staff prefer to hold them during pregnancy, as all participants can relax and celebrate rather than feeling anxiety about whether the process will work.

However, other professionals disagree. Dr. Elaine Gordon, among others, feels that meeting before the cycle commences gives all parties the right *not* to participate. Gordon reports that she gives donors and recipients each other's phone numbers, encourages them to talk and meet, and asks them to get back to her after the meeting. "Occasionally I'll get a call from either a donor or a recipient indicating that the person doesn't feel comfortable proceeding. When this happens—and fortunately, it is rare—it is my job to help the other party move on. It is important that no one feels obligated to do something with which they are uncomfortable."

Turn on your computer, click on to an egg donation website and you have access to program-recruited donors. Programs have become quite skilled at making this process "user friendly." Reasons for this are many and varied—programs want to run efficiently, they want prospective recipients to be able to access donors from all over the country, or even beyond its borders, and they want people to be able to make their decisions in the privacy of their own homes.

Mary Fusillo, Clinical Nurse Specialist in Houston, Texas, argues that donor photos do not belong on the internet. Although she recognizes the convenience this offers recipients, Fusillo feels that her program and others have a responsibility to protect the privacy of their donors. Fusillo suggests that websites be used to orient prospective recipients and to introduce them, in only the most general way, to the range of donors. She asks that actual matching occur in a more personal way. Making over twenty matches monthly, Fusillo meets with prospective recipients and goes over individual available donors with them.

Although egg donor programs can provide their prospective clients easy access to donors through the internet and other means, geography also pays a role in the "accessibility" of donors. Couples seeking donors are often advised, by their medical programs, to work with someone who either lives near the program or who is willing to travel and relocate for several days or weeks. This recommendation comes because egg donor programs and medical facilities have found it difficult to do oocyte donation with a donor who lives at a distance. The exquisite timing of two cycles, the need for close and consistent monitoring, and the increasing difficulties of long distance air travel are factors that have shaped this decision.

Cost

Program-recruited donation can be a costly undertaking, especially in states without insurance mandates. Putting the costs of medical treatment and perhaps even counseling aside, payments to a program, a lawyer, and a donor usually total over $10,000. If the first cycle doesn't work and there are no frozen embryos, the fee to the donor is repeated a second time. Or if the intended parents decide to move on to a second donor—or even more complicated, to another program— they may be facing a repeat of many of their program and legal costs. It is easy to see how program-recruited egg donation can cost a self-paying couple upwards of $25,000, and this is for the possibility—*not the guarantee*—of a pregnancy.

Fertility

As physicians often say, "The only sure guarantee of fertility is pregnancy." With program-recruited donors, as with *everyone* else, there is no "for certain" way to predict fertility. Nonetheless, it seems likely that a woman will produce "good" eggs if she has recently had a baby or recently donated her eggs in a cycle that resulted in pregnancy. Prospective recipients often choose a program-recruited donor because they feel that she offers them a better chance of success than do related or acquaintance donors, and some limit their choices to women who have previously donated, anticipating that is their best way to ensure a successful pregnancy.

The Child's Story

As we noted earlier, program-recruited donation can be open or anonymous–or something in between. From the child's perspective, an open donation is likely to be more comprehensible than an anonymous one. We have learned from children and adults conceived with donated sperm that donor offspring inevitably have questions about where they came from. Open donations will enable children conceived with a donor's egg to have most of their questions answered.

Thankfully, even an "anonymous" donated egg is not as truly anonymous as it once was. Not all that long ago, when medical programs recruited their donors, they matched their patients with these volunteer donors and offered neither party much information about the other. Today, even "anonymous" donation usually involves at least one photo, a written profile, and a medical history. Add an exchange of letters, a phone call, even an in-person meeting, and we can see how today's donor offspring will have the answers to many of their questions.

Donor offspring have questions about where they came from and they have other questions about how they came to be. It is this second set of questions that pose more challenges for parents through program-recruited donation. As parents, your part of this story will be the easy one: you wanted a baby very much and were fortunate enough to be able to have a baby. Part of your path to parenthood involved learning that you needed some help creating a baby, and thankfully, there was a kind woman willing to help you. That's the easy part of the story. The more challenging part comes when your child wants to know more about the helpful woman. "Why did she want to help someone have a baby?" "Why did she want to help strangers?" and the most difficult question of all, "Was she paid for donating her eggs?"

Donor sperm offspring have taught us that one of the most difficult parts of their experience has been grappling with the issue of payment. Many have been quite outspoken (Toronto conference, June, 2002) with their feelings about payment. They point out that the word *donation* implies a gift, not a sale. With ovum donation in the U.S. involving substantial fees to donors, often as high as $5000 and more per retrieval cycle, questions will likely arise about whether the donor "did it for the money." While some program-recruited donors provide clear and compelling evidence that their donation was not motivated by the payment, many donors state openly that they feel "It [egg donation] is a good way to earn money and do a good thing at the same time."

In a few moments (and again, in Chapter 11), we will address the ethical issues in payment to donors, but here we want to look at how the child will integrate payment to the donor as part of his or her story. Boston area therapist Peg Beck points out that there are many instances in life in which someone is paid for doing a good thing, and that the payment does not diminish the goodness of the work. Teachers, clergy, nurses and childcare workers are but a few of the occupations that are populated by deeply caring people who are paid for their caring and compassion as well as for other skills. Beck suggests that in talking with children, parents need not apologize for the fact that the donor received payment. "The exchange of money does not mean she didn't care."

Ethical Considerations

Program-recruited oocyte donation raises a number of ethical issues. In addition to questions regarding payment, there are questions about whether it is morally and ethically correct for a woman to take potent medications and undergo a surgical procedure in order to help a stranger, whether it is morally and ethically correct for women to be allowed/encouraged to donate multiple times, whether it is morally and ethically correct to intentionally create a child who will never know his or her genetic mother, and whether it is acceptable not to tell a woman who provides eggs whether a pregnancy was achieved.

Payment

Should egg donors/providers be paid and if so, how much? In England donors receive a token payment, something in the vicinity of $20, for their time and effort. In Australia they receive nothing. Caroline Lorbach, author of *Experiences in Donor Conception, Parents, Offspring and Donors Through the Years* (Jessica Kingsley Ltd., London 2003) and an Australian active in the Donor Conception Network, explains that in Australia, it is generally assumed that women donate eggs only for altruistic reasons. In 2004, Canada outlawed payment for donated eggs. In the U.S. program-recruited donation involves payment, and many people find this ethically acceptable since the process of donating is very time consuming and demanding and involves some physical pain and risk. The idea is that a woman is being paid for her time and effort and *not* for her eggs.

This argument—of being paid for time and effort—would be compelling if there were one standard fee for egg donation. Unfortunately, as of this writing (2005), there is no single accepted fee in the U.S. In some instances programs set fees and in other instances, donors set fees. It is this latter practice that we find especially problematic.

Although it could be argued that for one woman the injections, frequent tests and procedures should be compensated for at a rate of $3,000 and for another, at a rate of $6,000, differences in payment start to sound like "selling eggs." Some could surely argue that the payment differentials are because of the nature of the women's jobs (taking time off from work for appointments and travel will have more of an impact on one woman than another), the cost of living in their region of the country, and the effect on their family. However, it seems that women asking for higher payments are not doing it because the price of gas is higher in their state, but rather, because they are "more desirable" donors. Often included in this population are women who have donated before and are, hence, "proven" donors, women who consider themselves very attractive, and women with high SAT scores and/or academic records.

In the absence of one nationwide "usual and customary fee," some programs set a fee and advise all donors and recipients that that is what will be paid for time and effort, regardless of how many eggs are produced and how attractive the donor is in one way or another. Programs that practice in this way communicate what we feel is an important message: one woman's eggs are not more "valuable" than another's, and payment is for time, not eggs.

Chicago social worker Judy Calica observes that women "rarely do this for the money." Calica, who has interviewed several hundred donors, has found that although women are initially attracted by the offer of payment, those who proceed with ovum donation are motivated by other factors as well. Ms. Calica points out that, because the process of applying to be an egg donor is slow and arduous, it tends to eliminate women who do not feel a strong motivation to participate. She adds that when she has asked applicants what they plan to do with the money, she has received responses ranging from, "I'd like to donate it to someone" to "I'm planning to put it towards college or towards my children's future education."

Although Calica's findings—and those of others—are reassuring, we are aware that there are some women who "do it for the money." I (Ellen) had occasion to talk with one young woman who told me that she had donated several times *only* because she sought payment. This young woman also acknowledged having had emotional difficulties following the donation, difficulties she blamed on donation.

Is it ethically and morally correct for a woman to take potent medications and undergo procedures in order to help strangers?

Autonomy and beneficence are central principles of medical ethics. If we look at this question through a bi-focal lens of autonomy and beneficence, we see that a woman has a right to make decisions for herself, and egg donor programs have a responsibility to "do good." How does this play out when young women are "recruited" to donate their eggs? From our perspective, it comes down to the question of informed consent. If a woman has given careful thought to all of the ramifications of what she is doing, why shouldn't she be able to participate in oocyte donation?

How does a donor achieve informed consent? Responsible egg donation programs should accept only those women who are old enough and presumably mature enough to make educated, informed decisions about oocyte donation. But how is this determined? Many of us who counsel donors and recipients feel most comfortable with women who are mothers themselves, since we feel they are best able to consider what they are giving away. However, donor programs accept many women who are not mothers.

Short of motherhood, we turn next to age. Although many ovum donation programs will accept women as young as 21, 25 seems to be a more appropriate age. At 25, a woman is most likely involved in the working world and hopefully able to carefully examine what it might mean to her to donate eggs.

A responsible program should help her in this process, going to great lengths to make sure that she understands what is involved medically and emotionally in oocyte donation. This means reviewing the potential long term consequences of this decision, consequences which can range from medical issues including infertility to emotional issues about what it means to have a genetic child "out there." These issues should be reviewed when the prospective donor first approaches a program, and reiterated when she visits a medical clinic for evaluation. She should be reminded of them not only by program staff, but by the mental health consultant, and by physicians and nurses. We will further address how to find a good program later on in this book, in Chapter 7 on programs and Chapter 8 on attempting pregnancy.

As recipients, you have choices, both in the program you work with and in the donor you select. You can decide to look only at women who have children or perhaps limit your donor selection to women over 25. You can select a program that you feel works hard help a woman achieve informed consent. Given these choices, it seems to us that it is ethically and morally correct for a woman to choose donated eggs. As we saw in Chapter 3, there are many couples with a deep desire to bring a child into the world who are unable to do so without the gift of donor eggs.

Is it morally and ethically correct for a woman to donate multiple times?

In November, 2000, The American Society for Reproductive Medicine (ASRM) published a Practice Committee Report on "Repetitive Oocyte Donation." In it, ASRM addresses the two concerns that it has about repetitive oocyte donation—physical health risks to the donor and "inadvertent consanguinity. This refers to the possibility that two people, who were born through egg donation, will meet, fall in love and have a child together, unaware that they are half-siblings." We would like to raise a third risk not covered in ASRM's proactive committee report: mental health risks to all participants and to the offspring.

In addressing physical risks to the donor, the American Society for Reproductive Medicine notes "controlled ovarian hyperstimulation entails both known and theoretical risks… In the short-term, there is the risk of ovarian hyperstimulation syndrome (OHSS) which is reported to be associated with approximately 1% of cycles." The committee report goes on to acknowledge the on-going concern that controlled ovarian hyperstimulation might increase the long-term risk of ovarian cancer. This was first raised in the well known Whittemore article in which researchers Whittemore, Harris and Intyre from the Collaborative Ovarian Cancer Group (1992) studied the long term affects of infertility treatments. Although no subsequent study has found a causal connection between ovarian hyperstimulation and ovarian cancer, ethical concern recommends that it may take years for some troubling evidence to surface. In addition, the society notes that "the oocyte retrieval procedure itself also poses some risks for the donor." These risks include the risks of anesthesia, the small risk of pelvic infection, and intraperitoneal hemorrhage (Bennett, Waterstone, Cheng, and Parsons, 1993).

In addressing the issue of "inadvertent consanguinity," the American Society for Reproductive Medicine has advised an "arbitrary limit of no more than 25 pregnancies per sperm or oocyte donor, in a population of 800,000, in order to minimize the risks of consanguinity." (Curie-Cohen, 1980).

The society's guidelines lead us to our concern about the emotional consequences—to all involved—of multiple donations. It is all well and good for the society to recommend "25 pregnancies per 800,000," but we worry that this level of donation will lead to grave concerns in offspring and their parents about to whom the children are related. We are also concerned about what it could mean to a donor down the road when she reflects on all the children she may have helped create. When she encounters a donor who has donated more than two or three times, Dr. Elaine Gordon points out, "This is not a career path."

If women are going to donate multiple times, the only way to do this in a morally and ethically sound way is for all participants to agree to openness. From the start, the donor should agree to know each of the families to whom she donates and to enable them to know one another. Although we realize it is difficult for some families to commit to and follow through with this degree of openness, it appears to be the only way of sparing offspring the "genealogical bewilderment" they are likely to experience growing up as offspring of program-recruited oocyte donation.

Is it morally and ethically correct to intentionally create a child who will not be raised by his/her full biological parents?

Although many would argue that it is optimal for a child to be raised by his/her full biological parents, this is impossible in the case of gay and lesbian parents as well as others who do not have both eggs and sperm. Sperm donor offspring have reminded all of us, again and again, that the pain they experience does not come from being donor offspring, it comes from secrecy and anonymity. Based on what we have learned from them, and from the children of anonymous adoption, we feel that it is morally and ethically correct to create a child who will be parented by someone other than a full biological parent as long as that child knows the truth about his/her origins and has access to the donor.

Is it morally and ethically correct for a woman to be unaware whether her eggs helped create a pregnancy?

We believe that young women who donate their eggs deserve to know the outcome of their efforts. If they have helped to achieve a successful pregnancy, they should know when a child (or twins) is born and should know the sex of the child. We fear that withholding this information from a donor will leave her with unanswered questions which may last a lifetime.

In interviewing prospective egg donors, social worker Judy Calica found that these young women, although by and large an intelligent, capable and thoughtful group, did not always recognize the importance of knowing the outcome of their "donation." Some had been told by the programs they were working with that they might not learn whether pregnancy was achieved. Unfortunately, all prospective donors do not have the benefit of talking with someone like Ms. Calica, who can point out all the reasons why someone should know whether they have genetic offspring in the world. The following are but a few of the reasons why we feel that every woman who provides eggs should know whether a child was born as the result of her efforts.

1. Medical reasons include future infertility or medical problems in the donor's children,

2. Social reasons include questions the donors children may have about dating "half siblings."

3. Emotional reasons include feelings the donor may have about passing on something of herself in this world, especially if she is childless or should lose a child. Consider, for example, the story of "Charlie", chronicled in *Bio News* (January 2004). Charlie, the father of three, donated sperm 31 times between 1983 and 1985. Now, twenty years later, Charlie thinks of the "extra offspring" often and is haunted by the idea they may be searching for him. "I honestly don't think of myself as their dad. What I did to help create them counts for nothing compared to getting up in the middle of the night when they are sick. I would hate for any genetic child of mine to think of me as their father, par-

ticularly if there is a real father who raised them. But I would hate for them to wonder who I am or what I looked like and not to be able to find out. And honest, I am curious."

Our Family

Intended parents seeking a program-recruited donor tend to look at the profiles of prospective donors with a keen eye for who will "fit" in their family. For some, the emphasis is on physical appearance—they want to find a donor who resembles them, or, specifically, who resembles the intended mom. Other intended parents focus more on intelligence or personality style or ethnicity in their efforts to identify the donor who is right for them.

Couples seeking a program-recruited donor go about their decision making in a variety of ways. One couple found seven donors who seemed like potentially good choices and then they made a "rating scale," evaluating each donor along several parameters—appearance, personality, intelligence, age, motivation for donating, ethnicity. Then after compiling all of their ratings, they looked at each other, laughed, scribbled over all their charts and decided to "go on chemistry." For whatever reason, a particular donor, who hadn't scored all that high on the various charts, was the woman who "felt right"—the chemistry was there.

Shelley Smith observes, "Couples often fall in love with their donor. I see people go through a number of profiles and then have this 'aha' moment when they realize they've found her." What is it about a donor that can bring that "a ha?" Smith observes that we are a "visual society—it is usually something they see rather than something they read—perhaps her smile, or a photo of her hugging her two sisters, or a gentle, kind look."

Recognizing that the donor will never be a replica of the mom, some recipients choose someone who adds something to the family. One Christian woman, who is married to a Jewish man and plans to raise her children as Jews, was delighted to find a Jewish donor. "I don't want to convert, but I love the idea of my children being fully, authentically Jewish." And Nurse Clinical Director Mary Fusillo tells of recipients who have struggled with their weight and looked for thin donors in an effort to spare their children the same struggle. How nice, many couples feel, if the donor can bring something special to their family—a talent, an interest, particularly good looks or high intelligence.

Religion and ethnicity can be of critical importance to couples selecting a program-recruited donor. Italian intended parents tend to seek Italian donors, Jewish intended parents seek Jewish donors, Irish want Irish. It seems that many of us have a sense of being part of a larger "family" or "people" and we are comforted by the knowledge that someone is "one of our own." We can recall one man who got a list of Reform and Conservative rabbis and wrote to every one of them seeking a Jewish donor. And recently a Russian couple decided to move forward, "as long as we can find an Eastern European—preferably Russian—donor."

Elaine Gordon describes the process by which couples select donors as one of embracing. "I find that when people have found the person who is right for them, they feel ready to 'embrace' her. However, it's important to remember that this doesn't happen for everyone. Many prospective recipients benefit from talking with a mental health professional who is knowledgeable about ovum donation. This counseling or consultation may offer them new and helpful perspectives."

The high cost of egg donation prompts some couples to choose their donor primarily for her anticipated fertility. Although they would love to look for a donor to "fall in love with," their first priority is pregnancy. Such couples usually select someone who has donated before with a successful outcome.

For other intended parents, donor selection appears much more mechanical or antiseptic. They want someone who is fertile—"who has proven fertility"—and they usually want someone who is also intelligent, very attractive and sports a family history free from medical and mental health ailments. We'll admit that these couples sometimes begin to sound like they are looking for a "pedigree" rather than a person, and this can be worrisome.

I (Ellen) can recall one 52-year-old man who looked at several profiles and found something wrong with each donor. One woman's favorite books were ones that this man regarded as low brow. He was similarly disparaging of another donor's taste in movies. Within a few minutes, I understood why he had never married and I began to worry about any child that might come into his life as a result of donated eggs. Shortly after meeting him, I came across Michael Sandel's compelling article, "The Case Against Perfection," (*Atlantic Monthly*, April 2004). All pedigree-seeking would-be parents should read Sandel's article, paying particular attention to two "on target" comments, "The hyper parenting familiar in our time represents an anxious excess of mastery and dominion that misses the sense of life as a gift." And later in the article,

"We choose our friends and spouses at least partly on the basis of qualities we find attractive. But we do not choose our children. Their qualities are unpredictable, and even the most conscientious parents cannot be held wholly responsible for the kind of children they have. That is why parenthood, more than other human relationships, teaches what the theologian, William F. May calls an 'openness to the unbidden.'"

If you find yourselves inclined in the pedigree direction, we remind you that no one (including you) is perfect. More importantly, we want to be sure that you don't set yourselves up for wanting to create and expect the "perfect" child. Regardless of who the donor is, the hoped for offspring of her donation will be his/her own little person.

Meet Roberta and Mark…and Sandy

Roberta and Mark are two physicians who married in their late 30s and wasted no time in attempting pregnancy. Their older daughter, Rebecca, was born a year after they were married. Because Roberta was 39 at the time, she decided to nurse Rebecca for only a few months and then try for a second pregnancy.

Although they had done their best to beat the biological clock, Roberta and Mark did not succeed in having a second pregnancy. When it became clear that they would have to decide between remaining a one child family and having a baby through donor egg or adoption, they each thought a lot about their options. After many conversations in their own heads and with each other, Roberta and Mark opted for oocyte donation.

As physicians and as the parents of a young, curious child, Roberta and Mark felt it was very important for them to meet their donor and for their hoped-for child to grow knowing where he/she came from. Because they had no friend or family member who could donate, Roberta and Mark approached a large donor program requesting a donor who would meet with them and agree to stay in touch. They also wanted someone who was willing to enter into a legal contract saying that the family could contact her if there was ever a medical need for bone marrow. Roberta and Mark stipulated further that they were prepared to make a similar commitment—if a medical need ever arose for the donor or her children, she could contact them and they would do what they could to help.

Sandy, a feisty engineer with three children and a history of three prior donations, was only too happy to meet Roberta and Mark. She had met each of her other couples and remained in close touch with one family. Sandy welcomed another opportunity to know a recipient couple, and, as a mom, she was pleased to join in the commitment to be there for each other should medical issues arise.

Prior to attempting pregnancy, Roberta, Mark and Sandy got together for a two hour meeting. They asked a clinical social worker to be there with them in case the meeting proved awkward for any of them. As it turned out, there was no awkwardness. Rather, the meeting provided an opportunity for Sandy to share an array of family stories and family characteristics with Roberta and Mark. These stories became all the more meaningful and precious to the couple several months later when Roberta gave birth to the couple's second child. A boy. Alex.

....

And Meet Patty and Tim...

Patty and Tim are a couple who chose adoption over egg donation. They didn't have a family member or friend who could donate to them and both were troubled by the idea of Patty becoming pregnant with eggs from a stranger. As she put it, "It seemed like a weird idea—that physical matter would be removed from another woman—someone I did not know—and placed in my body. For me that was too strange. On the other hand, adoption didn't seem strange at all. I had known people who were adopted and we had friends who had adopted their children. So for lots of reasons, adoption seemed like the logical next step when IVF wasn't working for us."

Patty and Tim signed on for a domestic adoption and their son, T.J., arrived only a few months later. They were there at his birth, and from the start, he was the light of their lives. When T.J. was two, Patty and Tim began working on a second adoption.

To Patty and Tim's surprise, disappointment, and ultimately, distress, adoption did not work out for them the second time around. They were matched with a few expectant mothers considering adoption, each of whom changed her mind at birth or a within a few days of delivery. Eventually the couple got to a point where they felt they needed to look at other options—international adoption or perhaps, even ovum donation.

As they began to explore their options, Patty and Tim discovered that oocyte donation had changed dramatically since they had briefly visited it nearly a decade before. In addition to being much more available and accessible, program-recruited egg donation was no longer as shrouded in anonymity as it once was. Patty and Tim had met T.J.'s birthparents and felt strongly about meeting a woman who would help them conceive. And so they began looking at programs that offered open donation.

"It was like our second experience in adoption," Patty says. We began with clear ideas and lots of hope and then discovered that it wasn't going to be so easy. One program led to a second and one donor to another. " As things unfolded, Patty and Tim found themselves in territory they never expected to traverse: anonymous program-recruited ovum donation. To their surprise, they settled on working with a program that actually required that the process be fully closed—something previously totally anathema to Patty and Tim.

And so the couple who wanted a second open adoption ended up trying to conceive through an anonymous egg donor. This was a surprise to them, but it was dwarfed by the next surprise that came their way: Patty was pregnant. When she called for the results of her pregnancy test and was told they were positive, both she and Tim were floored. "I had never heard those words before. I had no idea what it would feel like when someone said, 'Yes, the test was positive and you are pregnant.'"

When interviewed, Patty was due to deliver within a month. Having initially chosen adoption, she and Tim had made peace with the idea that they would never share a pregnancy. Perhaps it was the relinquishment of that goal that has, in some ways, made this experience all the more sweet for both Patty and Tim. Again and again, they comment on what a "miracle" the pregnancy has been for both of them.

And so we see from Roberta, Mark and Sandy and from Patty and Tim, what we saw earlier in this chapter in the stories of Andrea and Margaret and of Carol, Mike, Laura and Herb, there are many different ways in which people participate in egg donation. Surely there are differences in their experiences, but there are also common themes. In addition to the ones we noted at the start of this chapter, we see that people's lives unfold in unexpected ways, that they choose to build their families in ways they never could have imagined, and that these unexpected journeys often offer them satisfaction and rewards they could not have anticipated.

As you move to the next chapter, we hope that you will feel encouraged by what you have read here. Patty and Tim never dreamed they could accept program-recruited oocyte donation and they could not believe that they would ever share a pregnancy. Now they are but a month away from delivery. Margaret, who faced life-threatening illness at 22, never dreamed she would one day be blessed with three children: one born to her through an anonymous donor, one born to her with the help of her sister and one who came half way across the world from China to join their family.

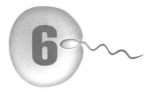

Lawyers and Mental Health Counselors

"The people you meet along the way shape your journey." This is one of the central themes of this book, and it is especially relevant to this chapter. Whether you use a relative or acquaintance as your donor or use a program-recruited donor found through a medical clinic or commercial program, you will surely meet and use mental health counselors and lawyers as you make plans to attempt pregnancy through donor egg. Their roles are distinct and very different from one another, but individuals in each category of "helping people" play significant roles in an egg donation journey.

Mental Health Counselors

First, a word about titles. We are identifying those who can counsel you about the emotional aspects of egg donation with the umbrella label of *mental health counselor*. The reason for this is that mental health professionals working in the field of infertility come from a range of backgrounds. They may be psychiatrists, psychologists, social workers, psychiatric nurses, etc. In certain instances it may be helpful for that person to be a psychiatrist or a psychiatric nurse, since they can help you make decisions about psychiatric medications. For example, some women are on anti-depressants and wonder whether to discontinue them prior to or during pregnancy. Others feel depressed or anxious and question whether they would benefit from some medication. Similarly, there are instances in which the skills of a psychologist—someone skilled in psychological testing—are called for. However, what matters for most people considering egg donation is that the mental health counselor(s) they speak with be compassionate, sensitive and well versed in reproductive medicine.

Women and men considering egg donation meet with mental health counselors for one of two reasons: the individual or couple proactively seeks counseling because they hope that someone can help them in some aspect of making the egg donation decision or in the process, or the individual or couple is instructed to see a counselor because their medical program feels it would be helpful. We will address both avenues to counseling.

Seeking Help

People considering or participating in egg donation seek help from a counselor for a variety of reasons. The following are among the most common "issues" of egg donor couples.

Loss and Grief

No one gets to advanced infertility treatment without experiencing loss. Your losses may have occurred years ago, perhaps when you were a young adult facing cancer treatment or recovering from emergency surgery that removed your ovaries. Or your losses were more recent—you tried to conceive, never anticipating a problem, and learned that you had premature ovarian failure. Possibly, you are one of the many people who "always wanted to have a baby," but didn't find a partner until your eggs were "too old." Or you may have experienced pregnancy loss, maybe even the devastation of a late loss or a loss of twins or triplets. Whatever the nature of your loss, it has to be there...part of what you carry with you as you move forward.

A mental health counselor can assist you with your feelings of loss and grief, and hopefully prevent them from interfering with the joy of parenthood through egg donation. Counseling can offer you the opportunity to talk about what you have been through, what it meant to you to have "your own biological child," what it means to move forward with egg donation knowing that a part of you will always ache.

Issues of loss and grief will differ depending upon whether you have had a biological child, whether you "always knew" you couldn't reproduce, whether you are filled with regret (e.g. for delaying parenthood), or with gratitude that this option exists.

The loss of a child that existed only in your hopes and dreams is a form of "disenfranchised loss"—one for which there are no rituals of mourning. A counselor can assist you in creating your own rituals. For example, you may choose to write a letter to the child you never had or plant a tree. You may bury all your fertility medications or find some other way of disposing of them, both literally and figuratively.

A counselor can help you find a way to accept that your sorrow and your joy can sit side by side. If you conceive through the help of an egg donor, you will most likely be thrilled, but you may also feel some sadness about what is not to be. Mental health counselors have found that those couples who most fully acknowledge their loss and grief over not having a full biological child (or a second) are often most prepared to fully enjoy and embrace egg donation. One couple who turned to egg donation after years of infertility and was now expecting their first baby captured the combination of emotions when they said, "We're 'over the top happy' and yet it is still very sad. We feel there has been a death in the family, but we are moving on with such joy and so much hope."

Decision Making

Your journey to parenthood has been a complicated one and it is not over yet. As you consider egg donation, there are decisions to be made. Is this the right option for you? If so, what type of donor do you prefer—family, friend, anonymous? How can you ask someone to donate? How do you select a contractual donor? Will you meet her? If so, should you wait until you are pregnant or meet her in advance? Would you prefer to talk with her by phone rather than meet face to face? If egg donation does not work, will you turn to adoption or, possibly, to combining egg donation with a gestational carrier? Or will you choose not to have children, or, in instances of secondary infertility, not to expand your family? A counselor knowledgeable about various paths to parenthood and the psychological processes involved in pursuing them can help you sort through these decisions and others that may arise.

The Couples Experience

Most people considering egg donation are part of a couple, either heterosexual or same sex. All couples face incredible challenges figuring out ways to keep their relationship strong while undergoing procedures which are stressful, intrusive, and sometimes physically painful and of uncertain outcome. Couples rarely move at the same pace through infertility treatment and egg donation, and they don't always agree about second choice paths to parenthood. Even those who do agree on what to do and when to do it may face differences about where to seek treatment, how long to try a particular approach, and, in the case of egg donation, which program to use and which donor. Additional areas of potential conflict include differences in who to talk with about egg donation, what to say, and when to say it.

Couples undergoing infertility and those pursuing egg donation or other options often find it helpful to have a counselor who can accompany them on their journey. Couples counseling for infertility, like individual counseling in this area, need not be weekly or even every second week. Rather, it can be helpful to know someone over time—to have her or him there and available as a resource. This counselor can help you listen more clearly to each other, avoiding such common Achilles heels of infertile couples as hearing "not yet" as "never," believing there is no potential for compromise and feeling that one's partner either "wants to talk about infertility *all* the time" or "*never* at all."

Relationships with Family, Friends, and Helping Professionals

Pursuing egg donation usually involves juggling a variety of relationships. You will be making decisions about what you say to family members and friends—whether you tell them you are pursuing egg donation, whether you share information about the donor, whether you decide to wait until after you are pregnant, or after you have your baby or later. You will also be navigating relationships with caregivers, some of whom may be responsive and sensitive to your feelings and others who may seem always to miss the boat.

A mental health counselor can help you sort through your reactions to and interactions with the cast of characters in your life. Someone who has talked with countless others facing similar struggles will understand what you go through when you learn your little sister is pregnant, when you are invited to yet another baby shower, when your cousin says something disparaging about egg donation, or when your mother tells you to "just adopt." The counselor can assist you in preparing for your conversations with people at work, with your physicians, and certainly, with prospective egg donors, whether they are family members, friends or strangers.

Preparing for Egg Donation

Chances are that you have been through IVF or some other high tech intervention before arriving at egg donation. Chances are that you also feel experienced with the procedures and hence, prepared for a donor egg cycle. What you may not have anticipated are the ways that this process can feel different from earlier treatment regimen. A counselor can help you prepare for any and all of the following:

Donor Selection

Selecting a donor can feel like an enormous responsibility. If you are deciding whether to work with a family member or friend, you will probably be grappling with questions about what it will mean to your relationship with that individual as well as with other family members or friends. You will also be wondering if your volunteer donor *really wants* to do this or whether she feels pressured or coerced. A counselor can help you explore your feelings about having someone close to you donate and she can be available to meet with your donor to help confirm that the decision is right for all participants.

If you seek a contractual donor, you will be most likely feel a great responsibility to "get it right." People play out this feeling in a variety of ways. Some conclude that they've "got it right" because they feel a powerful "chemistry" with the donor. Others attempt to "get it right" by carefully scrutinizing the donor's photos, SAT scores, interests etc, in an effort to select the best genes.

> Mary, 35 and deciding between her sister and a contractual donor, put it this way, "If my sister donates, we get what we get. I know who she is and I'm going into this assuming the child will inherit some of her characteristics. But if we go with someone we find on a list of donors, it will be my responsibility to pick wisely. It feels like too much control. What if I make a mistake?"

A counselor can help you sort through your feelings about different donors and she can help you make your way through donor profiles. She can reflect your reactions back to you and help you gain confidence in your ability to make a good decision. She can also help you keep the burden of this decision in perspective, reminding you that no one really has control of who their child will be.

Feelings about What the Donor—Whether Known or Anonymous—Is Going Through

People whose sister or cousin or friend is donating are often worried about "what we are putting her through." However, you are not the only ones concerned about the well-being of your donor. Couples working with contractual donors also find themselves concerned about their donor, both during the time she is taking the medications and especially during egg retrieval. A counselor is available to meet with your known or unknown donor, help her resolve her own feelings, and reassure you that her emotional needs are being met and that her feelings are normal and healthy.

A Resurgence of Feelings of "Failure" That You Can't Use Your Eggs

By the time you get to egg donation you will probably feel pretty convinced that you cannot use your own eggs. Hopefully, you will also feel that you have made peace with that reality. Hence, you may be surprised when you find yourself entering a cycle and still longing to use your own eggs. Counselors are experienced in helping clients move through these feelings.

A Resurgence of Ambivalence about This Decision

Ambivalence will be your traveling companion through this journey and will, most likely, accompany you into parenthood. It goes with the territory. Nonetheless, when you work so hard to make a decision and come to believe in the rightness of that decision, it can be terribly upsetting to encounter a resurgence of ambivalence. A trained counselor can help you work this through.

Profound Loss and Self Blame If It Doesn't Work

Couples work very hard to decide on egg donation, usually assuming that it will work. When a cycle fails or a miscarriage occurs, it is devastating. This devastation is often worse for a woman. You may feel it is the ultimate proof that your body does not work or worse still that you "are not meant to be a mother." You, who worked hard to move beyond the loss and self blame that you felt prior to egg donation, may feel catapulted back to that painful state. A skilled counselor can be invaluable in helping you deal with this renewed grief.

Stress in Your Marriage because You Feel That You Are "on Different Playing Fields"

Couples work hard to share egg donation but some still feel that they have unequal roles. Women who feel that genetic ties are more important than gestational bonds may enter into the process still feeling envy of their husbands and perhaps, a sense of unfairness. You may feel that you were beyond this and were ready to fully embrace motherhood through egg donation, but now you are tired, nauseous and feeling that your body is being taken over. It may all feel very unfair. Your husband or partner gets to have his biological child and you get to do all the work. Counselors serve as objective intermediaries in helping couples work through such differences.

Anxiety and Disbelief if the Pregnancy Test Is Positive

It helps to be prepared for the strong possibility that you will be flooded with anxiety and disbelief if the pregnancy test is positive. The anxiety will be about loss and perhaps, about fears that you're made a mistake or that there is something wrong with the baby. After all that you have been through to achieve an egg donation pregnancy, it is almost inevitable that you will have a complicated and perhaps, inconsistent, reaction to the news that you—or your wife/partner—are pregnant.

Feelings of Being "Fake" during Pregnancy

Egg donor parents are as "real" as parents can be, but that fact does not spare women pregnant through egg donation from feeling "like fakes." Time and again, women tell of how they felt they needed to camouflage the fact that they had help from an egg donor and that they felt deceitful when they were with other pregnant women. These feelings of inauthenticity can be terribly troubling, especially early in pregnancy when they tend to be most pronounced. Anticipating painful feelings does not eradicate them, but hopefully, reduces their intensity. A counselor who has been with your through this process can support you here.

The Blessing and Curse of the Meant to Be

As we noted in our introduction, people experiencing infertility, pregnancy loss and third party parenting often encounter the declaration "it was meant to be." While the words can be comforting when you have a wonderful baby through egg donation and cannot imagine loving any other child as much, they can sting when things do not go well. A pregnancy loss that "was not meant to be," can prompt you to feel that you forced nature. Although "it wasn't meant to be" can be a curse to anyone undergoing infertility, it carries with it special sting for those who turned reluctantly and with ethical, moral, and religious questions to egg donation. Sensitive professional support can assist with this.

Preparation for Talking with Children

Sadly, many parents through egg donation are afraid they won't be able to talk truthfully with their children. Specifically, they fear talking with their children about donor conception. An otherwise happy story, of a child wanted and planned for and loved, risks being transformed into a story of sadness and shame.

A compassionate, well-informed counselor can offer you enormous help in preparing for future conversations. Before a cycle it may be difficult to imagine you will ever become pregnant, let alone actually be a parent, so these practice conversations may seem remote. However, for many future parents, it is helpful to begin contemplating these conversations *before pregnancy*.

Group Counseling

Mental health counselors specializing in infertility and related areas often see people in groups, instead of or in addition to individual and couples' counseling. Meeting with others going through the same or a very similar experience as you are can be immensely reassuring. Groups can offer you camaraderie, companionship, shared humor, compassion and, often, valuable information. It is not at all uncommon for a group to continue to meet long after its stated "end point." People stay in touch when they have children and often groups evolve into parents' groups and perhaps, beyond that, into general women's or couples' groups.

Groups can be especially helpful to people considering or pursuing egg donation and for those who are already parents through this process. Unlike adoptive parents, who may easily locate one another, either because they adopted transracially or because they met at an adoption agency or adoption organization, parents through egg donation have no easy ways of finding one another. Joining a support group that introduces you to others who are parents through egg donation—or intended parents—will not only diminish your isolation. It will also provide you with valuable information as people will share their experiences with different medical and egg donation programs, as well as their experiences talking with others and with their children about egg donation.

Locating a Mental Health Counselor

Whether you decide to seek individual, couples or group counseling—or some combination—it is essential that you meet with someone knowledgeable about egg donation. Counselors specializing in this area can be located through RESOLVE, AFA, INCIID, IAAC, ASRM or through your medical program. Another route, although one that is probably less reliable, is to call your medical insurer and ask if there are people on their provider's panel who specialize in this area.

It is important that you feel comfortable with your counselor. You should experience her (or him) as warm, supportive, understanding and helpful. He or she should be someone you look forward to seeing, who provides you with a "safe haven" in which to express your fears, feelings, hopes and dreams.

As stated earlier, we are using the word *counseling* and not *psychotherapy* intentionally. In most instances, what you will be doing with a counselor will have very little to do with the distant past. Surely there are instances in which infertility resonates with someone's early life experiences and there may be a benefit in psychotherapy, but, for the most part, we are suggesting a present- and future-oriented counseling that, in many ways, resembles coaching. In fact, I (Ellen) often identify myself as a *fertility coach* as do some of my colleagues.

When Counseling Is Mandated

Although many people seek help from a counselor while they are in the throes of infertility treatment, or, perhaps, following a miscarriage, there are some who do not. If you are someone who feels "I can handle things on my own" or who is otherwise disinclined to use counseling or psychotherapy, you may be surprised when your medical program instructs you to see someone. You may even be a bit put off or offended, wondering if your physician or nurse is somehow questioning your stability.

So why does a medical program require someone to see a counselor? Sometimes this occurs because a patient lets the medical staff know that they are having a hard time. Perhaps you are calling the nurses frequently and expressing a great deal of anxiety? Possibly you are telling them of stress in your marriage or with your family or your job? Contacts like these may prompt staff to suggest to you that you talk with a counselor. Occasionally, people's upset or anxiety is so pronounced that staff require them to seek counseling before moving forward with treatment.

In most instances, a recommendation of counseling is not a commentary on your stability. Many programs require everyone going through assisted reproduction to have at least one meeting with a counselor. Counseling is most often mandated because you are undergoing a particular form of treatment. Many centers require that all IVF couples have one visit with a counselor either before or after the first cycle. More centers require counseling for third party reproduction. Even those programs which do not make pre-IVF counseling mandatory do, most often, require egg donor couples to have a counseling visit. And in instances of known donation—a family member or friend—there will probably be a series of required visits.

We know that most people don't like to be told what to do and that being instructed to see a counselor can feel paternalistic or judgmental. I (Ellen) can only say that there have been countless times when people sent to me have ended the session by saying, "I'm so glad we were required to do this. It was so helpful" or "I wish I had spoken with you earlier in this process." My sense is that many people are relieved to talk with someone who is very familiar with what they are going through, has information to provide, and understands things from an emotional perspective. It can also be reassuring to have someone you can call in the future, should you have questions or concerns that could be addressed in counseling.

The sequence and format of this counseling will vary, but the following are issues that should be addressed in counseling before you enter an egg donor cycle.

Volunteer Donors

Couples working with a family member or friend will be asked to participate in a series of meetings. The first meeting may be with the donor alone, it may be with the intended parents alone, or it may include both donor and recipients. Some counselors prefer to meet with the prospective donor first so they can help her make the best decision for herself. This may include helping give her "an out" if donation is not right for her at this time. Counselors who see the donor first feel this helps them as counselors to avoid feeling any obligation to the recipients. Other counselors prefer to meet with the recipients first in order to have some sense of history and a perspective on how this came about. These counselors feel they can remain open to helping a donor say no, if she feels she wants or needs to do so.

Regardless of who is seen first, the role of the counselor in meeting with recipients and with their volunteer donors is to try to confirm that everyone is entering into this with optimism and shared expectations. If the counselor senses that any participant (and this could be the donor's husband/partner) is uncomfortable with the endeavor, it is the counselor's responsibility to help the uneasy participant out of their dilemma. This assistance may take the form of additional counseling—to help participants either feel more comfortable with their decision or to make an alternative plan.

Regardless of whether you are moving forward with your volunteer donor or moving on to some other option, there should be at least one visit that includes both couples (assuming the donor has a partner). Either this visit will review why things are not proceeding as expected, or, more likely, it will be an opportunity to solidify your plans together. Assuming the latter, the visit will be a time during which participants can discuss their expectations for their relationships in the future and, specifically, their relationships with regards to the child or children that may result from the donation. It will also be important to talk about the possibility of disappointment—donors and recipients may do their best and still not achieve a successful pregnancy.

A conjoint meeting with a counselor will also provide everyone with a foundation for counseling in the future should any or all of you need to talk again. Something could come up either during a cycle, during a pregnancy or after the birth of a child that you will want to discuss with someone who knows the history of the donation.

Program-recruited Donors

If you are working with a program-recruited donor and have no plans to meet her, you may be asked to have only one session with a counselor. This session can assist you in donor selection, or it can focus on your feelings about the donor you have chosen. The session can address any couples' issues that might get in the way during a cycle, during pregnancy or later. You can also use the time to talk about privacy and secrecy as they relate to egg donation and you may want to explore the possibility of meeting your donor, if not before the cycle then during pregnancy.

If you plan to meet your donor, the counseling session can help you plan for and anticipate this meeting. The counselor can assist you in deciding whether you want to meet your donor prior to a cycle or only after a pregnancy test has been confirmed. She can serve as a sounding board if you are still struggling with uncertainty about which donor to pick and can help you as you grapple with the reality that there is no absolute "right" or "wrong" donor. You will be drawn to one woman for a particular reason and to another, for another. What matters is that you settle on a donor, feel good about your decision and feel optimistic as you move forward.

Because medical programs and donor agencies may have different arrangements with counselors, the counselor you meet with in advance of your donor-recipient meeting may not be the person who participates in the actual meeting. If this is the case, you should at least meet the counselor in advance. This will give you the chance to let him/her know what you hope will happen in the meeting and allow you to raise any fears or concerns. It will also give the counselor an opportunity to make some suggestions, such as encouraging you to bring photos and/or a small gift to the meeting. When all of you do get together, the counselor's role is usually just to "be there," listening attentively and prepared to "jump in" if there are some awkward moments. A skilled counselor can also contribute to the celebratory and ceremonial aspect of the meeting: it is a momentous time when people come together in the hopes of bringing a new life into the world. The counselor can honor and commemorate that time by taking a photo of the two/three of you together and, possibly, by recording a few words about the meeting.

Lawyers

In egg donation, as in many areas of life involving legal relationships, lawyers have two types of roles: one is to try to prevent problems, and the second is to step in when problems arise. Hopefully, your need for a lawyer familiar with egg donation will be limited to the first role, but we will provide you with information about the second as well.

We are grateful to attorneys Susan Crockin, Robert Nichols and Mark Johnson for helping us to introduce legal issues. Crockin is an attorney practicing reproductive law in Newton, Massachusetts and is the author of countless articles on reproductive law. She is the editor of *Adoption and Reproductive Law in Massachusetts* and co-author, with Machelle Seibel, of *Family Building through Egg and Sperm Donation*. Nichols is an attorney practicing reproductive law in Norwood, Massachusetts. Mark Johnson is an attorney practicing reproductive law in Atlanta, Georgia. Crockin, Nichols and Johnson have all had extensive experience with the legal issues involved in egg donation.

A Legal Overview

Internationally, egg donation is governed by a variety of laws, ranging from those in Italy, which bans all forms of egg donation, to those in

Canada, which prohibits payment to egg donors. In the U.S. the right to procreate is one of the central rights protected by the U.S. Constitution, as a recognized part of the right to privacy. These constitutional protections extend to both individuals and couples seeking to become parents through third party reproduction.

Marriage, divorce, child custody and adoption have traditionally been the domain of individual states, all of which have statutes regulating each of these areas. In addition, thirty states have their own laws regarding sperm donation and, as of this writing, five states (Florida, North Dakota, Oklahoma, Texas and Virginia), have laws concerning egg donation. There are no statutes preventing people from participating in ovum and embryo donation, but there are laws that prohibit and criminalize payment for human organs, tissues or babies. Since states vary in their definitions of *organ* and *tissue* and in the activities they permit and restrict, paid oocyte donation could, in some instances, be deemed illegal.

Court rulings in adoption, surrogacy and sperm donor cases may also have relevance to egg donation. Laws in the United States and worldwide applying to egg donation and other areas of human reproduction are ever unfolding, and lawyers with practices in reproductive law must pay keen attention to them.

Do I Need an Attorney?

To avoid legal conflicts related to oocyte donation, it is essential that all participants in the process seek legal counsel. By *all participants* we mean not only the donors and recipients but also their medical and donor egg programs.

While an attorney is not "required," the procedure is one of the more important undertakings a couple would ever consider. "You should be aware that there are considerable risks in egg donation. Disease, genetic disclosure, informed consent of medical risk and maternity determination are but a few," explains Mark Johnson. "Another important consideration is to assure that the egg donor is in no way exploited. A bankruptcy judge was asked if debtors could represent themselves in a bankruptcy. He replied that it was possible, but so is whitewater kayaking, blindfolded." In other words, while you do not legally need an attorney, it is wise for both donors and recipients to consult one.

Egg donor arrangements do not require either court involvement or a formal adoption. However, few states have statutes specifically dealing with ovum donor arrangements. Some of the most favorable in the nation are in Texas. Those statutes allow the transfer to the wife of an infertile couple either a donated egg (fertilized by her husband's sperm) or an embryo (no biological connection to the infertile couple). Any resulting child is then treated as the child of the infertile couple without the necessity of an adoption or other court involvement. While courts in other states may rule similarly in cases which come suit, few states have enacted such laws.

An attorney cannot represent both sides in any transaction, and egg and embryo donation is no different. Therefore, independent counsel should see all donors and recipients before entering into any donor agreement. In addition, all parties should consent in writing to the arrangement.

How Do I Find a Lawyer?

To identify an attorney with expertise in reproductive law, you should contact your local RESOLVE chapter, AFA, IAAC, or ASRM. And since many lawyers specializing in reproductive law come to this area with a background in adoption law, the American Academy of Adoption Attorneys may also provide you with a good referral. In addition, you can ask your physician to recommend a lawyer.

What Will a Lawyer Do?

Lawyers advise that recipient couples and their donors—whether known or anonymous—enter into a legal agreement regarding all aspects of the donation. The intended parents should be represented by one lawyer and the donor, by her own independent attorney. These contracts, which may or may not be legally binding, depending upon the state, will address a range of matters including clearly defining the child's parentage, identifying the specific medical procedures to be undertaken, acknowledging the risks involved, making a genetic disclaimer, and specifying plans for disposition of "extra" embryos. The contract should also detail when the eggs cease to "belong" to the donor and who controls the disposition of frozen embryos now and in the future.

Another goal of the ovum donation agreement is to establish the parties' intent that the resulting child or children will be the legal children of the biological father and the intended mother. The agreement will establish that the donor is relinquishing all parental rights for any child who is conceived through the donated eggs.

The written egg donation agreement should provide protection to all parties against claims brought by the other party for complications resulting from the ovum donation procedure. Risks should be identified and allocated fairly. Ideally, insurance is available and purchased by the recipients for any medical complications. For example, the donor could claim damages for illness or injury during the donor cycle or even for emotional harm following donation. Similarly, without a written agreement concerning these issues, the intended parents could claim damages for complications during pregnancy or for genetic or congenital defects in the child.

In addition to providing certain safeguards, lawyers note that the process of negotiating a formal written agreement often serves to raise issues that the participants may not have fully considered. It is preferable for these issues to arise prior to the egg donation process rather than during a cycle, or worse still, during a pregnancy. If the participants cannot reach agreement on any sticking points, it usually makes sense for the intended parents to seek a new donor (or vice versa).

Formal oocyte donation agreements are advised regardless of whether the donor is known or anonymous. Lawyers assure clients that the agreement can be done while maintaining complete anonymity between the parties. Each party signs one copy of the agreement and the attorneys each retain a complete set.

Lawyers advise medical and donor egg programs to prepare their consent forms and other documents with the guidance of a lawyer who practices reproductive law. Consent forms must specify who makes decisions about eggs and embryos, medical risks and matters of privacy and confidentiality.

What Should Be Included in a Contract?

Contracts between ovum donors and their recipients must cover a range of issues that include who "owns" the eggs, establishment of maternity, who will pay the various medical and legal costs, at what point their ownership is transferred, and what will be the disposition of cryopreserved embryos. Attorney Mark Johnson provides us with the following outline of the central features of an egg donation contract.

- Identification of the Parties Involved—It is important to clearly identify each of the participants by role. For example, a contract may say, the "mother/recipient" and then explain she is "the woman who shall carry the child and ultimately be deemed it's 'mother.' "

- Establishment of Maternity and Paternity—The contract should clearly establish who will be the parents of the child, spelling out that it is the mother/recipient and her husband (in the case of married, heterosexual couples) who will be the child's parents.

- Relinquishment of the Donor's Possible Rights—Since in most instances it is the genetic mother and father of a child who have parental rights and this is not the case in egg donation, the contract should include a relinquishment of the donor's rights.

- Establishment of Procedures to be Undertaken—The contract should outline the medical procedures that will be involved in oocyte donation, including ovulation induction, egg retrieval and embryo transfer.

- Informed Consent—The contract should identify the short and long term medical and psychological risks associated with egg donation for all participants.

- Genetic Disclaimer—The contract should indicate that certain diseases or conditions may be known to exist in the donor's family, or may be found within certain populations or ethnic groupings. These conditions should be divulged and the risks assumed by the recipient couple. In order to assist the attending physicians of the child or children to be born, medical and genetic history of donor and donor's relatives should be provided from the ovum donor.

- Embryo Storage—The contract should specify whether embryos will be cryopreserved and if so, where they will be stored, at what cost and to whom and for what duration. It should also confirm that the cryopreserved embryos are available to the recipients for future pregnancies.

- Embryo Disposition—The contract should address the intended parent's plans for the disposition of extra cryopreserved embryos. Since many intended parents may not be able to predict their feelings in the future, all options available to them should be listed as possibilities: donation to another couple (if the egg donor has consented to this), degeneration or donation for scientific research.

- Costs—The contract should identify the costs involved in egg donation, including the fee provided to the donor as well as any costs for medical insurance for the donor and of embryo cryopreservation and storage. In addition, the contract should clearly address who will be responsible for these costs. In almost all cases, the recipient is completely responsible for all costs associated with the ovum donation process, including those pertaining to the donor.

Specific Legal Questions to Be Addressed in Contracts between Donors and Recipients and in Program Consent Forms and Contracts

Payment for Time and Effort, not Eggs

To ensure that egg donation is never identified as the "buying and selling of eggs," Attorney Crockin recommends that "payments to donors be clearly structured to reflect the expense, inconvenience, time involved and, according to ASRM guidelines, 'to some degree' the risk and discomfort undertaken. Payments are typically structured over the course of a donor's efforts, with payment at the end of those efforts." (ASRM Guidelines for Gamete Donation, 1993).

Can a Donor Gain Parental Rights?

Prior to July 7, 2004, there was no case on record of an ovum donor seeking custody of a child or children created from her eggs. However, in the "brave new world," the following was reported (www. post-gazette.com, July 18, 2004).

> A 62-year-old man, James Flynn of Cleveland, Ohio, and his 60-year-old fiancé, Eileen Donich, sought parenthood through an egg donor and a gestational carrier. Following the birth of triplets, the gestational carrier, Danielle Bimber and the egg donor, identified as "J.R." both sought custody of the children. Bimber argued that she was the one who has provided the most care for the children, gestating and delivering them, and then, when Flynn failed to produce legal documents to secure custody, Bimber cared for the infants for eight months. Meanwhile, "J.R.", the egg donor, who is reportedly a college student, filed for custody. According to Attorney Steve Litz, the director of Surrogate Mothers, Inc, J.R. is involved in a scam with Flynn. Litz claims that J.R. does not want to raise the children, but is cooperating with Flynn.

Aside from this case, which illustrates, in so many ways, the grave need for regulation in egg donation, there have been no reported cases in which an egg donor, either known or anonymous, has sought parental rights or responsibilities following egg donation. The eight states with statutes regarding ovum donation all relieve the egg donor from all parental rights and responsibilities and specifically transfer them to the intended mother. Attorney Crockin advises us to look to the history of sperm donation for further guidance and to predict legal developments in this area.

Although the statutes in the thirty states that have regulated sperm donation vary in many ways, all presume that a child born to a married couple is the child of that couple. According to Crockin, "These laws should, in most states and situations, protect a child and its presumed parents from a sperm donor later attempting to assert parental rights to a child born from his genetic material." However, Crockin goes on to say that there have been no reported cases of a previously anonymous sperm donor asserting parental rights and "only a few cases in which a known sperm donor has challenged his status and asserted a claim for paternity." In fact, the many lawsuits that have involved children born through sperm donation have involved efforts on the part of the legal father to avoid child support. Crockin notes that these have been uniformly rejected by the courts.

Susan Crockin tells us that things have been somewhat different with some of the known sperm donors. She recounts a small number of cases, including two involving lesbian couples whose known donors argued that they had intended to have a role in the child's life. In the earlier of the two cases, although his paternity suit was initially denied, an appeals court granted the donor parental rights because it noted that the three adults had never recorded their understanding in a written memorandum. More recently, in a similar factual situation in Florida, the courts ultimately denied the donors paternal status.

On May 14, 2004 an appeals court in Seattle (*Seattle Times*, May 13, 2004) ruled that a sperm donor did do not have any rights and responsibilities of fatherhood when he did not sign a consent as required by that state. The case involved Michael Kepl, a man who agreed to give his long-term girlfriend, Teresa Brock, a sperm donation through a University of Washington Fertility clinic. Kepl was married and shielded the affair from his wife. Brock gave birth to a son in 1998 and Kepl paid monthly unofficial child support, took out a life insurance policy benefiting the baby, and signed a sworn statement of paternity. But the couple did not sign a legally recognized consent from stating that Kepl accepted legal responsibility for the child. The affair crumbled in 2001, Brock went on to have a second child with Kepl's sperm and the two ended up in court. The trial court focused on the consensual nature of the affair and dismissed Kepl's argument that he was only a sperm donor and that Washington state law shields sperm donors from the legal duty of fatherhood, except when couples sign a specific agreement at the time of insemination. However, the Appeals Court reversed the trial court decision and said that sperm donors can't be forced to accept the rights and responsibilities of parenthood without complying with the statute.

The case may be very significant because it can shield women from donors who later want to intervene in their child's life and it protects sperm (and presumably ovum) donors. According to Lisa Stone, executive director of the Northwest Women's Law Center, "If you provide sperm, you're not the father unless there's a separate piece of paper that says this person will be the father and donor."

The well known California case of Johnson v. Calvert,(19 Cal Rptr2d 494 [5.Cal 4th 84] 1993) in which a gestational carrier sought recognition as the "mother" of a child she carried for a couple, sheds light on the ways that courts might respond to an egg donor attempting to claim parental rights. The California Supreme Court ruled that "she who intended to procreate the child—that is, she who intended to bring about the birth of a child she intended to raise as her own—is the natural mother under California law." Crockin comments that this reasoning—one that focuses on the intention to parent rather than on genetics, "may extend to egg donor situations as well." She adds "the difference between egg donation and sperm donation may enhance the intended mother's rights over that of her male counterpart. Unlike a man, a woman can be biological parents in two ways: she can gestate the child or provide genetic material for it. Arguably, an egg recipient, because she both gestates and intends to parent the child, is in a stronger legal position than the husband of a sperm recipient, who would be biologically limited to solely an intended parent role."

Although it is highly unlikely that a donor would ever seek parental rights, let alone be granted them, it is important that the legal contract with your donor clearly state your intent to parent the child that results from ovum donation and the donor's clear intent never to seek parental rights.

How Should Donors Be Legally Protected?

Just as you need to know that your donor will never seek parental rights, so also does she need to know that she will never be held liable for child support or any other maternal obligations to a child born through egg donation. Susan Crockin recommends that recipient couples agree in writing not to seek such support and "to indemnify a donor if the state were to seek such support." In addition, she notes that donors and recipients "can specifically name their beneficiaries in their wills in addition to any general class description (such as 'my children') to avoid any unintended inclusion or exclusion of a child."

The donor needs to be protected in other ways as well. It needs to be made clear precisely when she is donating her eggs and to whom. Even with anonymous donation, you can be designated as the sole recipients of her donation. She has a right to be reassured that you will not pass her ova on to another couple either in the form of oocyte or as embryos.

You will want to know that your donor is also protected financially should she have complications from the procedure that require additional medical treatment. Susan Crockin reports that there is one reported case of a donor insisting a program cover the cost of a complication, despite the fact that she had insurance, as she was concerned about her future insurability. She adds that specialized donor insurance may be available and is helpful in addressing these risks.

Legal Work in Response to Problems

What Happens in the Event of Divorce? Are There Special Custody Issues Related to Egg Donation?

Two reported cases regarding egg donation involved divorcing couples. Crockin reports that in a New York case, MacDonald v MacDonald, [MacDonald v MacDonald, 1996 AD2d 7, 608 NYS2d 477 (1994)] a husband attempted to gain custody of twins because he was "the only genetic and natural parent available to them." His claim was rejected because the court found "that the couple's intention to jointly have and rear offspring made the recipient woman the 'natural mother of the children'". She was granted temporary custody. In the second case of an Ohio couple, Ezzone v. Ezzone, a divorcing father claimed that since his wife's sister donated the ova, the wife was not the natural mother of her children. The court ruled against the husband, "analogizing his situation to sperm donation and finding an even stronger connection for a woman because she gestates the donated gamete." Crockin goes on to say that the court concluded that to treat a woman differently than a man who used donor gametes "would violate both state and federal equal protection laws."

On June 12, 2004, *New York Times* writer Leslie Eaton told the bizarre story of Zack Hampton Bacon III, 51, and Diandra Douglas, 48, an unmarried couple who sought to have children through a gestational carrier and egg donor (the article does not acknowledge the ovum donation but we can only assume given Ms. Douglas' age!). The surrogate became pregnant with twin boys and the couple, who had been together since 2000, split up after Ms. Douglas refused to marry Bacon unless he would pay her the hundreds of thousands of dollars she would lose in alimony from her ex-husband. In addition, Ms. Douglas "was unhappy that the babies were both boys, according to Mr. Bacon's court papers," and just prior to the twins' birth, "she announced she was planning to adopt a baby girl from Kazakhstan." When the twins were born three months premature, the couple entered into a coast-to-coast custody battle, with Ms. Douglas arguing to be able to raise the boys in California and Mr. Bacon, in New York.

Although the Douglas-Bacon case has not yet been decided, Eaton's article concludes by saying that if it remains in California, the fact that Ms. Douglas is not the biological or genetic mother of the twins is unlikely to make a difference. She quotes Attorney Leslie Ellen Shear of Encino, who says that California law emphasizes "intent" when deciding who is a legal parent.

When a Partner Dies

What happens if a couple has frozen embryos following infertility treatment and one of the biological parents dies? In general, decisions concerning whether or not to have a child have been considered a private matter and a fundamental right of individual adults, but there is limited precedent on how this might be expressed or respected after one's death. According to the ASRM's Policy on Posthumous Reproduction, if an individual designates the use of stored frozen gametes or embryos that can be used for posthumous pregnancy, either for the use of a spouse or as a donation to others, it would seem to be totally appropriate to honor this designation after their death in the absence of any adverse consequences to the living participants in the pregnancy or any expected children. The gestating woman and/or the rearing parent(s) must be fully informed and in agreement with the process.

Many programs for assisted reproduction have consent forms that stipulate the disposition of gametes and embryos, including disposition after death of one or both gamete donors or after a certain period of time. If donation after death is declined, this should be honored. Whether a time limit should be put on how long after death such gametes or embryos might still be used is problematic. It is not clear how the interval between death and use would affect the process and the outcome, but the general presumption is that such use should occur within an interval of no more than a few years.

Programs are urged to insist that donors make their wishes known. If no decision on disposition after death has been made, one would expect that in most instances this would preclude any posthumous use. The ASRM cautions, however, that if both partners die, there is less certainty of the impact on the child. More caution should be exercised for posthumous reproduction that occurs with the use of donated gametes from unrelated individuals who are not living and may have been deceased for several years, as may occur with the use of commercial banks as a source for sperm, frozen embryos, or ova. There is little legal precedent for this occurring, however.

What If Our Insurance Won't Pay for Egg Donation?

As we have noted throughout this book, a relatively small number of states (fifteen as of this writing) have laws mandating insurance coverage for fertility treatment. The specific treatments that insurance companies are required to cover also vary widely from state to state. In most instances, insurance companies are authorized to adopt reasonable guidelines to define what will be covered and what will be excluded. Accordingly, coverage for particular procedures can vary substantially from company to company. Attorney Robert Nichols urges his clients to talk with an infertility specialist at their insurance company.

Nichols reports, "Very often, company representatives who are assigned to answer general calls do not have the experience to answer very specific questions regarding infertility. In addition, you should ask to see written language in the policy or in on the company's website to back up any answers given by your insurance company representative. In most cases, you may not know whether you actually will receive coverage for a donor ovum cycle or any other type of infertility treatment until your doctor submits a formal request for insurance approval. Those requests almost always require a certain level of testing to prove that you are eligible for the coverage. For example, in Massachusetts, there are currently two main reasons why people get denied insurance coverage for a donor egg cycle. 1) Prior miscarriage and 2) elevated FSH levels after a certain age. The prior miscarriage denial is based on the definition of infertility in the Massachusetts mandate since it defines infertility as the inability to conceive or maintain a pregnancy within a one year period and therefore does not meet the definition of infertility. The second issue is an attempt by the insurance companies to define the difference between a woman who is medically infertile and a woman who is menopausal. If the insurance company can say that a woman is menopausal, that is a naturally occurring event and not a medical condition and therefore, there is no coverage. Many insurance companies have used FSH and age (usually somewhere between 40 and 46) to determine whether there should be coverage. Every insurance company has detailed guidelines as to where they will draw the line. If you do not meet these guidelines, you will most likely be denied. Once denied, you have the right to appeal to a review board within the insurance company to overturn the decision. If you are not successful at that level, most policies provide for an external review either through a state agency or an independent review agency under federal law. Chance of success on appeal is very much tied to the specific facts of your case. You may be able to pursue the appeal successfully on your own with the help of your physician or you may consider working with an attorney experienced in insurance appeals regarding infertility."

Even in states with mandates, there are insurance carriers that do not offer coverage for fertility treatment. Under the federal Employee Retirement Income Security Act of 1974 (ERISA), self insured health plans are exempt from state regulation. In addition, state law may also may exempt certain employers based on size or some other feature.

Attorney Susan Crockin comments that the Americans with Disabilities Act (ADA), the Civil Rights Act of 1964 and the Pregnancy Discrimination Act of 1978 may all offer patients some potential federal statutory protection in their quest for parenthood. Crockin adds that in the 1998 case, Bragdon v. Abbott, the U.S. Supreme Court held "that reproduction constitutes a major life activity under the ADA." (Bragdon v. Abbott, 524. U.S. 624, 118 S. Ct. 2196 [1998]). This case involved an HIV positive woman who alleged discrimination in the denial of dental care. The Court reportedly found HIV to be a "disability" that substantially limited a major life activity, reproduction. Crockin observes that even though this decision did not directly involve infertility or insurance coverage, "it may be argued to apply in the context of employer-sponsored health insurance discrimination against those with infertility."

Crockin adds that people denied access to infertility treatment can also seek protection under Title VII of the Civil Rights Act of 1964 and the Pregnancy Discrimination Act. The Civil Rights Act prohibits "employment practices that discriminate against an individual with respect to his compensation, terms, conditions, or privileges of employment because of such individual's race, color, religion, sex or national origin." (Saks v. Franklin Covey Co. 3`5 F 3d 337 [2nd Cir. 2003]), This prohibition includes discrimination in providing health insurance and benefits. Crockin explains that the Civil Rights Act was amended by the Pregnancy Discrimination Act (PDA) in 1978, an act that forbids discrimination based on "pregnancy, childbirth or related medical conditions." However, she adds that some courts have included infertility in the protections of the PDA and others have not.

What Happens If the Medical Program Makes a Mistake, such as Transferring the Wrong Embryos or Giving Eggs to the Wrong Recipient?

Although our hope, in writing this chapter, is that you and your medical program will always be on the same side of the law, there have been instances when this has not been the case. Specifically, physicians have been accused of mishandling gametes and embryos in their care. In one well publicized instance, physicians at the University of California at Irvine were accused of having mishandled hundreds of gametes, creating embryos without the knowledge or consent of the gamete providers. (Stone V Regents of Univ. of Cal. 77 Cal. App. 4th 736, 92 Cal. Rptr. 2nd 94 [1999]). According to Attorney Crockin, the University agreed to pay claimants nearly $17 million to settle claims and at least six children were reportedly born to couples from "erroneously-created or mistransferred embryos, using gametes from patients who allegedly never consented to their 'donation' to another couple."

Another embryo mix-up occurred in the twin pregnancy of Donna Fasano, who learned that a vial of embryos from the Rogers family had been transferred to her along with her own embryos. The amniocentesis revealed that one of the fetuses was genetically related to the Fasanos, but the other was the Rogers' biological child. The Fasanos initially attempted to parent both children. Following birth, the Rogerses filed suit and successfully obtained legal and physical custody of that child (Perry-Rogers v. Fasano, 276 A.D. 2d 67 [NY 2000]). In addition, each family sued their doctors and the laboratory for mixing the embryos (Fasano v. Nash, 723. N.Y. S 2d. 181 [App. Div. 2001]) and additional suits for negligence and medical malpractice.

In addition to illustrating the legal responsibility that medical programs and their laboratories have to ensure that their patients receive only those gametes and embryos that are theirs, either through biology or donation, the case is also significant for that fact that the court overturned the common law presumption of maternity for Ms. Fasano and gave custody to the genetic parents. It illustrates how critical it is that intent be clear in gamete donation so that no donor can ever claim to have donated "unintentionally."

Another widely publicized case involved a sperm bank that allegedly failed to inform recipient couples that a donor had disclosed a family history of kidney disease (Johnson v. Sup. Ct. of LA, 101 Cal. App 4th 869 [2002]). A family whose child through sperm donation had kidney disease brought suit against the sperm bank and their physicians. The California appellate court found in favor in the sperm bank and physicians, stating they did not cause the child's genetic abnormality. Similarly, the Utah Supreme Court rejected a case in which a couple who had healthy triplets sued the sperm bank for "negligent infliction of emotional distress" by inseminating the wife with the wrong donor sperm. The parents alleged that they selected a particular donor based on his blood type and hair color, but after birth the children were found to have a different blood type and physical appearance.

Again, we hope that you and your medical providers will always be on the same side of the law. These cases of clinic mistakes and of disappointed parents are included not as cautionary tales but rather, to illustrate just how careful medical and donor egg programs must be. When you are asked to sign lengthy and complex consent forms you will have some idea how and why they came to be.

How Do I Find Out about Reproductive Laws in My State?

Only eight states have a law covering ovum donation. As the law stands now, many state laws determine that a woman who gives birth to a child is his/her parent. To find out about your state, you can do an Internet search, or contact your State Bar Association. However, we recommend talking with an attorney practicing reproductive law. Yes, it is expensive, but this surely seems like one of those times when it is better to be safe than sorry.

Legal Reform

Some patients and physicians are concerned that there will be state laws created in the future that will be in direct disagreement with contracts drawn up now. Attorney Johnson explains that there are there are generally proscriptions against retroactive or ex post facto applications of law. In other words, the legal agreements you draw up now will most likely stand the test of time regardless of future changes in the law.

And so we see that egg donation presents a range of psychological challenges and legal puzzles. Because this is such a new frontier, so unique and constantly changing, it is important that you find a mental health counselor and a lawyer who devote their practices to assisted reproduction. They need to be able to provide you with expert guidance during some of the key parts of your journey to parenthood through oocyte donation.

Recruited-Donor Programs

It wasn't all that long ago that a couple seeking an ovum donor had limited choices. If you didn't have a family member or friend who was willing to donate, you needed to figure out a way to find a contractual donor. For this, some people turned to advertising—on the internet or in newspapers or magazines—while others waited patiently for medical programs to eventually find them a donor. Everything changed in the late 1990s when a number of oocyte donor programs developed throughout the United States.

As we have mentioned several times throughout this book, egg donation is an unregulated industry. The American Society for Reproductive Medicine publishes guidelines for its members, but they are just that—guidelines. There is no requirements that member physicians and clinics adhere to them. By and large, then, programs are left to set their own standards. The result is a range of programs. Some seem to be ethically driven, striving to provide safe, ethically sound, legally secure services to both donors and recipients and attempting to serve the best interests of children created through egg donation. Sadly, there are other programs which appear to pay less attention to the well being of the participants, and whose practices could be seen as primarily profit driven.

In the United States, programs making available contractual donors come in a variety of sizes, shapes and colors. According to Dr. Andrea Braverman in her article, "Agency vs. Clinic: Choosing the Best Fit," (*Family Building*, Summer 2004) a Google.com search for "egg donor agency" brings about 50,000 links. Braverman reassures her readers that there are not 50,000 programs, but there are a vast number of programs offering egg donation services. These programs are of two types.

There are programs that are part of medical clinics offering egg donation as one element of a much broader medical treatment program.

An ART center may hire an a person to serve as an ovum donor co-ordinator, whose job is to recruit donors for the program. Such programs range in size from the fertility center that brings in a few donors here and there to centers that include large, active donor recruitment programs. Though oocyte donation programs are not regulated by the states, all medical programs are staffed by doctors and nurses, who are accountable to their licensing boards.

There are also a large number of independent donor "agencies." These are businesses which have as their sole purpose recruiting, screening, and counseling donors and then working in collaboration with a medical program, usually one that is in the same geographical area, to make matches between their donors and potential recipients. These businesses are unregulated and unlicensed by any governmental or professional agency. These programs also vary in shape and size, from large ones, working with a few hundred donors and utilizing a web site that is up-dated daily, to small, hands-on matchmaking services, some of which focus on services for specific ethnic or religious groups.

Potential recipients are not limited to agencies and clinics when seeking an ovum donor. They can work independently or with an attorney to find an egg donor on their own, mainly through advertising. This option also has the potential to be costly, relies on the recipient couple's ability to work independently, and leaves them potentially vulnerable, especially if they become emotionally attached to a prospective donor before she is medically and psychologically screened. For these reasons, together with the fact that so many people considering oocyte donation have already traveled such a difficult journey, we prefer to focus on programs—either free standing agencies or clinic based—rather than on more independent routes.

It is beyond the scope and purpose of this book to provide a comprehensive guide to egg donation programs. Things are changing too rapidly in the field and within the programs themselves for us to say whether it is to your advantage to work with a medical program that finds its own donors or to find your donor independently, through an attorney, or through an agency that then works in collaboration with your medical program. Decisions such as this one will be affected not only by changes with the programs, but also by where you live. As of this writing, there appear to be significant geographical differences as to where and how people find their donors. In some cities, most of the medical programs find their own donors, leaving couples little impetus to go outside them, but in other cities it has become common practice for medical programs to rely on patients using donor-recruitment agencies, often local, to find their donors.

What we can offer here that we believe will be of value to you are some general guidelines for selecting a program. Whatever the size, shape and flavor of your program, we suggest that you select one that maintains ethical standards of practice and which operates in an efficient, effective, and responsible way.

Qualities of a Program That Has Ethical Standards of Practice

The Program Truly Cares about Its Donors and Makes Every Effort to Help Them Achieve Informed Consent

You are the prospective recipients, so you will want a program that cares about *you*. You are also the paying clients, so the program should be motivated to tend to *your* needs. We understand your desire to be supported and cared for, and we encourage you to work with a program that approaches you with compassion. Nonetheless, it is important to remember that it is the donors who are more vulnerable. These are healthy women who are being recruited to undergo a medical procedure that carries with it some risks, both psychological and physical. We most respect and appreciate those programs who feel their first responsibility is "to do no harm." For example, Dream Donations of Newton, Massachusetts will not accept college undergraduates as donors. Director Katrina Twomey, RN says, "When young women—under 25—apply to us to be donors, we pay particular attention to their understanding of the egg donation process and encourage them to take a careful look at what they are doing and why they want to do it. We want to make sure that they fully understand the short and long term ramifications of egg donation and that they are not acting impulsively. We also go to some lengths to make sure they understand they can change their minds along the way."

Helping prospective donors achieve informed consent is a challenge and a responsibility for all ovum donor programs. Dr. Elaine Gordon, a psychologist in Santa Monica, California, has interviewed hundreds of prospective donors. She believes that the only donors who can truly give full informed consent are those who are already mothers themselves. Gordon feels that all other donors "are unqualified to give informed consent by their not having experienced pregnancy and birth before. When I am interviewing these women I go to special lengths to do due diligence. I make every effort to encourage a childless woman who is planning to donate to try to anticipate how she will feel when she has children and how she might feel if she is unable to have children in the future." Gordon and others emphasize that good practice means making every effort to encourage a young woman who is planning to donate to try to imagine where she may be in her life 10 or 20 or 30 years hence. It may help to remind her that women seeking donated eggs are often people whose lives unfolded in unexpected ways. Her future, also, may be different than she imagines it.

One tool used in trying to help a prospective donor achieve informed consent is a discussion of "anticipatory regret." The mental health consultant interviewing a prospective donor goes through a number of "what ifs" with her:

- What if you one day have a child and begin to think more about the child that resulted from your donor cycle?

- What if you one day face infertility?

- What if you suffer a pregnancy loss or if you do not marry and decide not to pursue pregnancy as a single woman?

- How might you feel if your mother expresses sadness that she is not a grandmother or if she talks about "her grandchildren" that resulted from ovum donation?

No one expects a young donor to have answers for all of these questions, but rather the hope is that she will "visit" each of them. These "visits" should remain with her in the future and hopefully help her to diminish or eradicate feelings of regret should they begin to arise.

Another issue with informed consent involves comprehending the arduousness of the medical experience. Even donors who are very enthusiastic about donating find the process to be emotionally and physically exhausting (Raoul-Duval, Letur-Konirsch, and Frydman, 1992.) It is the responsibility of the medical programs to review the physical process (including side effects and risks) with donors, but it is crucial as well that the donor program provide counseling that helps prepare donors for the challenges of the procedure.

Judith Bernstein, MSN, (Crockin and Seibel, 1996) recommends engaging prospective donors in a risk-benefit analysis. Bernstein advises that donors also be encouraged to take a close look at the risks. It can be helpful to engage her in a discussion that explores the long term advantages and disadvantages of donating. Bernstein observes that "egg donation can provide beneficence, or benefit, in the form of gratification through altruism, increased self-esteem or fulfillment of a desire to re-work a negative past experience with a better outcome, such as a donor who has had an earlier abortion helping a couple have a child through egg donation." In the face of these potential "abstract and non-essential" rewards, Bernstein advises that donors also be encouraged take a close look at the risks.

The Program Does Not Entice Women to "Sell" Their Eggs

Countries that ban payment for egg donation do not have to worry that women will be drawn to egg donation because they will receive substantial sums of money. However, in the U.S., where there is no regulation of the egg donation industry, there are programs which recruit women with high fees. While some would regard the most common current fee—$5000—as so high as to be enticing, we acknowledge that the egg donation process is time consuming, uncomfortable, intrusive and involves some physical risks, so that $5000 does not seem to be an extraordinarily high figure for all that is involved.

Unfortunately, there are programs which either do not set a standard fee for their donors or perhaps set a fee that is higher than the "going rate" of $5000. Either way, money is likely to play a bigger role in a woman's decision to donate.

The lawyers tell us that fees for ovum donation must be payment for time and effort, not eggs. The mental health professionals remind us that there may be grave consequences to a child who learns his genetic parent "sold her eggs for money," and consequences, down the line, for the woman who essentially "trades oocytes for money." The ethicists join in and say that a childless young woman cannot truly achieve informed consent in egg donation and should not be enticed, in any way, by payment. Nonetheless, there are programs that allow donors to request high fees because they have excellent SAT scores, or are very attractive, are highly athletic, belong to a minority ethnic group, or have exceptional fertility. We feel that once donors can request special fees for special attributes, they are no longer receiving payment for time and effort—they are being paid for eggs.

We are especially troubled, then, by those programs that offer "an elite" or "Ivy League" or "premier" group of donors, since these programs offer some women substantial sums of money. If payment is for time and effort, not eggs, it is hard to explain why women would receive higher fees if they are very pretty or have high SAT scores or have donated successfully or are of a particular ethnicity. We see no justification for higher fees for one donor over another within the same program except in instances where a donor will have to travel a great distance or be otherwise seriously inconvenienced in order to donate

We know that many people wonder why a woman would ever decide to provide her oocytes for a stranger. It is natural to suspect that these program-recruited donors are driven by the payment involved. We know also that these questions and suspicions make it difficult for many prospective recipients to move ahead with program-recruited donation feeling proud and confident about what they are doing. We offer some observations that we hope will reassure you. Contrary to what you might expect, women who become involved in contractual donation are often described as kind, compassionate, capable and emotionally secure women who are determined to help others experience the joy of parenthood.

Chicago social worker Judy Calica, who has interviewed several hundred donors, says of the donors, "They're an extraordinarily impressive group—they are well functioning, capable women who have a strong sense of themselves. I have loved talking with them and have found their desire to help others to be very affirming of the human condition." Calica goes on to say that many prospective donors are women who make volunteering an important part of their sense of self. "These are often former candy-stripers, women who donate blood regularly and who feel that they have some responsibility to make good use of their eggs that would otherwise go to waste."

Ms. Calica has other interesting observations about the women who apply to donate ova. "They range in age from late teens who haven't been to college to a physician in her thirties. I've found that many are fascinated by the science involved. Sometimes I feel that in another life, these women would be our astronauts." Calica adds that many of the women she has interviewed have children, some have completed their families, and there are others who have decided not to become parents but want to pass on a piece of themselves in this world.

Dr. Adele Kauffman, Program Psychologist at the Reproductive Science Center in Lexington, Massachusetts, echoes Ms. Calica's observations and adds, "A large percentage of the donors I have seen come from families where divorce and remarriage have occurred. Many of these women have experienced significant relationships (such as step parents, step siblings, half-siblings) that have not been based on shared genes, but rather on shared experiences." Kauffman continues, "These women have grown up in a technological world, a DNA world. Many feel that it is great that technology is available to make egg donation possible. Often potential donors are mothers themselves and cannot imagine what their lives would be like if they had not been able to have children. Others have known someone who has gone through the pain of infertility."

The Program Is Concerned about the Welfare of the Offspring

Program directors and counselors are not gate-keepers in a position to decide who should and who should not be parents. We imagine that any program that tried to turn people away because they deemed them "unsuitable" to be parents would face a law suit claiming discrimination. However, a lawsuit of this type would probably not be fruitful since there are no national guidelines which clearly determine who can participate in egg donation. Still, we do feel that ovum donor programs have a responsibility to the children they help bring into this world. This responsibility includes making sure that those children will have access to information about their genetic history, including extensive medical information, and, ideally, to information about other children who were conceived with eggs from the same donor.

The Program Avoids Coercive Practices

Although independent egg donor programs generally do not work with infertile women hoping to finance the cost of their own treatment, some medical programs offer "deals" which we regard as extraordinarily coercive: a woman, desperate to be a mom, who is undergoing IVF receives her treatment at a reduced fee—or perhaps, at no cost—if she agrees to relinquish or "donate" extra eggs. What if the recipient becomes pregnant and the donor does not? What if both conceive and the woman, whom we call *the involuntary donor*, finds herself grieving over "a child of mine out there?"

We are told that this practice began at a time when cryopreservation of embryos was not readily available and women undergoing IVF sometimes preferred donating extra ova to discarding them. However, now, with all medical programs offering cryopreservation, there will be only a few women seeking homes for extra eggs. This group will include only those women who oppose both discarding and embryo donation. Should they choose to donate it should not be for a reduced fee nor for any other form of coercion.

There are programs which allow or encourage women to donate to two couples at once. The idea behind this is that fertile young women often produce several eggs. By splitting the "batch" of eggs in two parts, the program can reduce the costs to recipient couples, since each will not have to pay the full donor fee. Because your relationship with your donor is a special one, we cannot support this system. Even if the two of you never meet, you will know that this young woman has chosen to generously give of her time, effort and physical comfort in order to make a difference in your life. To ask her to donate to two women simultaneously and to ask you to participate in such an endeavor, certainly changes the nature of the donor-recipient relationship.

Although we are concerned about the adults involved in ova sharing, our primary reason for opposing this practice is what it means for the children. In addition to making sense of the fact that the donor donated to two women simultaneously (so this child came from an egg that could have easily landed with another couple), the child will face the reality or possibility of having half siblings who are very close to him/her in age.

If a program does practice egg sharing, it should certainly do so in an open manner. Recipients have a right to know when their children have half bio-siblings and if so, whether the families live nearby. In addition, the egg donor program should make sure that recipients receive counseling in advance of the donation regarding the potential long term impact of being part of a shared egg donor cycle. This impact can range from medical implications (if children have siblings and one needs bone marrow or some other medical help from another) to psychological (if one recipient becomes pregnant and another does not, the one that is unsuccessful may live with regret for having participated in a shared cycle or self blame for not having conceived when someone else did).

The Program Supports Contact between Donors and Recipients—When They Want It

We understand that not all donors are open to contact with recipients, nor are all recipients eager to meet their donors. Furthermore, we are not taking a position regarding long term, ongoing, open contact between contractual donors and recipients. We do, however, encourage you to work with a program that recognizes the benefits that can come from meetings between the parties around the time of selection and birth. These are benefits not just for the donors and recipients, but most importantly, for the offspring. It could be reassuring and grounding for your child to know that you met and talked with your donor. You will be able to describe her and to tell your child a little about her family. Perhaps you will be able to take a picture of your donor, or better yet, have a photo of the two of you together.

In terms of benefits to you and your donor, think about how affirming it could be to be able to look each other in the eyes and talk about why each of you has chosen egg donation. Any mystery about motivations will vanish as you speak openly and frankly about what brought you to this point. You will have an opportunity to say thank you and your donor will have the pleasure—first hand—of knowing she is making a real difference in your lives and in your family for generations to come.

Having a connection to the donor as a whole person and a real person appears to serve recipient couples in the future as well as in the weeks and months leading up to donation. Parents and expectant parents who met—or who learned a great deal about their donor—seem to approach parenthood with the confidence that their child is coming from a good place. In addition, they appear to be more comfortable watching the child's identity unfold. One mother through egg donation, who did not want to meet her donor but did so at the donor's insistence, told us, "Thank heaven we met. Now that our son is born, I can't imagine what it would be like to look at him and not have seen her face. I think that I would be spooked by any features that were not my husband's. Meeting her helped me feel whole. It reassured me that three good people were pulling together to bring our child into this world."

We contrast this to the poignant story of a mother who has lovely twin girls whom she adores. However, the twins were recently rejected from a very prestigious private school, an event which devastated their mother. Sadly, she "blames herself" for failing to pick a smarter donor. She is quick to add that in her eyes, her daughters "couldn't be any better," but says that it was her responsibility to "pick good genes." Shelley Smith, LMFT, Director of the Egg Donor Program in Los Angeles, and others shift the focus from "selecting good genes to finding a good person."

Although there was a time when some medical programs had the notion that they were doing both their donors and their recipients a service by keeping them separate, we believe that that time has passed. Professionals involved in oocyte donation have learned from sperm donor offspring, as well as from generations of adoptive families, that "closed" adoption and "closed" sperm donation leave people grappling with long lists of unanswered questions. In recent years, there has been increasing appreciation of the benefits of openness in all forms of third party family building. Nonetheless, there remain programs that encourage closed donation, promoting it under the euphemism of "confidentiality." We strongly suggest avoiding programs that *deny* you the opportunity to meet your donor and worse still, those that communicate a message that donors and recipients should be hidden from each other. In addition to depriving all participants of valuable contact, this approach fuels the feeling that you and your donor are engaging in some sort of shameful activity.

We caution you against working with a program that advises you to have a completely closed relationship with your donor. It may be that this is what your donor wants and requests and you may feel so certain that she is the right donor for you that you may choose to abide by her wishes. However, this is different from working with a program that explicitly says that "confidentiality" —i.e. secrecy—is a good thing. We've said it before and we'll say it yet again, secrecy breeds shame and misunderstanding. Simply think, for a moment, about how different it would feel to respond to a child who asks about the donor with, "She's a really nice person. Her name is Jane. We met and talked about how much Daddy and I wanted a baby. Here's a picture of all of us together" rather than, "We don't know her name. We have some pictures of her and some things she wrote about donating her eggs, but we never met her nor talked with her."

We were especially troubled to hear from one donor egg recipient who is pregnant with twins from a split cycle with a donor who has previously donated four times, all with successful outcomes. This woman, although delighted to be pregnant, is now deeply troubled to feel so in the dark. She has asked her program for some information about the donor and the other recipient families and was told she cannot have it out of respect for others' confidentiality.

The Program Offers Chances, not Promises

The *New York Times* magazine section and airline magazines among others feature an advertisement with the headlines, "Have a baby in a year or your money back." This particular program makes entering into egg donation sound similar to buying a vacuum cleaner. If you are not satisfied, they will offer you a money back guarantee.

Responsible programs make no such offers. They know that ovum donation may or may not work and that indicating otherwise to you is unfair. Their goal is not "to get you pregnant," but to help you bring a child into your family in a loving, proud, confident and secure way. They understand that in some instances, that may mean moving on to an adoption after a few unsuccessful cycles with the donor you really like. Like any good medical practice working with infertile people, they appreciate the fact that there are many kinds of successful outcomes and all do not include pregnancy.

Although egg donation helps create many happy families, much can go wrong. In addition to failed cycles and pregnancy losses, there are problems that arise before a cycle even commences. Work with a program that helps to prepare you for disappointment and that assists you when it happens. Katrina Twomey reports having had would-be do-nors who tested positive for cystic fibrosis, donors who were diagnosed with premature ovarian failure themselves, and donors who realized, perhaps after meeting with the mental health counselor, that donation was not right for them. When this happens, Twomey talks with the couple and explains the situation. She has found that when told in a gentle, compassionate way, recipients can accept and understand what has happened and move on.

Qualities of an Efficient, Effective Program

The Program Has a Track Record of Successful Pregnancy and Birth

Having just said that all good outcomes do not necessarily involve pregnancy, we know that everyone turning to egg donation does seek pregnancy. So you do want to work with a program that offers a number of donors and has a good success rate. Success will depend, in large measure, on the medical programs that the program is either a part of or collaborates with. It will depend also on the donor program's ability to assess donors, not only on the basis of their personalities, character etc., but also on their ability to comply with the medical protocol and to participate responsibly before and during a cycle.

"How do we know how well a program is doing?" you might ask. Unlike traditional IVF programs, which must report their results to the Center for Disease Control, egg donor programs have no reporting responsibility. Nonetheless, responsible programs do keep track of their on- going pregnancies and should be able to tell you what percentage of their recipients succeeded in having a child through ovum donation. In a sense, this information should be more valuable than the information you would get if you were a "regular IVF patient," seeking information about a program's IVF statistics. Since there are many diagnoses that bring people to IVF, an IVF program may have great statistics because it turns away people whose chance of success is small. Donor egg programs tend to be on a more even playing field—most people who come to donor oocyte do so for the same reason: they need eggs.

The Program Is Well Organized, Responsive and Offers Personal Attention

The Internet can provide recipients and donors with a great introduction to a program, as well as to one another. Since egg donation is a complex, deeply personal decision, it may be very comforting to be able to visit a website in the privacy of your own home. There you can familiarize yourself with a program and its donors without feeling that anyone is watching, evaluating or pressuring you. However, the flip side of this is that the internet is impersonal. We believe that, ultimately, people do need human contact when making such a personal decision.

In selecting a program, you should look for one that will offer you personal attention. We don't mean immediate responses to ten phone calls a day, but for a decision as important as this one, you should be able to talk with real people who can answer your questions, provide you with some counsel and refer you to other professionals when appropriate. "Ours will never be a big program," according to one program's director, Katrina Twomey. Twomey goes on to say that if her program grew much larger than it is (it does around 200 matches yearly) they would lose the opportunity to respond promptly and patiently to phone calls and emails from donors, prospective donors, former donors and all recipients. By contrast, Shelley Smith, whose program has a database of over 250 donors at any given time, feels she succeeds at offering personal attention because she is personally involved with all her clients and works closely with her "large, cohesive staff, many of whom were former donors."

The Program Offers Recipients Extensive Information about Donors, and Assists Those Recipients Who Request Help In Making a Decision

Although there was a time when recipients of egg donation received virtually no information about their donor (one woman we spoke with said she was told only that her donor was "American with yellow eyes"), times have changed. Recipients have come to expect extensive information about donors. This information often includes three generations of medical history and three generations of genetic history in the donor's family, her academic background and SAT scores (if available), information from a lengthy questionnaire she completes and from her personal interviews with program staff, and her own and her family's mental health history.

We have found that couples choose donors for a variety of reasons. Most seek a donor based on a physical resemblance, an interest, a personality style, an ethnic heritage, or a combination of these. Some clients are essentially looking for a "stand in" for the intended mom—someone who appears to be like her in some critical way.

All couples cannot afford to seek a donor based on love or chemistry. Shelley Smith reminds us that some of her clients are stressed financially by donor egg costs and need to find a donor who seems to be very fertile. Specifically, Smith recommends that those couples look for someone who has donated before and whose donation helped create a large number of high quality embryos.

Although it happens infrequently, there are couples who select a donor and then it doesn't work out with her for some reason. She may not stimulate well or all may go smoothly but the recipients don't have a successful pregnancy. A very difficult situation that arises occasionally is when a donor becomes pregnant just prior to commencing a cycle.

When couples who have been disappointed seek a second donor, they sometimes approach the process from a different perspective, possibly focusing more on fertility than "chemistry" or with some added emotional distance "because it was too painful to fall in love with one person and have it not work with her."

How much time do you have to decide? Choosing a donor is a big decision and most people don't want to feel terribly rushed or pressured in the process. At the same time, however, programs cannot function smoothly if people put someone "on hold" for more than a few days. Smith observes having a time frame limits people's ability to "obsess."

Yes, this is, in many ways, one of the most significant decisions they will ever make, but what can they learn about someone on day six or seven that they don't already know within hours, if not minutes, of receiving donor profiles?

The Program Carefully Evaluates Its Donors and Values Them for Reasons Other Than Beauty, Brains and Proven Fertility

There will be several steps in screening a potential egg donor. Screening will be both psychological and medical. In most instances, efforts are made to first confirm that a woman is prepared emotionally, socially and logistically for ova donation and only then, to refer her on for medical evaluation.

Although each program has its own way of bringing potential donors into its system, there are some features that many have in common. Often an initial phone call or other early contact is used as a first screening measure and one that can gracefully discourage those women who are likely to be unsuitable for donation. These include women with serious medical or mental health conditions, high body mass index (over 30 is considered high), and troubling psychosocial problems such as a very recent divorce or break-up of a relationship or unemployment.

Screening phone calls are usually followed by a longer assessment. For example, Twomey provides an approximately 45-minute-long telephone orientation for its prospective donors. This call, which the program likes to postpone for a few weeks after the donor's first contact—in order to be sure that she has reflected on this decision—is an opportunity for the program staff to get to know the young woman and for her to get to know the program.

Women who go from this longer assessment to a physician for medical evaluation should do so with full understanding of the risks and side effects of the medications and of the egg retrieval. They need, also, to understand the potential emotional consequences of this decision. Although the prospective donor will later meet with a mental health counselor, during this initial longer assessment, the program wants her to begin to think about such questions as: How she will feel if she is never able to have children of her own, how she anticipates she will feel years from now as she looks back upon this decision, how she might feel when she has her own children, knowing they have a half-biological sibling (or more). In addition, the program should ask prospective donors about significant others in their lives—husbands, boyfriends, parents and siblings—reminding women that they will need the support and understanding of their loved ones if they undertake egg donation.

Early assessment should also confirm that a donor will be able to work with the program she has contacted. First and foremost, the staff and the donor need to like one another. If prospective donors are difficult, unreliable, intentionally misleading in the orientation, it is unlikely things will improve when they become more involved in egg donation. Responsible programs prefer to screen these women out at the start. Also screened out are those who have some condition or life situation which will render them inappropriate for donation. Included in this group are women who may be going through a difficult time in their lives and who are receiving counseling and medication to assist them (such women may donate appropriately at another time). Programs should also make every effort to eliminate those prospective donors who may have donated several times at another program and may be hopping from one place to another in an effort to donate more than the recommended upper limit of five to six donations in a lifetime (see ASRM guidelines).

It is during the assessment period that donors should be introduced to the advantages—primarily for potential offspring—of donors and recipients meeting each other. Prospective donors should then be asked if they are interested in having an in-person meeting and/or a phone conversation with their recipient couple. They learn that this option, which is available to them but usually not required, does not have to include any identifying information. Staff should explain that some donors appreciate being able to meet the recipients, because the meeting offers them the reassurance that their eggs are going to "good people" and it offers them a chance to give the intended parents, and eventually the child, the gift of personal stories and family history. Most of the time donors learn that if they choose to have contact with their recipients, it will be on a first-names-only basis, and the meeting will be facilitated by a mental health professional.

Psychological evaluation with a mental health professional is an in depth process. In their article "Psychological Counseling and Screening for Egg Donation," psychiatrist Mara Brill and social worker Susan Levin provide the following list of essential components of the psychological evaluation:

- Demographic information
- Motivation for egg donation
- Current level of functioning
- Mental health status including competence and intellectual ability to understand procedures and possible risks
  - Past adaptation to developmental stages
  - History of alcohol or drug abuse
  - Psychiatric history
  - Previous trauma (e.g. sexual abuse, rate, early parental losses and adaptation to them
- Previous pregnancies and outcomes, as well as adaptation to pregnancy losses
- Family history, including alcohol or drug abuse, medical or psychiatric history
- History of how she has dealt with previous major decisions
- Time and availability for the cycle
- Ability to follow through on major life decisions
- Attitude towards medications, medical procedures and recuperative phase
- Support systems and who knows of the decision to become an egg donor
- Ability to think about the impact of the donation on herself, her spouse and her children in the future

Psychologist Kauffman adds, "I am interested in why the donor wants to donate. Is there financial coercion? If a donor is in a desperate financial situation, her judgment may be compromised. I want to engage the potential donor in a discussion of what it means to give someone your eggs. What does it mean to her to have a genetic connection to another person? Can she live with the unknowns that an anonymous donation entails? It is important to explore how she may feel at different points in the future. In five years, ten years, when she starts her own family, etc. What if she finds herself having difficulty conceiving when she is ready? I wonder with them whether they can 'let go.' Will curiosity or worry about the child created from the donation intrude in their lives later on?"

At some point in the evaluation process, donors should be asked to undergo psychological testing. Programs use different psychological tools, the most common being the Minnesota Multiphasic Personality Inventory 2 (MMPI-2). This widely respected psychological assessment tool is employed for two reasons—to help the program screen out women with serious psychological problems and to better familiarize the caregivers with the prospective donor's personality, psychological strengths and weaknesses.

The MMPI-2 is always evaluated by an experienced psychologist, who can identify women who are trying too hard to look good, as well as women who suffer from serious psychopathology such as schizophrenia, bipolar illness or a personality disorder. Occasionally, women who appear to be trying too hard will be asked to re-take the test and to answer more spontaneously and with more candor.

The information provided by the MMPI-2 is only a small part of the psychological assessment of prospective donors. A mental health clinician should meet with the donor and attempt to confirm that the woman has given careful consideration to ovum donation, is not likely to regret this decision, and has done all that she can to achieve the goal of informed consent. The psychologist/social worker/psychiatrist will explore the donor's motivation for donating as well as any issues in her current life or in her past that might make donation inadvisable or in-advisable at this time. The mental health professional will talk with the donor about her experience with or plans for motherhood and about the fact that any child that results from this donation will be the half biological sibling of the donor's children. The clinician will remind the donor that her children may have feelings about having half bio siblings "out there," especially with regards to medical issues and to dating and marriage.

Psychological assessment of the donor also includes looking at her general mental health. In addition to trying to confirm that egg donation is right for her at this point in her life, the clinician tries to determine whether this is a woman who is prone to depression or anxiety, both of which can be genetically transmitted. Does she have a history of serious mental illness such as serious depression or anxiety which may be genetically transferred? By doing a comprehensive psychological evaluation, the mental health clinician is attempting to protect several people: the donor from doing something she is not truly prepared to do, the recipients from passing on "bad genes," and potential offspring from being created for parents who are not really prepared to parent them.

Ironically, the women whom physicians consider ideal donors are not the ones that we consider optimal. From our vantage point, an ideal donor is a woman in her late 20s or early 30s, who has (hopefully) completed her family and who wants to donate eggs because she wants to help someone. Her youth and the fact that she has had a child or children in recent years suggest that her eggs are still good. Often she is someone who has seen friends or family members struggle with infertility and she wants to help others in similar straits. Perhaps she, herself, had a miscarriage or some difficulties conceiving. To this donor, payment is incidental to the donation. She may put the money to some good use, but it is not what brings her to donation. Our ideal donor is prepared to meet the recipients, plans to donate to only one family and will keep the donor program up-to-date on her medical and mental health for many years to come.

It is probably fairly obvious why we regard this woman as an ideal donor. As a mother, she knows how she feels about genetic and gestational connections and can make an informed decision about "giving away her genetic material." Since her family is complete, we are spared concern about how she will feel if she is unable to have children in the future and yet has helped someone else have a baby. We like the fact that she plans to donate to only one family and that she is prepared to meet the parents since these factors will spare their child—and the donor's own children—the genealogical bewilderment that can come when someone does not know to whom they are related.

Unfortunately, many physicians and some donor programs do not hold our ideal donor in such esteem. They seek even younger women, "because they are likely to be 'more fertile'," and women who have donated before, "because they have proven fertility." The maturity, ability to give informed consent, and understanding of infertility that we value are less important to many than a beautiful face and high SAT scores.

We remind readers that the story of how he or she joined your family will be important to your child. Knowing that a mature, kind, well intentioned and informed woman made a decision to help bring a new life into this world and into his/her family seems to us to be a greater gift to a child than good looks or high intelligence.

The Program Works Closely with Physicians—Either as Part of the Same Program or in Collaboration

Medical evaluation usually follows psychological assessment. A reproductive endocrinologist should assess a woman who plans to donate from two perspectives: is it medically safe for her to donate eggs at this point in time, and is she likely to produce several "good" eggs? The first part of the medical assessment is simpler than the second.

The physician looks at a would-be donor's general health, trying to determine if there are any medical reasons which might be inadvisable for the donor to take fertility medications or undergo an egg retrieval. If the physician finds no contraindications to a woman donating eggs, he/she will move on to the more challenging evaluation: is she likely to be a fertile donor. Since there is no definitive test of a woman's egg quality, the physician must rely on the tests that are available: the FSH, Inhibin B and other measures of presumed fertility. FSH helps predict the quantity of eggs a woman will produce and Inhibin B measures ovarian reserve. Although past performance is no guarantee of future success, a history of successful donations is often seen as a good sign. When a woman has donated previously at another medical clinic, the physician will request records of that donation.

Medical evaluation of a donor will include some assessment of her genetic history. In addition to being asked about personal and family history of a range of potentially hereditary medical and psychological conditions, the donor may also be assessed for certain autosomal dominant and autosomal recessive disorders, especially if there is a question of genetic disorders in her family history or in the family of the intended father.

Although there is no definitive way to predict a woman's fertility, the physician will look at the would-be donor's FSH and do an ultrasound of her antral follicle count in the hope of gaining some valuable information about her likelihood to produce viable eggs. FSH helps predict the quantity of eggs left in the ovary and from this, a woman's responsiveness to fertility injections can be inferred. However, as Nurse Practitioner Carol Lesser cautions, this is dose dependent and dependent on how an individual woman responds to medication. Antral follicle count measures the small follicles early in a woman's cycle and hence, offers some prediction of the number of recruitable oocytes after gonadatropin stimulation.

Although many couples seeking egg donation are already working closely with a reproductive endocrinologist, people often travel for egg donation. In some instances, recipient couples travel internationally for egg donation. When this is the case, a well run program will regard the coordination of medical services as part of its role. It will make sure that its clients see physicians who are skilled, supportive of ovum donation, sensitive to the loss issues involved and respectful of both donors and recipients

The Program Works Closely with Legal Consultation

As we made clear in far more detail in Chapter 6, we believe that legal consultation is essential for donors and recipients and programs.

A responsible program will require all of its donors to have a legal consultation. Katrina Twomey explains that this is to protect the donor from any assertion by the recipients or their offspring that the donor has parental responsibility, from the possibility that her eggs will go to anyone other than the recipient couple and from the possibility that the couple will donate resulting embryos. Prior to donation, the donor signs a legal agreement regarding the donation.

The following is a sample of an attorney opinion letter that attorney Melissa Brisman of Park Ridge, New Jersey, sends to agency programs and medical clinics on behalf of clients participating in egg donation. While she "represents the recipients" –at least in this letter—it is clear that the letter also protects donors from some unintended outcomes of her donation:

Dear Donor Program/Dr. John Doe:

This office represents Intended Parents, Mary and John Smith, matched with Donor 123. This letter serves as legal clearance to proceed with ova donation referenced in this matter as the parties have signed a legal agreement regarding the donation.

Please note that the parties have agreed that Intended Parents shall have ownership, custody and control of all retrieved ova. However, the parties have agreed that Intended Parents shall not donate embryos to another couple and/or individual for their use in conception and /or parenting of a child without the written consent of the donor.

Further, the parties have agreed that if both Intended Parents should die after retrieval but prior to fertilization of the ova, ownership, custody and control of the retrieved ova shall revert back to the Donor. However, if the ova have been fertilized prior to the death of both Intended Parents, the remaining cryopreserved embryos shall be destroyed.

Further, as this is a designated donation between the respective parties, Donor has not and will not execute any conflicting documents pertaining to the retrieval procedure with anyone, including the physician, fertility center or hospital wherein the ova are donated to anyone other than the designated Intended Parents in this matter.

Signed…Melissa Brisman, Esq.

Prospective recipients of egg donation are also required to have legal consultation and to enter into a contract with her even when the donor is anonymous. This contract serves to protect all participants from unintended consequences of the donation and unintended outcomes.

For the recipients, the lawyer wants to be sure that their parental rights are secure and that they are equal. It is important that in the event of a divorce, a mother through ovum donation be treated no differently than a mother who gives birth to her full biological child.

The lawyer also wants to protect the recipients from any claim on the donor's part that she has any parental rights or other rights to the eggs. As of this writing, only eight states have passed statutes defining the status of children born through egg donation. All transfer parental rights and responsibilities to the recipient and relieve the donor of any parental role. However, lawyers in other states can write contracts that explicitly state that the donor relinquishes any parental rights to the ova upon donation. It is important for the contract to specify whether donation occurs at the time of retrieval or transfer.

The legal contract should also protect the recipients from any unintended use of the eggs or resultant embryos by the egg donation program or by the fertility clinic. Specifically, the ova and embryos should become the property of the recipient couple and as Attorney Brisman's letter indicated, cannot be offered to another couple. In addition, since the donor has consented to donate to that couple and not to others, the recipients should be permanently restricted, in the contract, from voluntarily donating ova or embryos to another couple.

We hope that you will return to Chapter 6 for a more detailed discussion of legal issues.

The Program Is Well Versed in Insurance Issues

Egg donation is an expensive proposition. There are fees to the donors, fees to the programs, fees to lawyers, and, in states without insurance mandates, substantial medical costs. Donor programs need to do all they can to help their patients utilize all the benefits of their existing insurance, and, when possible, help them locate insurance that will better serve them. In addition, the program's financial staff should make sure that neither their donors nor their recipients incur additional expenses as a result of medical complications. To this end, responsible programs require recipients to purchase secondary insurance. This is usually in the form of a Blanket Accident Insurance Policy which offers coverage that begins as soon as the recipients sign the program agreement and continues for ninety days following retrieval.

The Program Is in Close Contact with the Donor during Her Donation Cycle and Remains in Contact in Years to Come

Since the process of donating is demanding, both physically and emotionally, a program's staff should remain in close contact with their donors throughout the cycle, making sure that they feel comfortable with the way things are going. Effort should be made to confirm that the donor is being supported by the fertility center staff as well as the key people in her personal life. The program should also make sure that she has a way of getting to her retrieval, has a ride home and that there is someone to be with her when she is recovering from the procedure.

In order to best serve all participants, an egg donation program should require all of its donors to remain in contact with the program for eighteen years regarding medical information. In addition, donors should be invited to keep in touch with program staff. In addition to paving the way for donors to provide recipients with significant medical up-dates, having donors remain contact lets them know that they are not simply providing a service and then being dropped. Staff remain interested in and concerned about donors in the weeks, months and years following their donations.

The Program Knows When and How to Offer Psychological Counseling

No one pursuing egg donation wants to feel they are being judged or evaluated, but there will be times when prospective recipients would benefit from some psychological assistance before proceeding with their family building plan. A program needs to have a staff that can deal with this sensitive situation and refer the following groups of people—as well as some others—for counseling.

Individuals and Couples with Lingering Grief

There are people who turn to oocyte donation without having grieved the loss of their full biological child. There is no formula for this grieving, but Smith and others have found that lingering grief can really derail an egg donor process. It expresses itself in anger (at staff, at themselves), in dissatisfaction with the donor or the donor agency's process, with severely heightened anxiety before procedures. A skilled counselor will listen carefully to confirm that the recipient couple is really ready to welcome and celebrate a donor egg pregnancy. Some of the other reasons why a couple might be referred by their donor program for counseling include:

Couples Who Are Not Experiencing Synchronicity

It is said that opposites attract, and some of the happiest couples are rarely in sync in many areas of their lives. Still, it is important that partners not be too far apart regarding egg donation. Surely there are some instances in which one partner would prefer adoption, but has agreed to go along with the other's preference for donor egg. Or there can be significant differences within the couple regarding donor selection, number of embryos to transfer and even about when to do the cycle. When a program staff member spots troubling differences within a couple, she should encourage them to pursue additional counseling before commencing an egg donor cycle.

Donor Selection Problems

As we indicated above, when requested, a responsible program will provide couples with some assistance in selecting a donor. However, there are couples who have considerable difficulty choosing a donor. This may be because they seek someone who is a member of a certain ethnic, cultural or racial group where there are few—if any—donors available or their difficulty may be related to emotional issues concerning egg donation. Counseling may help them understand why they are having difficulty with this process and assist them in gaining confidence and a clearer perspective in decision making.

Conflicts in Parental Confidence and Feelings of Legitimacy

As we have said throughout this book—and so, we'll say it again—parents through egg donation need to feel confident in and proud of their decision. They also need to feel "legitimate." Some couples are referred for counseling because it seems that they need some help gaining confidence and a sense of legitimacy.

Your choice of an egg donation program is an important one, so you want to take some care in making it. In this chapter, we have tried to give you some characteristics to look for and what to avoid in making this important decision. As you search, we encourage you to visit programs in person if you possibly can. Geography may make this difficult, and both the internet and the phone will provide you with extensive information, but there are many times in life when there is no real substitute for a face-to-face conversation. This may well be one of them.

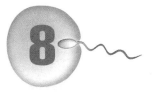

Attempting Pregnancy—
A Collaborative Effort

The medical process in most kinds collaborative reproduction—gamete donation, surrogacy, etc.—is an unusual one. Where else in medicine do three people enter treatment together to resolve one problem?! In looking at the next step in your journey to parenthood, we will focus on what you, as a recipient of donated eggs, can expect when you locate a medical program and undergo an egg donation cycle. But since you are not the only patient in this situation, we will focus, as well, on what your husband/partner's role is and on what your donor—whether known or not—will be going through. While clinics vary in exact protocol, we want to you be prepared, know what to expect, and have enough information to allow you to ask your health care provider educated, pertinent questions about your course of treatment.

Can We Even Afford Egg Donation?

Egg donation is a big financial commitment, bringing with it bills that can total tens of thousands of dollars. For many individuals, egg donation is not covered by insurance and must be covered out of pocket. While medical costs vary from clinic to clinic, in 2005, an egg donation cycle with a known donor's ova typically costs about $20,000-$25,000, while an egg donation cycle with a program-recruited donor can cost $25,000-$30,000 or more. Although costs vary regionally in the United States and throughout the world, these figures usually include the following:

- The donor's fertility medications ($3,000)
- The donor's cycle fees, i.e. ultrasounds, blood work, pain medications, antibiotics, etc. ($2,500)

- The donor's egg retrieval procedure, embryology lab costs and embryo transfer ($3,000)
- A facility fee ($1,500)
- Initial embryo freezing ($750)
- Recipient cycle costs, i.e. ultrasounds, medications, blood work, lab work, cycle management, sperm preparation, follow-up care, etc. ($12,000)
- ICSI, if needed ($1,500)

In addition to these costs, most medical clinics who recruit donors pass along to recipients donor fees ranging (conservatively) between $2500 and $5000 per retrieval cycle. Many medical clinics have done away with recruiting egg donors themselves and have moved to using outside egg donation agencies. And if you are in a special circumstance (such as you also need a sperm donor or your egg donor lives in another state), there can be additional costs as well. Also, there will be costs associated with legal fees and counseling fees for both donor and recipient. These vary widely from state to state and even clinic to clinic. These costs are normally not included in the initial price for the egg donation procedure. It is important to remember that *all* costs associated with the egg donation process are the financial responsibility of the recipient.

As you can see, there are many costs associated with ovum donation, making the process a financial burden for many. Your next step should be to consider your financial resources. For many of you, this may mean talking to a financial planner about taking money out of savings or retirement plans. Or perhaps you are considering checking out several banks about taking out a loan, such as a home equity loan against your home. You may even be thinking about asking close family members for financial assistance. In addition, some infertility clinics accept major credit cards, which might allow you to spend more than you can actually afford.

Allocating substantial amounts of money to ovum donation is not without risks. Since egg donation is not a sure bet, you want to be sure to avoid depleting your resources to such a degree that you are unable to afford adoption should the egg donor cycle not prove successful. You also want to avoid compromising your family's financial future in some other way. The costs of raising the child you are trying so hard to conceive are high, too.

So what can you do? First of all, call your insurance company and find out exactly what is covered and what is not as far as infertility treatments are concerned. To validate your coverage, get a copy of your insurance policy to review. Some couples are pleasantly surprised that insurance may cover a portion and in some cases all of the costs associated with egg donation. It can't hurt to ask and know exactly what your policy includes. As mentioned in an earlier chapter, a few states now mandate that insurance companies either pay for or at the very least offer policies to employers that can cover the costs of infertility treatment. Whether you live in one of the states with an insurance mandate can influence the affordability of ovum donation for you.

Egg Donation in a Mandated State

Even with the insurance mandate, using donated ova involves some significant costs. For women under 40, the medical treatment will almost certainly be covered, but any fees to the donor, a lawyer and a donor agency will not be included. For recipients in their 40s, many insurance companies will seek some evidence that the need for donor eggs is not the result of natural aging. In the absence of that evidence, they will not cover egg donation.

Egg Donation in a Non-mandated State

With no insurance both egg donation and "regular IVF" are very costly. On top of the $10-20,000 for the IVF cycle, there will be fees for medical and psychological evaluation of the donor, legal fees and in the case of program-recruited donors, fees to the donor and to her program.

With the realities of your insurance coverage (or lack of it) made clear, next talk to your fertility clinic. Most fertility clinics have a financial person on staff. You are not alone, and just about everyone considering egg donation is in the same boat as are you. Fertility clinics are used to answering questions about finances and may be able to provide you with more detailed information matching your specific situation. Also, they should educate you about all the costs involved and what type of payment structure they offer. Some clinics require that you pay up-front before any procedures begin, while others offer payment plans so that you can pay off what you owe over several months. Additionally, it is important that before you start any type of procedure you get clarification from your fertility clinic about exactly what is covered by the stated pricing structure and what is not. Sometimes advertised costs do not include "hidden" costs, such as the price of the fertility medications or costs associated with any complications that may occur, which can also be steep.

After you have gathered all of your information about the costs of egg donation and know how much you will be responsible for, you should sit down and plan a budget. How much can you really afford to spend on this particular option to have a baby? Keep in mind that once you start, it is very easy to get caught up in all the reproductive technologies that are available that might enable you to become pregnant. After all, you may say to yourself after some unproductive cycles, you just spent $50,000, what's another $10,000 or $20,000? What types of changes and sacrifices will you have to make in your life and lifestyle in order to attempt egg donation? What will you do if oocyte donation does not work?

As with any major financial decision, it is not uncommon for couples to seek out professional financial advice as to how to organize their money. Egg donation is not just a difficult emotional journey, it can also have a long-lasting financial impact, so we encourage you to make educated decisions in order to protect your future.

Choosing a Fertility Clinic and Assembling the Medical Team

Many people considering ovum donation are already connected to a physician and fertility clinic that they like and trust. If you are among this group, your selection of a medical program may be already completed by this point. However, if you are among those individuals or couples who come to egg donation without a history of fertility treatment or if you have relocated or want, for whatever reason, to find a new program, there are decisions to make.

In the United States, there are over 400 fertility clinics, most of which participate in egg donation. Not all clinics are created equal. There is great diversity in quality and traits of each clinic and its staff, from large university-based programs within hospital settings to one-physician clinics in small towns. You want to find a clinic that not only has significant experience with oocyte donation, but also offers thorough, attentive and compassionate care.

Most high quality programs participate in SART (Society for Assisted Reproductive Technology) and adhere to its reporting and staffing regulations. In choosing your clinic, you may want to seek SART statistics by contacting the American Society for Reproductive Medicine (ASRM) in Birmingham, Alabama. In addition, all programs using donated eggs (and sperm and embryos) are now required to register with the Food and Drug Administration. The FDA's regulations, "Eligibility Determination for Donors of Human Cells, Tissues and Cellular and Tissue Based Products" include the regulations that all clinics must adhere to for screening potential donors for infectious diseases, criteria for donor eligibility, specifics about quarantine and storage of reproductive cells, specifics about maintenance of records and the establishment of standard operating procedures.

In selecting your program, you will not only want to look at SART and FDA guidelines and participation. You may want to turn to fertility organizations and support groups, such as RESOLVE or AFA or IAAC, which have lists of recommended fertility clinics. Beyond these sources, people talk with friends, fellow infertility patients and physicians to see which programs they recommend and why.

You need to find a clinic with which you feel comfortable. Remember, this is a big commitment, both in time, effort and money, so you want to feel confident that your communication with staff will go well. You will trust these people with your already fragile emotional and physical well-being as you work together to create a much desired baby. You want to feel free to ask questions and voice concerns. This may mean interviewing several clinics or physicians to get a better understanding of their backgrounds, their style, and the way the staff works together and with clients before making your decision.

It is important to find a clinic that is convenient for you. Remember that you will have to visit the clinic many times over the course of at least several weeks for treatment and examinations. You have to be able to get there easily, and often, if necessary. For those who choose a clinic that is far away, many couples decide to stay in a hotel or with friends close by the clinic during the course of the treatment. Some clinics are used to out-of-town patients and can offer you additional information about treatment scheduling and accommodations.

Since there is no standardized reporting of egg donation success rates to which you can refer, you need to ask the clinic about their pregnancy rates as well as actual birth and multiple birth rates as a result of egg donation. Remember that all this data is self-reported by the fertility clinic, and it is in their best interest to show strong success rates. As a result, all statistical information will have to be taken with a grain of salt. Even in the best case scenario, be realistic in your expectations and know that your chance of taking home a baby are probably fifty/fifty. Many programs report a 50% pregnancy rate per cycle and then there is the 1 in 4 to1 in 5 chance of miscarriage. So we're assuming that your "take home baby rate" is about 50% if you try two times. Knowing this will help you better cope if failure occurs. Despite these weaknesses, assessing any egg donor program's statistics should give you some indication about how experienced the clinic is with the procedure and will provide you with opportunities to ask additional questions and get to know the clinic better.

Another important factor is gathering information about your medical team. You want to know as much as possible about the specific medical team that will be assisting you. Although most IVF centers are run by reproductive endocrinologists (REs), you should confirm that is the case with the clinic you are considering. An RE is someone who was first trained as an obstetrician/gynecologist and then completed a two to three year fellowship in the field of reproductive endocrinology and infertility. When choosing an RE, seek someone who has good communication skills as well as expertise in the medical and surgical aspects of reproductive medicine. E. Scott Sills, MD, of Atlanta, Georgia, underscores the importance of this combination when he says, "One of the most gratifying parts of my work is talking with patients. I have found that it is crucial to take time to really listen to people—to hear their concerns, to respond to their questions, to convey to them that they are not simply numbers. Patients need to know that they will see their physician most of the time and that he or she will be available by phone." Sills goes on to recommend that people seek a clinic with low physician turnover, since it is important that your physician be familiar with and an integral part of the nursing and laboratory teams.

Because so many aspects of egg donation are laden with ethical and moral concerns, you want to find a physician whose beliefs and value system complement your own. Everyone has different limits as to what they want to try and what they do not. You do not want to place yourself in a situation where your physician may try to overtly encourage or deny you certain treatment options. It is good to know up-front what you can expect and avoid any judgment conflicts later on.

All IVF centers have trained embryologists and follow the SART guidelines that detail the staff requirements that are necessary for IVF units. A qualified embryologist typically has a degree in biology with additional training in embryology. This additional training varies and can include certifications or advanced degrees such as a master's or even a doctoral degree in embryology. As with the physicians, you want to a clinic with a well-trained embryologist who has had several years of experience with techniques used in egg donation.

In addition, you should feel comfortable with the nursing staff. They will be your primary contacts during your treatment. You need to make sure that they are sensitive and compassionate to your situation and that you feel comfortable talking to them. The nursing staff should have significant experience with dealing with infertility issues and people experiencing infertility. You also need to have information about your continuity of care. Will you be assigned one nurse or a nurse coordinator who will oversee your treatment plan, or will there be someone different each time you come in for an office visit? As with all other clinic staff, long-term employees—ones who have been there several years, enjoy their jobs and have experience working in the field of infertility—usually ensure competence and confidence. These factors will say a lot about the quality of your clinic.

The clinic you choose should also have a mental health professional on staff or should be able to refer to a list of qualified counselors who specialize in working with couples struggling with infertility. As we have stressed before, the egg donation process brings with it many emotional and psychological issues, many of which should not be dealt with alone. A good counselor can help guide you through these difficult situations and assist you in making important decisions about the long-term impact of your ovum donation.

Remember that egg donation is an intensive process. Your egg donor must take potent fertility medications and your cycle must be synchronized with hers, so your medical team should be attentive to you at all times. You will need to be closely monitored to avoid complications and to increase you chances of becoming pregnant. Since issues can arise at any time during an egg donation cycle, you should find a clinic that has staff available to return phone calls or emails during evenings, weekends and holidays in case you have questions or need to be seen right away. In fact, there are many people who choose a particular clinic or decide against one based on how easy or difficult it is to schedule an appointment. Maybe you do not mind talking to a machine, but remember that there will be many times during your treatment experience when you will need to talk to a person.

The Initial Infertility Work-Up

In most instances, couples have already endured numerous fertility tests, medications and procedures before approaching egg donation. However, others of you may be new to ART—you may come to egg donation having known for a long time that donor eggs were needed. For this last group, all of the lingo of ART and all of the medical procedures are unfamiliar.

Regardless of where you are in your infertility journey, however, before beginning an egg donation cycle, you will undergo extensive testing to confirm that you are in good health, that your uterus is prepared to accept an embryo and grow a baby, that you are unlikely to have a problem carrying a baby (twins are more challenging) to term. If you are in your 40s, additional testing, such as mammogram, glucose tolerance test and an electrocardiogram will probably be requested. In addition, recipients might also be asked to complete basic pre-conception testing such as Pap test, blood count, kidney and liver function, rubella screening, blood Rh factor, and thyroid function, in addition to tests for HIV, hepatitis, gonorrhea and chlamydia. Meanwhile your husband or male partner should also complete another semen analysis to ensure that his sperm will be able to fertilize the donor's eggs, as well as having HIV and hepatitis tests to avoid spreading these diseases. Finally, a test will be performed to confirm that the uterine cavity is normal. This can be accomplished by a hysterosalpingogram, sono-hytserogram or hysteroscopy.

Although you will have several exams and tests, most likely your donor will be assessed even more extensively. Whether she is a program-recruited donor or a family member or friend, she will be asked to complete an extensive individual and family medical history questionnaire. This will be followed by physical exams that will focus on both her reproductive and her general health. Physicians will pay particular attention to her hormone levels, especially FSH, and they will follow FDA regulations, which require blood tests for HIV types 1 and 2 hepatitis B and C, syphilis, gonorrhea, chlamydia and human transmissible spongiform encephalopathy (TSE, or Creutzfeld-Jakob disease). In addition, your donor's genetic history will be evaluated The American Society for Reproductive Medicine recommends that donors be excluded for any of the following conditions: a major Mendelian disorder, a major multifactorial or polygenic malformation; a familial disease with a major genetic component, a chromosomal rearrangement, a carrier of an autosomal recessive gene know to be prevalent in the donor's ethnic background for which her carrier status can be detected; or advanced age (over 35). The Society also recommends that donors be rejected if they have a first-degree relative (parents or offspring) with any of the following: a major autosomal dominant or x-linked disorder with late age of onset; an autosomal recessive disorder (if the disorder has a high frequency in the population), or a chromosomal abnormality, unless the donor has a normal karotype. (Cohen, 1996). Your donor will be encouraged to report personal or family history of conditions such as high blood pressure, heart disease, deafness, blindness, severe arthritis, diabetes, alcoholism, schizophrenia, manic depression, epilepsy, Alzheimer's disease, cleft-lip or palate, heart defects, clubfoot, spina bifida, color blindness, cystic fibrosis, hemophilia, muscular dystrophy, sickle cell anemia, Huntington's Disease, polycystic kidney disease, glaucoma and Tay-Sachs disease.

In addition to genetic problems, your prospective donor could be rejected by the physician because she is significantly overweight, because she smokes or because she or a first degree relative have a history of mental illness. Or the program mental health counselor may reject her because of a variety of psychological issues, including the recent break-up of a relationship, the death of a loved one, and, possibly, a history of sexual abuse. Overall, about 20 percent of potential egg donors are rejected for at least one of these reasons.

In order to encourage the best chance for success, you, your partner and your donor will be instructed to notify the clinic of any medications that are being taken as well as to avoid smoking, alcohol, caffeine, weight loss programs, vigorous exercise, hot tubs, and saunas before and during the egg donation process.

Cycle Synchronization and Ovarian Stimulation

With ovum donation, both recipients and donors must take fertility medications for several weeks. Recipients must take several different types of fertility medications in order to prepare the uterus and synchronize their cycle with the donor. Consequently, your uterus, more specifically your uterine lining or endometrium, will be ready as soon as the embryos are ready for transfer.

Likewise, your donor will be taking fertility medications in order to stimulate the follicles in her ovaries to produce multiple eggs. Even if your donor ovulates regularly, she will still need to take these hormones in order to produce many eggs rather than just one which is typical under normal circumstances. This is often referred to as super-ovulation. This ensures a higher number of good quality ova for donation and will maximize the chance that fertilization and optimum transfer.

The actual fertility drug combination varies depending on a number of factors, such as patient's age and weight. Also, each doctor has his own specific protocol based on his or her own experience, and depending on your and the donor's reaction to this protocol, changes might have to be made. Although every doctor has a slightly different method of achieving the same result, basic general approaches to stimulating egg production are used. Here we will walk you through a sample protocol so you can gain a better understanding about what to expect, both for you and your donor. Because medications are being developed rapidly and trade named forms of many drugs are available, we have chosen not to use trade names in describing medications you might expect to see used in your protocol. Instead, when we feel that it would be important to name a drug, we will use its generic name.

Before the real egg donation process takes place—typically during the month before the actual cycle—you may be asked to participate in a "mock cycle" with the donor to ensure that hormone levels of each of you can be successfully manipulated with medications. While not as common as it once was, some physicians still recommend an endometrial biopsy during this mock cycle on the actual day transfer would have taken place if this were a real cycle. This biopsy will help to confirm that the lining is maturing to allow implantation to occur. However, many physicians bypass this test since it has been shown to be unreliable. More often today, physicians will perform an ultrasound after 10-12 days of estrogen to measure the thickness of the endometrium. An endometrium greater than 7 mm insures that the estrogen dose is optimal. If everything checks out during this mock cycle, you will be given the go-ahead to attempt a real cycle next time.

Next, it is important for your cycle to correspond perfectly with your donor's cycle. In order to accomplish this, certain fertility medications or low dose birth control pills are often prescribed to the donor and the recipient.

In 2005, one such fertility medication that is often used to synchronize the menstrual cycles and to prevent ovulation from occurring naturally is leuprolide. Both recipients (if you are still ovulating) and donors begin to taking this about a week or so before their periods are expected. Leuprolide is a gonadotropin-releasing hormone (GnRH) antagonist which suppresses the release of the luteinizing hormone (LH) by the pituitary gland, a gland located within your brain. The pituitary gland normally triggers the eggs to mature within the ovaries by releasing LH. By suppressing the pituitary gland, a temporary menopause-like state is created. As a result, fertility specialists are able to inhibit egg production while maintaining the menstrual cycles with other medications to ensure that the recipient's uterus will be ready to receive the embryo created by the donor egg.

Leuprolide is taken every day for about two-and-a-half weeks, or until the eggs are ready to be retrieved from the donor. Leuprolide is administered through daily subcutaneous (also called sub-q) injections. For subcutaneous injections, a short needle is used to deliver the medication to the tissue just under the skin. As an alternative, researchers are working on a daily nasal spray or a long-lasting single injection which may be soon be available to some. Other forms of GnRH antagonists are available and sometimes used.

In order to prime the uterus, you will also begin taking estrogen a few days after your period has started. Estrogen helps get the uterus and uterine lining ready for embryo transfer and should be taken every day until the embryo is transferred. Estrogen can be taken in the form of injections, patches or by mouth. The estrogen should be natural, not synthetic.

Additionally, you will begin taking progesterone a few days before the embryo transfer is scheduled. Again, this helps to mature the lining of the uterus to allow implantation. Progesterone levels are very critical for all pregnant women during early pregnancy in order to maintain the pregnancy. To ensure adequate progesterone levels, most fertility specialists recommend that donor ova recipients continue progesterone supplementation throughout the first trimester of the pregnancy. After the first trimester, the placenta takes over maintaining appropriate hormone levels for the baby.

Progesterone should be natural, not synthetic, and is taken most often via intra-muscular injection; however, sometimes a vaginal suppository, vaginal gel or pill form may be recommended. Side effects of progesterone sometimes include vaginal dryness, bloating, breast tenderness, depression, and mood swings.

What's happening with your donor during this time? Once her menstrual cycle begins, she starts taking medications to stimulate her ovaries, such as human menopausal gonadotropin (hMG) or follicle stimulating hormone (FSH). Forms of hMG are obtained from urine that is extracted from post-menopausal women. Current forms of FSH are genetically engineered, making them purer and more uniform and much more potent. As a result, FSH is commonly the medication of choice today in order to stimulate the donor's ovaries. These medications encourage the development of many egg follicles, allowing the fertility specialist to retrieve as many mature eggs as possible. This process significantly elevates a donor's fertility at this point, so donors are asked to abstain from sexual intercourse to protect against unintended pregnancies while in the midst of trying to donate their oocytes.

Either FSH or hMG is typically taken every day for about nine days and is administered through injections, which can be either subcutaneous or intramuscular. After a few days of administering this medication, donors will have a blood test taken to measure the estrogen level and will undergo a transvaginal ultrasound to assess the development of the follicles which are the fluid filled cysts that house the eggs. Once it is determined that the donor's follicles have matured, she will receive an injection of human chorionic gonadotropin (hCG). HCG is very similar to LH, which is a hormone that matures the egg during a natural cycle and forces ovulation to occur. Approximately 40 hours after the hCG injection, ovulation will occur. Therefore the egg retrieveal will be performed about 36 hours after this injection.

You will be busy at this time too. At about the time of egg retrieval of the donor, periodic transvaginal ultrasounds will be performed on you as well. This is to ensure that the endometrium is developing appropriately. To provide the best chance for embryo implantation, the endometrium should be about 6 mm thick and should have an appearance of three layers stacked on top of one another.

In order to maximize the effects of the medications, it is recommended that all medication, except acetaminophen and prenatal or multi-vitamins, be avoided. If you are on any other type of medication, discuss this with your physician before the treatment cycle begins. Also, avoid smoking, alcohol and caffeine during treatment as well as any changes in diet or weight loss. Typically, normal exercise is not prohibited; however, you many want to avoid hot tubs and saunas. Both recipient and donor should be monitored regularly to ensure neither is experiencing adverse reactions to the medications.

Administering Injections

Both you and your egg donor will be giving yourselves injections, sometimes daily, for several weeks. Although giving yourself an injection can be daunting, many women find that practice makes perfect. To begin, find a clean, quiet and comfortable place where you will not be disturbed for ten to fifteen minutes (roughly the amount of time that it will take you to do your injection). Gather and organize your supplies, including your medications and any fluids that you will need to dilute your medications, syringes, needles for mixing the medications (usually larger needles), needles for injecting the medications (usually smaller needles), alcohol swabs and a container to safely dispose of used needles and syringes.

Some medications need to be mixed or diluted. This is done by mixing a powder which contains the medication with sterile liquid. On the other hand, some medications may be drawn directly from the vial in which they are provided or from a glass ampule. With ampules, you must break off the top of the ampule to get the medication. When you receive you medications, you should talk with your pharmacist about the best way to prepare each type of medication and any specifics about storing them properly.

Next, choose an injection site. For subcutaneous injections (which are similar to insulin injections), the medication is delivered just under the skin by a smaller 27 gauge or one-half inch needle, and can be administered to your belly (although the area directly around your belly button should be avoided), the back of the arm, or the top of the thigh. Intramuscular injections require a longer (one to two inch or 22 gauge) needle that delivers the medication deep into the muscle such as the mid-thigh or buttock area.

Make sure you clean the injection site with alcohol and allow to air dry before you attempt the injection. After the injection is complete, you should safely dispose of any needles or syringes in a sharps container rather than in the trash can in order to prevent others from being stuck accidentally.

Your physician or a nurse should explain the medication schedule. You will have to administer injections every day for several weeks. Timing of the medications is important. Make sure you do not miss a dose or forget to administer the injection. While it is desirable to take the medication at roughly the same time every day, an hour or two earlier or later probably will not make a difference. Make sure you completely understand your medication schedule and do not be afraid to ask questions if you are unsure. Also, make sure you know whom to call if questions arise once you get home.

What If You Cannot Give Yourself an Injection?

You might want to recruit a close friend or family member, such as your husband, to give you these injections. The person you choose should feel comfortable with doing this and should also talk to the pharmacist or physician to make sure they understand how to handle and prepare the medications. Another option is to find an urgent care or drop-in clinic to administer the injection. Because such a clinic would charge a small fee for their services, this may not the answer for the long term for most patients. However, this might be an alternative when you are in a pinch and you cannot find anyone to help you.

Can You Hurt Yourself When Giving an Injection?

Probably not. Giving yourself injections, or having someone else do it, is relatively safe. It is possible to hit a blood vessel, which could cause bleeding or bruising, or a nerve, which could be painful. However, you are very unlikely to seriously hurt yourself by administering an injection improperly.

Cycle Monitoring

As with all medications, some of the fertility medications may have side effects. This is why it is so important that both donor and recipient are monitored very closely throughout the process. Some side effects that occur in about ten percent of women can include pelvic pain, nausea and vomiting, hot flashes, bloating, abdominal cramping, mood changes, breast tenderness, blurred vision, and rashes or hives. It is vital that recipient or donor call your clinic immediately if either experiences any of these side effects at any point in treatment.

For your donor, some of these side effects may be early warning signs of Ovarian Hyperstimulation Syndrome (OHSS) since her ovaries are being prepared to produce many eggs at the same time. OHSS occurs in about one or two percent of donors. It occurs when too many follicles are stimulated, causing the ovary to become enlarged. If left untreated, OHSS can worsen quickly and develop into a serious medical condition. Again, we stress that if a donor experiences any adverse side effects or if she suspects that she could have OHSS, she should call the doctor right away. It is much better to be safe than sorry.

Cycle monitoring is also important in order to perfectly time the egg retrieval and embryo transfer. Both recipient and donor will have to come in several times (sometimes even on a daily basis for some weeks) for monitoring to ensure the coordination of exact timing for egg retrieval and embryo transfer.

Cycle monitoring usually consists of blood tests and ultrasounds. Blood tests are used to monitor hormone levels, while ultrasounds are used to look at follicle and egg development in the donor and to gage the thickness of the uterine lining of the recipient. Transvaginal ultrasounds are typically used. With these ultrasounds, a hand-held cylinder-shaped instrument called the transducer is inserted into the vagina. The health care provider will move the transducer within the vagina in order to get a good picture of the reproductive organs. For the most part, this is a quick process and is no more painful or uncomfortable than a regular pelvic exam.

Egg Retrieval

Once it is determined that the ova are ready for retrieval, your donor will come to the clinic for the egg retrieval process. This is often referred to as a follicle aspiration procedure. While laparoscopy through a small incision made in the abdomen was once the common route to retrieving oocytes, this process has been replaced for the most part by a less invasive, minor surgical form of egg retrieval that can be performed on an out-patient basis and takes five to ten minutes to perform. Depending on the clinic, a light anesthesia is used during the procedure. Additionally, some women experience nausea during this procedure, so an anti-nausea medication may also be recommended.

A transvaginal ultrasound is inserted into the vagina to help the physician position the ovaries on the other side of the vaginal wall. He or she guides a suctioning needle into the follicle and the fluid is removed. The fluids are then examined by an embryologist who identifies the eggs. Following this egg retrieval process, the donor usually remains in the clinic for one to two hours before returning home. An antibiotic is typically prescribed to prevent any possible infection, and a follow-up exam and ultrasound are scheduled for one week later.

Most often, between ten and twenty eggs are retrieved from a donor. Sometimes, donors have more eggs, occasionally upwards of forty.

If your donor is your sister or cousin in her mid-30s, there may be fewer eggs. Less than 10 may compromise the ability to create good quality embryos for transfer. Although greater numbers of eggs generally bode well for ultimate success (since you are likely to have frozen embryos available for future transfer) having fewer eggs does *not* mean you will not achieve pregnancy.

We know that egg retrieval—for both donor *and* recipient—is a very stressful time. You will be worrying about what your donor is going through— especially if she is your sister or someone else close to you—and you will be focusing on the outcome of the retrieval. Try to remember that this is all a process over which you have no control. Be fair to yourself and don't hold yourself responsible if your donor has an uncomfortable procedure or if only a small quantity of oocytes are obtained.

It is important to remember that even though egg retrieval does not involve any incisions, it is considered surgery. While relatively rare, some donors may suffer damage to organs that are within close proximity to the ovaries. Other complications may include trauma to the ovaries, infection, vaginal bleeding, and lacerations. These complications may necessitate a hospitalization and possible surgery. Your egg donor must realize that a consequence of a complication is that it may impact her future fertility. Fortunately, serious complications are rare and the vast majority of egg retrievals proceed uneventfully.

Your ovum donor will need to have someone drive her home after the procedure, and she is usually advised to rest for the remainder of the day. Again, if she is someone close to you, it is likely that you will be with her, tending to her discomfort and letting her know how much you appreciate what she has been through. If she is a program-recruited donor with whom you are not in contact, you will surely be thinking of her, perhaps sending her flowers or a small gift. Know that responsible programs will make sure that she is well cared for after retrieval. It is also their job to stay in close contact with her to be sure she is recovering uneventfully, both physically and emotionally.

Sperm Samples

Before egg harvesting, your husband or male partner will have to provide a sperm sample. The two of you should talk to your fertility specialist about the best time to collect the sample. Fresh sperm obtained on the day of egg retrieval is usually most desirable for fertilizing the ova. However, many couples feel uncomfortable waiting until the last possible minute and risking the chance that the male partner may feel too stressed about the pressure to produce a sperm sample on demand. While not ideal, it is possible that the sperm sample can be provided early and frozen until the eggs are retrieved and ready for fertilization.

In order to increase the chances that a good sperm sample is provided, men are asked to notify the clinic if any illness involving a fever or a sexually transmitted infection having occurred in the last few months. They are also asked to avoid hot tubs, saunas, drugs, alcohol, smoking, and vigorous exercise. Men are encouraged to abstain from having intercourse for at least two days before the sample is given.

Fertilization—Creating an Embryo

After the ovum is identified, it is placed in a nutrient culture media in a small Petri dish, which is then placed in an incubator. In the early afternoon, the prepared sperm sample is added to the eggs. The following morning the eggs are checked to see if fertilization has occurred. At the end of 48 hours, the fertilized eggs (called embryos) should have already divided into two or four cells. Three days following the egg retrieval, the embryos should have divided to 6-8 cells. It is at this point that embryo transfer into the recipient's uterus is possible. Sometimes fertilization is more difficult. As a result, many physicians opt to use a micromanipulation technique called Intracytoplasmic Sperm Injection (ICSI) to enhance the chance of fertilization. ICSI is almost always used for men who have experienced issues with male factor infertility, when sperm that has been frozen is used, and if pre-implantation genetic diagnosis (PGD) is planned. However, despite previous semen analysis, whether or not ICSI is used depends on how the quality of the sperm sample is on the day of fertilization. It is fairly common for ICSI to be recommended even for men with no history of problems with their sperm.

ICSI is performed immediately after the egg(s) are retrieved or soon after if fertilization has not occurred. In cases where the sperm may have trouble penetrating the eggs, the embryologist will use ICSI to directly inject a single sperm into the ovum. Obviously to do this, the embryologist must be highly skilled. After this procedure, the eggs are placed in Petri dishes and placed in the incubator. After about fourteen hours, the embryologist will check to see if the fertilization was successful.

There is no guarantee that any of the eggs undergoing micromanipulation will fertilize or that embryos will implant. With ICSI, there is no way to know for sure which are the best sperm to choose for injection. There are risks to the ICSI procedure. The procedure could render the eggs non-viable—this occurs 1-2% of the time. If the ICSI procedure is performed for a very low sperm count, (<5 million sperm/cc) there is a slightly increased chance that the baby could be born with a chromosomal imbalance involving the sex chromosomes.

Embryo Quality

Your physician will want to select the best embryos for transfer in order to maximize your chance for pregnancy. All embryos are graded by an embryologist to assess their quality. This grading assesses cell number and what is called *fragmentation*. Embryo fragmentation refers to the problem of cells of an embryo splitting off into small fragments. This is considered normal and is expected to some extent among all embryos. However, an excessive amount of fragmentation is indicative of a lower quality embryo. The goal is to identify the six to eight cell embryos on Day 3 of embryo development that have minimal fragmentation.

Although we hope and expect that you will have had a conversation with your physician at the start of the cycle about how many embryos to transfer, it is possible that there will be additional discussion at this point. Since the goal, in almost all clinics, is a singleton pregnancy, with twins but no higher order multiples being an acceptable outcome, most physicians recommend transferring two high quality embryos. This practice is common because transferring two high quality embryos usually results in no greater than a twin pregnancy There have been, however, occasional instances in which an embryo splits. For example, I (Ellen) have an egg donation patient who had two unsuccessful transfers and on the third frozen transfer, two thawed embryos resulted in a triplet pregnancy that included identical twins. You will probably be planning on transferring one or two high quality embryos, but what if you have only three "mediocre" ones. Your physician may encourage you to transfer all three, knowing, of course, that you run the risk of a triplet pregnancy. About one in four of all ART pregnancies results in multiple gestation, the majority of which are twins.

Preimplantation Genetic Diagnosis

Preimplantation Genetic Diagnosis (PGD) is a procedure developed in order to test embryos for genetic disorders before the embryo is transferred to the uterus. PGD can be used by couples undergoing any type of ART who have significant concerns that a genetic disease may be passed to their child, leading to pregnancy loss or the birth of a severely ill child. PGD has been performed since 1990, initially for genetic disorders such as Fragile X syndrome, Down syndrome, Tay-Sachs disease, muscular dystrophy, hemophilia, Turner syndrome, and cystic fibrosis, and, more recently, to help couples with unexplained infertility determine whether they have a previously undetected genetic or chromosomal problem.

What role does PGD have in egg donation? Most often, there is little indication for PGD since egg donors are carefully screened for genetic disorders and male partners should be screened as well. However, there will be occasional situations in which PGD can be helpful. These are most likely to occur in intrafamily donation—if your sister is your donor and there is a question of some genetic disorder in your family and in your husbands, you may want to consider PGD.

PGD is usually performed on day 3 of embryo development. Once the embryo is isolated, a single cell is removed from each embryo and evaluated under a microscope for the presence of genetic disorders. A diagnosis is provided within a day or two, and only unaffected embryos are transferred.

As of this writing, only a limited number of fertility clinics offer PGD as an option. PGD is expensive. Costs for this procedure are usually more than $5,000 and are not covered by insurance.

Embryo Transfer

Physicians vary in their opinions about the optimal time for embryo transfer. Some recommend transferring the embryos on day 3 (after the egg retrieval) while others like to wait until 5-6 days when the embryo has reached the blastocyst stage (approximately 50-75 cells). This is an area of controversy, and a real catch-22 situation. On one hand, if you transfer the embryos early, you will have more to transfer in hopes that one will make it. On the other hand, if you wait until the embryos have had time to further develop, you might have very few, if any, embryos still available to be transferred. However, each of these embryos will have a higher chance of success than less developed embryos. Because this is such a difficult decision and there are no definitive answers, you should talk with your physician about his/her perspective. Every clinic has had different experiences with embryo transfers and the physician might suggest a slightly different protocol based on his or her personal experiences and your specific situation. This decision should be well-informed and made on a case by case basis depending on how your embryos are growing and reacting in the laboratory.

Embryo transfer is an outpatient procedure, and typically, you can have a family member or friend stay with you during the entire procedure. If someone close to you is your donor and you were with her before and after her retrieval, you may both want to share the experience of embryo transfer—hopefully, it represents the beginning of your pregnancy. The transfer requires no anesthesia and involves placing the embryo(s) into your uterus by means of a small plastic tube, or catheter, which is inserted through the cervix into the uterus. An abdominal ultrasound is also usually used in order to view the uterus and locate the best position in which to place the embryos.

After embryo transfer, you will be taken to a recovery area to rest comfortably on your back for about two hours. You may also be given an injection of hCG to help maintain appropriate hormone levels. Then you will be sent home to wait and wonder "Did it work?" Once home, you will be advised to rest for the first 24 hours after the embryo transfer and engage in only limited activity. After about 24 hours, you will be told that you can resume normal activities. However, for many women this is easier said than done. Up until this point you have had virtually no control over the outcome of the cycle. In fact, what you do or don't do probably still has no impact on what happens, but now it feels different. Live embryos have been placed inside you, and you are likely to feel responsible. Your donor did her part. Your husband did his part. Your physician and embryologist did their parts. Now it *feels* like it is up to you. Not surprisingly, some recipients are tempted to go to extremes, avoiding all exercise and exertion, eating an exemplary diet, trying to stay calm and relaxed by meditating.

Try to remember that as far as anyone knows, there is really nothing you can do to increase your chances of a successful outcome. All depends on the quality of the embryos and the post-transfer hormonal support, neither of which you can control. Therefore, if you can, you should go about your regular daily activities without worrying that you will harm a potential pregnancy. If this is difficult—and we expect it may be—try to remember that staying active helps distract you a bit and this can help reduce stress. While we are not saying that stress prevents implantation, stress *does* make the experience more difficult for both you and your partner.

Extra Embryos and Cryo-preservation

One of the benefits of a fertile oocyte donor is that she is likely to produce several high quality eggs, hopefully resulting in several good quality embryos. If there are more good quality embryos than can be safely transferred at one time, there are several options to consider. It is important to think about your decision before you are faced with it. Many counselors bring up this issue during the pre-screening counseling session. All of these options for dealing with extra embryos bring with them important concerns.

Many couples have extra embryos frozen, or cryo-preserved, for later use. It is not unusual for a first cycle to fail and for a couple to achieve pregnancy on a frozen or "thaw cycle." It is also not unusual for couples to have a child, wait a year or two or three and return to have frozen embryos transferred in the hope of a second pregnancy.

Embryos are frozen in small protective straws at about -40 degrees Celsius and are kept in a liquid nitrogen tank. Research has shown that good quality embryos often freeze well, and that there are no significant differences between fresh and frozen embryos. It is unclear exactly how long embryos can be frozen. While there are still embryos out there that have remained frozen since the dawn of IVF over twenty years ago, most researchers suggest using embryos that have been frozen for less than five years. Additionally, not all embryos will be suitable for freezing. The embryologist will carefully evaluate the embryos and eliminate the poor-quality embryos that will not be able to survive the freeze and thaw procedures. Many clinics charge couples yearly or monthly storage fees for storing embryos. For those couples who cannot afford these on-going fees, maintaining frozen embryos might not be possible.

But what do you do if you complete your family during your first cycle or decide for some other reason not to use your frozen embryos? As of this writing, you have three options.

One option is to donate embryos to scientific study, such as stem cell research. This is not always easy to accomplish, but some clinics do have arrangements that facilitate donation to science. In a June 23,

2002, *Boston Globe* article, "A Worthy Gift, a Difficult Task," I (Ellen) told of Mark and Carla, a couple who worked long and hard to donate their embryos and, who, with the help of Dr. Steven Bayer of Boston-IVF, were able to donate them to a program at Harvard University for Parkinson's Research. Carla and Mark, devout Catholics, came to this decision because, "We wanted to help others but we could not imagine someone else raising our biological children."

Other couples choose embryo donation—donating embryos to another infertile couple. Although we have had limited experience with couples choosing to donate their embryos, we suspect that it is a different experience for those whose donor is a family member or friend rather than a program-recruited donor. When a sister or close friend has donated her eggs, our sense is that the embryos may feel more like a personal gift that needs to be kept in the family. In contrast, this option makes sense for egg donor parents who worked with program-recruited donors. The embryos are already partially from someone outside their genetic family so why not pass them on to someone who needs them. However, this decision brings many ethical and some legal issues, including the intent of the donor when she donated her eggs to you.

Finally, there is the option of allowing degeneration to occur. Thawed embryos usually degenerate in less than a day, and continued growth is impossible without placement into the uterus. Most often this is done in a laboratory setting; however, a few women have chosen to place these embryos into their vaginas in order to provide a more natural environment within their bodies for the embryos to degenerate. There is no chance for pregnancy to occur using this method, since the embryos cannot travel from the vagina to the uterus.

A recent development in reproductive medicine is egg freezing. On September 21, 2004, the *New York Times* reporter, Sally Wadka, reported that 100 babies have been born worldwide as a result of egg freezing. Most of these were conceived in Italy. However, egg freezing is becoming increasingly available in the U.S. As of this writing, success remains limited. Unlike sperm and embryos, eggs are difficult to cryopreserve. Eggs are filled with fluid, making it difficult to freeze them without damaging them. New advances are using a cryoprotectant formulate that helps dehydrate the watery eggs so that they can be safely frozen without forming damaging ice crystals. As of this writing, the procedures are still experimental. Dr. Marc Fritz, spokesperson for ASRM, states in the *NY Times* article, "The ASRM feels it's premature to openly market this now, but these technologies are quickly evolving and the limited body of evidence we have is encouraging. Research is also currently being conducted to find a way in which ovarian tissue or the entire ovary can be frozen in order to preserve the eggs for later use. Only time will tell if this will be successful or not."

For parents who have gone through complicated measures such as egg donation to have a child, it may be difficult to part with our embryos and decide their eventual fate. Cheryl Meyer, author of *The Wandering Uterus* (New York University Press, New York, 1997) explains that for some couples the choice may be out of their hands. Some states and countries prohibit the destruction of embryos, and others severely restrict the use of embryos for research. However, for the most part, couples with frozen embryos will eventually be forced to contemplate the fate of their "could-be" children.

Pregnancy Testing

Sophisticated blood tests make it possible to know that you are pregnant less than two weeks following transfer of embryo(s), when blood tests may be obtained to insure normal hormone levels and to detect pregnancy. Most women find the two weeks between the embryo transfer and pregnancy testing to be excruciating. Terri, age 42, explains, "I felt I was on pins and needles for the whole two weeks. I would ask myself a hundred times a day, Do I feel pregnant? Do my breasts hurt? Do I feel nauseated? I was so pre-occupied that I couldn't do anything during those two weeks except wonder if I was pregnant."

It is difficult to determine if you are actually pregnant before the initial pregnancy test. It is a cruel fact that you are still taking fertility medications, particularly progesterone, which has side-effects that mimic the early symptoms of pregnancy. So you really do not know if it is the progesterone that is making you feel sick to your stomach and bloated or if it could actually be the pregnancy that you are hoping for. As hard as it is, the best thing to do is to try to stay calm and wait for the pregnancy test.

Pregnancy is determined by analyzing the hCG level in your blood or urine. If hCG is detected, you are pregnant. The hCG level may be repeated—the value should double every 2-3 days. An ultrasound is performed 4-5 weeks after the transfer to assess the growing embryo and perhaps see a beating heart. Egg donation pregnancies are subject to the usual risks, and these risks are unrelated to the egg donation treatment. While women who have become pregnant through egg donation still may experience miscarriage, the rates for miscarriage are not any higher for the general population. This is due largely because the ovaare from younger women, typically those under 35 years old. However, if eggs from a woman over the age of 35 are used, this could increase the chance of having a miscarriage. So far, it does not seem that simply having an older uterus contributes to miscarriages although there has not been much research in this area.

And so you come to the end of an ovum donation cycle. Hopefully, this ending is also a new beginning—the beginning of your pregnancy. Or, it may represent yet another of the difficult junctures in your journey to parenthood. We hope that those of you who are not pregnant after one cycle will have embryos available for subsequent transfer or that you will feel prepared to travel down a different path. We hope, most of all, that you feel good about the efforts that you and your donor made and satisfied that you can move on without feelings of regret.

As we said earlier in this book chapter, decisions are made sequentially. What feels like the right choice for you today may not be right for you tomorrow. We remind you, again, that all you can do is make the best decisions you can at the time you make them. You may be able to revise them in the future or you may need to live with them, knowing that you did what you could, when you could, to act wisely.

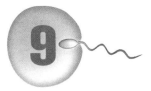

Pregnancy with Donated Eggs

You are standing in line at the ATM machine and notice that the woman in front of you is at least seven months pregnant. She looks content and cute in her maternity Capri pants and turtleneck. You leave the bank feeling sad and envious. As you are getting into your car, you see a woman walk by pushing a twin stroller. Seated in front of her are her two little boys—perhaps 7 or 8 months old—seated upright and apparently enjoying the ride. Then you drive off convinced there is practically a conspiracy of parents—they are planted everywhere to plague you.

Consider this. The woman at the ATM may be carrying a baby conceived with donated ova. The twins could very likely be donor offspring. Last week when you were in church or synagogue and a baby was christened or named, did you stop to think that those families, also, may have been helped along by other women?

We hope our point is clear: families built using donated ova look like everyone else and, in most aspects of pregnancy and parenthood, they are like everyone else. The mom you see on the playground, tirelessly pushing her little boy on the swing or the dad you see teaching his daughter to ride her first "real" bike may be parents through egg donation. The physiology of pregnancy is the same whether the child was conceived with the mom's eggs or with donated eggs; the day to day format of parenthood is the same whether the child was a spontaneous "accident" or the reward that came after months upon months of planning, cost and the coordination of two women's cycles.

In this chapter, we will begin with some of the feelings you may encounter as you make your final plans for egg donation. Then we'll move on to pregnancy and parenthood after ovum donation and will focus, because of the subject matter of this book, on the aspects of these experiences that are altered, in some way, because of egg donation. However, we remind you, yet again, that a pregnancy is a pregnancy, regardless of the ingredients that went into conception. A mom is no different a tooth fairy nor a dad, a carpool driver, because their child came to them through oocyte donation.

Before the Cycle Begins

Your journey towards parenthood continues. We're assuming that at this point, you have made a decision to move forward with egg donation. Still, questions, doubts, uncertainties and fears linger. Let's talk about them…

What You Can Do to Prepare Physically

As you approach your egg donation cycle, you will probably be wondering what control you have—if any—of its outcome. While there is nothing you can do to ensure that you will have good embryos to transfer, there are ways you can prepare for pregnancy.

"Preparing for pregnancy" may sound like a strange notion, especially if you have never been pregnant. But that is, indeed, what you are doing when you enter into an egg donor cycle—you are taking your first step towards pregnancy. What are some of the other steps you can take?

Folic Acid and Other Nutrients

Adequate intake of folic acid has been found to be an essential ingredient of a healthy pregnancy. Many obstetricians now advise that women begin taking folic acid supplements even before a pregnancy test is confirmed. Why not begin taking a pre-natal vitamin prior to embryo transfer? Doing so may help create an optimal environment for a fetus.

Diet and Nutrition

Along with vitamins and folic acid you will want to maintain a healthy diet during pregnancy. This is crucial not only for your hoped-for baby's health, but also for your own. This may feel especially important to you if you are an older expectant mother and are approaching oocyte donation with concerns about your age. A diet rich in fruits and in brightly colored vegetables, as well as in protein and calcium, can assist you in maintaining your general health. This is so helpful for active motherhood, and it will help your baby get a good start in life.

Exercise

Women undergoing fertility treatments are often afraid to exercise. Somehow they have the feeling that if they move too fast, "the embryo will fall out." Although marathon running and other strenuous exercise have been implicated in infertility because rigorous training can interfere with the menstrual cycle, there is no evidence that more moderate exercise interferes with conception. In fact, to the extent that exercise promotes general health and emotional well being, it might even help conception.

Our recommendation is that you not initiate a vigorous new exercise regimen when you are trying to conceive and that you talk with your physician about the exercise you are already doing. Most likely, he/she will encourage you to keep swimming, walking, cycling and advise caution about any exercise that involves overheating or heavy lifting.

What You Can Do to Prepare Emotionally

In addition to preparing physically for pregnancy through egg donation, you should be prepared emotionally as well. It may be helpful to anticipate feeling some—if not all—of the following…

Ambivalence

"Do we really want to do this?"

You thought you were sure. You thought you'd put doubts behind you. Now they creep in again and you wonder what they mean. Does this mean that you don't really want to attempt pregnancy through ovum donation? Does this mean you haven't "resolved" your infertility?

Please remember that it is okay to be ambivalent. In fact, it is difficult for us to imagine anyone moving forward without ambivalence. This is a huge decision you are making. Anyone who attempts pregnancy—whether on their own or through donated gametes— is making a lifelong commitment to a total stranger. How scary is that?! When you think of it that way, can you imagine someone feeling 100% convinced that they are doing the right thing?

Fear That It Won't Work

"Egg donation has great success rates." That's what you have been hearing for a long time. Now that you are about to begin a cycle, you wonder, "But what if it doesn't work? What will this mean about me if I can't even become pregnant with a donated egg?" Egg donation does not always work and when it doesn't, women tend to feel very responsible and very much to blame. They are also left feeling betrayed by their bodies, which "don't seem to work at all—even with 'good' eggs."

Women whose sisters or friends are donating to them have additional motivation for wanting a cycle to work. "After all we are putting her through, I will feel terrible if it doesn't work." If this is the situation you are in, try to remember that your sister, cousin or friend is donating because she wants you to have a chance to have a baby. The counseling she has received has amply warned her that her donation in no way guarantees a successful pregnancy.

Fear That You Will Feel Like a Fake

You've worked hard to make sense of ovum donation and to feel confident that if it works, you will be a full and legitimate mother. Still there is that old nagging fear that this hoped-for pregnancy won't feel "right," that others will somehow identify you as different, that you will feel obliged to tell everyone who notices your growing belly that "it's a donated egg."

We remind you, yet again, that you have a right to privacy and to authenticity. Your child will need to know the truth about his or her origins and he has the right to tell others his personal story. But beyond this, you have no obligation to tell anyone how you conceived. Think of it, do your "fertile friends" tell you their getting pregnant stories?

Loss

No one grows up looking forward to having a baby through egg donation. No matter how you got here, there have been losses along the way—failed cycles, pregnancy losses, perhaps the loss of your ovaries due to serious illness. Regardless of how much you may want to do it, oocyte donation is a second choice.

Looking around you at other women going through ovum donation, you are likely to notice different reactions to loss. Those of you who were older when you married or began to attempt pregnancy probably spent many years fearing that you would never have a child. For you, the opportunity for pregnancy through egg donation may feel more like a *miracle* or a *gift* than a loss. Your journey has been decidedly different from fellow travelers who may have experienced premature ovarian failure and arrived at the choice to use donated ova somewhat "shell shocked" by what happened to them. There are also those aged around 40, who come to egg donation only after years of fertility treatment, failed cycles or pregnancy losses.

Regardless of what brought you to oocyte donation, loss is part of your experience. As you move forward, loss will travel with you. We hope that your egg donor cycle will lead to the joyous arrival of a baby you will love and cherish. Still, this will not be your genetic child.

> Nancy, 37, who is eight months pregnant through donor ova put it this way, "This baby is our dream come true, and yet, I still feel that someone has died."

Your feelings of loss will shift as you make your way along your journey. The woman who spoke of such profound loss when she was eight months pregnant was giddy with delight when her son was born. Her reaction is a common one: women are relieved and thrilled when they finally give birth to a healthy baby. But things change again. Mary Fusillo, who has led a fifty member support group for donor egg moms has observed, "Feelings of loss tend to vanish after the baby arrives but return when children are around 3 years old. At that time, they've 'lost' their 'baby' and are dealing with an active toddler. Looks are solidified. Personalities emerge, and parents sometimes think 'who is this little person?'" Fusillo reminds her group participants that most parents feel some loss when their child moves out of the "baby stage," and that here, as in so many other aspects of parenthood, parents should not feel that there is something wrong with them.

Hope and Anticipation

It has probably been a long time since you have felt hopeful about pregnancy. You are now at a point where hope is appropriate and anticipation makes sense. Egg donation isn't a sure bet, but it does bring many, many babies into the world. You have reason to hope that yours will be one of them.

Pregnancy

> I wasn't able to create my baby, but I realized, as soon as I learned I was pregnant, that I would do everything in my power to make sure he had a good start in life. I had taken good care of myself with my pregnancy with my daughter years earlier, but this time I was hyper-vigilent—no caffeine, no vigorous exercise, milk ten times a day, and enough broccoli, carrots and tomatoes to feed an army of vegetarians. —Kathy, 37.

"Taking good care of my baby." These are the watch words of women pregnant with donated eggs. In addition to the caution, appreciation and sense of wonder felt by all infertile expectant moms, donor egg moms-to-be feel an added responsibility: to grow their babies well. Like Kathy, they couldn't create their children, but they can do all they can to take care of them.

Why does it feel so important? Why do women pregnant through ovum donation regard eating right and sleeping right and thinking right and moving right to be such a sacred responsibility? It is important to note that these are the feelings of many women pregnant after infertility. However, they are made all the more powerful for ovum donation moms, who feel that if they can't "create" their child, they want to do all they can to "grow him well" during pregnancy. So what can you do to help your baby get a good start in life? We turn here to common medical and emotional questions.

Obstetrical Care

You found a good reproductive endocrinologist, you worked well with him/her and now you are pregnant. At some point early in your pregnancy—usually around week 8 or 9—you will "graduate" to an obstetrician. Although congratulations are very much in order, it is not always so easy moving on. Your reproductive endocrinologist may be someone you have been working with for years. He/she knows you well, knows how special this pregnancy is, how vulnerable you feel. He/she is sensitive to privacy issues. It may have been this physician who helped you through a pregnancy loss or with the decision to turn to your sister or a friend or an anonymous donor for eggs. But reproductive endocrinologists don't usually offer obstetrical care. It's time to find a doctor who does.

Some of you may be returning to a physician you know well. Your Ob may have been your gynecologist for years. He/she may have delivered your first child, if you have secondary infertility. Or perhaps it was this doctor who did your initial infertility testing. He/she may be the one who found your reproductive endocrinologist for you.

But for those of you who do not have an Ob that you want to return to, we have some suggestions for how to choose an obstetrician:

- Talk with your RE about whether you should see a high risk Ob, and if so, whom. If you are over 45 or carrying multiples, you may well be referred to a high risk doctor. However, if you are younger, carrying a singleton and have no risks such as diabetes, you are probably headed for a regular Ob. This makes sense medically, but does it also make sense emotionally? This pregnancy is very precious to you, and you may benefit from the added attention that comes in a high risk practice.

- Seek a physician who delivers at a facility in which you have confidence. Child birth services vary from one hospital to the next, and not all medical centers have neonatal intensive care units. In addition, there are different levels of neo-natal care, with only a limited number of hospitals offering the highest level. While we hope that you deliver a full term, healthy baby, it can be reassuring to know that there is the highest level of neo-natal intensive care available, should you need it.

- Seek a physician with whom you can be open, honest and vulnerable. Obstetricians are busy, and the current medical malpractice climate has made their practices stressful. Still, there are many dedicated obstetricians who love their work and who genuinely enjoy accompanying women through pregnancy. It will be important for you to find someone who is comfortable with egg donation and who will convey to you a sense that your pregnancy, while very special, is a "regular" pregnancy.

- Pay attention to your Ob's staffing, especially around coverage. If your Ob is a sole practitioner, you will want to know who will cover for him/her should you need to call during a vacation or on a weekend. Who will deliver your baby if your doctor is unavailable? If he/she is in a group practice, you should ask whether you will be seeing different doctors for each visit, and what the chances are that one of them will be delivering your baby.

- Look also at the efficiency and lines of communication in the practice. Do you get a machine with several prompts each time you call, or do you get to talk with a real person? This may sound trivial, but if you are bleeding or have some other concern about your pregnancy, you will want to know that you can reach someone and have a prompt response to your concerns.

Prenatal Testing

You will, most likely, be undergoing some prenatal testing regardless of the age of your donor, your husband, genetic family histories etc. Hopefully, this testing will be reassuring. Ultrasound monitoring is an integral part of contemporary obstetrical care. Ultrasounds will offer you an opportunity to see your baby grow and should help make him/her more real to you. Blood tests that indicate assorted levels are within normal range should provide you with additional assurance that things are going well.

It is also possible, however, that this "routine" prenatal testing will prompt concerns. If one of the practitioners caring for you notices something that concerns him or her, additional testing may be suggested. Should this occur, it will be upsetting, but we hope that the outcome will be as it was for my (Ellen's) friends. They are both very short people, and their donor, a sister, is quite petite. During month 7 a routine ultrasound indicated the baby was "small." After a flurry of tests, the doctors concluded that there was no reason for alarm, at which point the expectant grandfather, himself a pediatrician, said, "I wished they had looked at the height of the parents before worrying that their baby was small."

During your pregnancy some of you will face questions about prenatal testing. Perhaps some concern is raised by an ultrasound or blood test. There may be another reason for testing, such as a genetic disease in the family (this will depend on the nature of the genetic disorder and of the chances that the donor, as well as the expectant father, are carriers) or because the donor (perhaps a sister or friend) is over 35, or because the expectant father is in his late 40s or 50s.

Before deciding to undergo any of the "invasive" pre-natal tests such as chorionic villus sample (CVS) or amniocentesis, you will want to carefully consider why you are having the test. Would you ever terminate a pregnancy? If so, under what conditions? If you would not, is there a reason to have the test? Some of you may feel that you would want to know, in advance, that you were expecting a child with a particular condition so that you could feel more prepared. However, you will need to consider whether the added preparation is worth the potential risks involved with prenatal testing. Each procedure carries with it some risk of pregnancy loss, a risk that will vary depending upon the test, the skill of the person performing it, and the timing of the test.

Nutrition, Exercise and General Health

As we noted earlier, you will want to take very good care of yourself during pregnancy. Remember, though, not to go overboard. Women who have gone through years of infertility and those who choose oocyte donation often make promises along the way. "If I am ever pregnant, I will eat lots of fruits and vegetables." "If I am pregnant, I won't drink or have a lot of caffeine." "If I am pregnant, I will cut back on my running, perhaps shift to walking or swimming." These may all be good ideas, but try not to take them to an extreme. Eating lots of vegetables doesn't mean ten servings of broccoli daily, nor does it mean removing every last french fry from your diet. Staying away from alcohol doesn't mean you can't drink a little champagne at your sister's wedding or enjoy some chicken cooked in wine. And limiting rigorous exercise does not suggest you should lie on the couch and meditate during the time you usually run or play tennis.

You are looking for balance. You have entered into pregnancy in a strange, high tech way, but now your body is finally doing something it was made to do: grow a baby. If you eat a good diet, get adequate rest, exercise in moderation, and take pre-natal vitamins, you will be doing what you can to give your baby a good start in life. Remember that it will be good for you and for the baby to regard this pregnancy as a natural process rather than as a scientific project.

Finding a Pediatrician

Yes, if this is your first child, you will need to find a pediatrician. This should not be a difficult task logistically, since pediatrics seems to attract some of the brightest, kindest, easiest to relate to physicians. Good pediatricians, with privileges at good hospitals, abound. Nonetheless, it may not feel so easy to make a few calls so that you can visit a few pediatric offices.

You may feel that you are being presumptuous calling a pediatrician before you have a baby. If you have had pregnancy losses along the way, it may be especially difficult. Remind yourself that this is how it's done—expectant parents (and you are one of them!) do contact pediatricians several months before their due dates. After all, your child's physician will need to examine him or her shortly after birth.

What To Look For

- Your pediatrician should be affiliated with a hospital or medical center with an excellent pediatrics department.

- Your pediatrician should have a well run office that you can get into and out of without expecting to wait hours in the waiting room.

- Your pediatrician or his staff should be available for a call back for an urgent phone call.

- Your pediatrician should have a nursing staff that is accessible, answers questions and helps you with routine concerns.

- Your pediatrician should take time with you, answer questions, and help you feel like a competent and informed parent.

- You should be able to talk comfortably from the start about donor conception. You should tell prospective doctors your history on first meeting. Doing so will accomplish two things—you will know, right then and there, if this is someone you can feel comfortable with; and second, you won't have a secret that you might someday have to "reveal" to your doctor.

This leads us into the other part of the pregnancy experience—your feelings.

Who Am I Expecting? And How Much Will This Baby Be "Mine"?

All parents have ideas of what their children will be like. Most base these expectations on their own appearance, interests, abilities. Tall parents expect tall children, engineers expect little engineers, women with curls expect babies with curls, and neatness is expected to beget neatness. Rarely, if ever, do parents get the children about whom they fantasize. Almost always, parents come to accept and often celebrate the ways their real children differ from their fantasy children.

Women who know their donors inevitably assume that their children will in some way resemble the donor. After all, if you didn't expect the donor's appearance, intelligence, personality and health to express themselves in the child, you wouldn't care where the egg came from. But you *do* care and you *do* expect to see the donor in your child. If she is your sister, this will generate one set of feelings, and if she is someone you found through a donor agency, selected from her pictures and questionnaire and met only once, other feelings will arise.

What if you never met your donor? Never spoke with her by phone? Although openness is becoming increasingly common, there remain many women who carry babies created from the eggs of strangers. If the donor is a stranger, you may wonder if the baby, also, will feel like a stranger. One woman, who had a child from a donated egg several years ago and never saw a photo of the donor recalls having images of something out of the movie *Alien*. The film was popular at the time and she remembers thinking that an alien would "pop out of my stomach."

Women pregnant with a child through egg donation often describe going through a process of questioning the "mine-ness" of their baby. They describe wondering, especially at the beginning of the pregnancy, whether this can really be their baby. Fortunately this question, which can be torturous for some, seems to diminish over time.

In the words of Sandra, 38 and an expectant mom, "*Mother* has taken on a whole new wonderful meaning for me. It is not about conceiving anymore. It is not about genes. It's about nurturing a child, it's about my blood supply, what I eat, how my body takes care of the child growing within it. Yes, this will be my child."

Marriage and Family Therapist, Carole Lieber Wilkins observes, "*Mother* and *father* and *parent* are verbs as well as nouns. We become a parent by parenting. A father is only a dad when he fathers, not when he donates sperm."

Therapist Peg Beck observes that women expectant with a donated egg go through a process of what she calls, "making the baby theirs." Beck feels this often comes when the woman experiences pregnancy symptoms, especially the uncomfortable ones such as nausea. She smiles and says, "A few nights in a row of throwing up go a long way towards convincing a woman that she is the mom. This little being that is wreaking such havoc on her life is indeed her baby."

Nurse Clinician Mary Fusillo offers some intriguing ideas about how a mother through ovum donation makes the baby hers. Fusillo tells the story of meeting two women who had the same donor, a woman Fusillo had also met. The two recipients were as different from each other as anyone could imagine. One was very tall, large-boned, with bright red curly hair. The other was short, petite, with straight dark hair and dark eyes. As luck would have it, the tall red head gave birth to twin boys and the petite, dark haired woman had twin girls. In each instance, the children bore a remarkable resemblance to their mom.

How does this happen? When asked, Fusillo offers explanations that range from the divine to the scientific. "I have different ways of understanding and explaining it. I am a person of faith, and I feel the Lord acts in amazing ways. God gives each person the child they were supposed to have. But I also feel there may be some scientific explanation. I'm thinking specifically about mitochondrial DNA. It's in every cell in our bodies. So think of it—a baby grows in a woman's uterus, shares her body and connects with her cells for nine months. Something goes on there. I know the scientists would 'poo poo' it but I think that the baby may really take on some features of the mom."

In fact, some children conceived through donated eggs have a strong physical resemblance to their mothers and others do not. What we feel is most significant about Fusillo's observations is that they speak to how much parents and their children belong together. In my work with adoptive parents (Ellen), I have had Caucasian parents of Chinese children tell me that people comment on how their daughter looks like them and I can remember one fair haired mother of a dark skinned child from Colombia who said that other parents in her daughter's 3rd grade class were surprised to hear she joined their family through adoption. "But she looks just like you," this mom remembers them saying. What these comments do, we believe, is reaffirm the bonds of family and the "rightness" of particular people being together.

Bonding through the Donor

Whether the donor is a sister, a friend or a stranger you have met once, your positive feelings about her will help you bond in utero with your child. Shelley Smith, Director of the Egg Donor program in Los Angeles, observes, "I see people falling in love with their donors and then, when they become pregnant, their hearts expand to love their unborn child as well."

. . . .

Meet Carrie...

"We're excited, and I think meeting Lisa, our donor, helped a lot in getting us there. The first few months of the pregnancy were difficult, because it was so scientific and so " step by step." First, Lisa had to pass all her screening tests. Step Two "was having her take the medications. Then Step Three, the retrieval. Step Four, fertilization. Step Five, embryo transfer. Step Six, first pregnancy test. And it has continued from there...more pregnancy tests, an ultrasound, then another. Only in recent weeks have I begun to feel really excited. Our daughter has been moving a lot, and when she does, I fast forward to her birth, to holding her, to naming her. I think it helps a lot to have met Lisa. Because I met her, I am able to picture a real baby, to anticipate her arrival with joy, to truly believe that this little girl growing inside me will be a totally lovable little girl."

This is Carrie. She's five months pregnant with her first donor egg baby. Carrie was a career woman. Big time. The fourth of five daughters from a spirited Italian family, Carrie went to New York City following graduation from college and set her sights on a successful career in advertising. Through a lot of hard work and a little luck, Carrie rose in her career. By the time she was in her mid-30s Carrie was earning a high salary and she was celebrated and respected in her field. At that time in her life, Carrie, who had always assumed she would be a mother, gave little thought to getting pregnant or to finding a husband, for that matter.

Along came Carrie's late 30s and things began to change. "I wasn't really conscious of it at the time," Carrie recalls," but I was thinking more seriously about the men I dated. In the past, I had simply been interested in a good time, but when I met Franklin I was looking for something more, whether I knew it or not!" Franklin is Carrie's husband. They met at a tennis club, in the lounge after Carrie had won a very competitive match.

"He said to me, 'You look wiped, can I buy you a drink?' And the rest is history."

Well, not exactly. The history of Carrie and Franklin's courtship and subsequent marriage is pretty straightforward. They began dating immediately after the tennis club lounge encounter and were married a year later. Within weeks of their wedding, Carrie discovered she was pregnant. When she went to her doctor, she learned that she was actually further along than she'd thought. "I guess I was so caught up in the wedding plans that I didn't notice my period hadn't come. Or I assumed it was late because so much was going on. When the doctor told me I was nearly twelve weeks along, I wasn't all that surprised. In lots of ways it fit. I'd been tired and queasy around the wedding, but figured it was the wedding. I'd had a little trouble fitting into the top of my wedding gown but figured I had been eating too much because I was stressed. And yes, I'd been 'peeing' a lot, as well, but again, I chalked it all up to wedding stress. My first trimester, wedding stress!"

Sadly, Carrie's pregnancy ended in a late miscarriage at 15 weeks. Following this loss, baby fever struck. Carrie remembers it being somewhat like a lightening bolt. Suddenly, the executive turned devoted wife was feeling that she needed a baby.

Franklin was reluctant. The couple was only recently married; they had spent their entire married life either expecting a baby or dealing with pregnancy loss. He was not so eager to try again so soon. "But I had just turned 40," Carrie says, "And there was no waiting."

Carrie prevailed, and the couple began trying actively to have a child. Although Carrie knew that her advanced age could be a problem, she assumed it would not be because she had conceived the surprise baby so easily. What Carrie and Franklin could never have anticipated, as they began trying on their own and eventually moved on to a fertility specialist, was that they would devote a good portion of their time and energies over the next three years to high tech infertility treatment. Their efforts would include four IVF cycles, three of which would result in early pregnancy losses.

"When my doctor first mentioned using a donor's eggs, I thought she was crazy. Why would I possibly want to have a baby through egg donation? I had conceived a baby, and as far as I was concerned, I could do so again. Remember, I'm a very determined person and I'm used to working hard for what I want. *I'll try harder,* I quietly thought to myself. *I'll figure out a way to make this work.*"

It didn't work. Carrie, the determined former career woman, confronted the lesson that torments so many people going through infertility: becoming pregnant probably has nothing to do with hard work (or being deserving or fairness or…). After Carrie's third miscarriage, she and Franklin began talking about trying to identify a "Plan B." Was adoption the way to build their family, or should they visit the subject of oocyte donation, something Carrie had initially vehemently opposed?

"When we began talking about it, I was surprised by my reaction. Very surprised. I'd assumed that it would seem totally weird—something I could not imagine ever doing. But when Franklin pointed out to me that I would get to carry his baby, that I'd be pregnant, that I'd get to nurse the baby, and that I would be the one bringing a new life into the world, it felt different. I can't say I jumped right into egg donation, but I was certainly more prepared to give it a careful look."

Carrie and Franklin did take a careful look at ovum donation. They did a lot of talking together and they talked with couples who had children with the help of donors. They talked about whether there were any family members they could ask to donate, and when they concluded there were none, they looked into program-recruited donation. "We knew it was important to us that our child be able to know where he or she came from. So we looked only into programs that would allow us to meet or contact our donor."

Carrie and Franklin were lucky. They identified a program they liked, found a donor—Lisa—and met with her for two warm and sharing hours just prior to beginning the cycle. Medically things went well. Carrie conceived on the first cycle, and her pregnancy proceeded uneventfully. The couple learned, several weeks ago, that she is carrying a girl.

But what about expectant moms who don't get to meet their donors? How does the anonymity of their situation impact bonding? It seems that the most important ingredient is positive feelings about the donor. You don't have to meet her to feel that she is a really good person and for you to feel your child is coming from a good place.

> I loved the way she wrote about her family and particularly, her close relationship with her sister. There were other prospective donors who looked more like me, but we chose this particular donor because family is so important to me and this was something I wanted to have in common with her. —Helena, 43 and 6 months pregnant

Privacy Issues

When you are the midst of infertility treatment, you give up all privacy. As Lucy, 33, put it when she was introduced to yet another physician in her infertility clinic, "Now I guess there is no one left in all of Minneapolis who has not seen my vagina!"

Her comment illustrates two things: women, in particular, feel like they are surrendering all physical privacy when going through infertility treatment. The other message she conveys is that it helps to keep laughing!

Being pregnant means being very public about a very private matter: you are having a baby. Being pregnant with a donated egg raises new questions of privacy. Does anyone need to know the origins of your pregnancy? If so, who? We feel that your obstetrician and your child's future pediatrician will need to know. Probably your family and some close friends. But does the woman next to you in prenatal yoga class, or the couple you stop to talk with on the way out of your childbirth class need to know? Would you be inclined to tell them other private information?

Karen, 40, pregnant with a donated egg, told her family she was pregnant. When her father asked, "Is it donor egg?" she replied, "Does it really matter?" Her father said, "No" and discussion ended there.

The challenge for those who become parents using donated eggs comes in claiming a right to privacy, but distinguishing it from secrecy. We would venture to say that there is no reason why someone visibly pregnant should feel compelled to tell people who comment on the pregnancy or congratulate her that she conceived with donor egg. It is simply a private matter.

On the other hand, your obstetrician and your child's pediatrician should know the origins of the pregnancy. Why? Because the physician who treats you will make certain assumptions based on who you are and on your health. For example, the physician who recommends an amnio because you are 40 years old, would probably have a different recommendation if you told her your pregnancy came from eggs of a donor who was under 30. Similarly, the pediatrician will seek family medical history in order to offer informed care for his/her new little patient. You will want to explain to the pediatrician that you are providing your donor's medical history. Don't be surprised, however, if he/she also wants some medical history on your side as well. As an adoptive mother (Ellen), I once had that experience and asked the physician about it. He answered that he feels environment, nutrition, lifestyle all influence health and disease.

The Impact of High Tech Conception

Women pregnant after IVF, whether it be with their own eggs or with donated eggs, are often surprised to find that the old adage, "You can't be a little bit pregnant" doesn't seem to pertain to them. In fact, from the time that there are fertilized embryos in a lab, they feel "a little bit pregnant." They are "a little bit more pregnant" when there is a positive pregnancy test and this "little bit" increases as their pregnancy hormones rise. Often by the time the first trimester has passed, they can drop the "little bit" and finally think of themselves as "pregnant."

Conceiving through donated eggs may contribute to the sense of disconnect that women feel early in an assisted pregnancy. Just think of all the steps one goes through to achieve an egg donation pregnancy and it is easy to see why the news that a pregnancy test is positive may feel like yet another small step forward towards a goal.

The good news is that women do begin to feel "really pregnant" somewhere along the way. Best we can tell, it is usually around the beginning of the second trimester that women pregnant with donated eggs really begin to think, "Yes, I am pregnant. Yes, there may really be a baby at the end of this journey." Many women report that the pregnancy feels real to them when they feel the baby move.

One of the reasons that the role of technology diminishes as the pregnancy progresses is that pregnant women are referred on from reproductive medicine programs to obstetrics programs at around week 9 or 10. Most who are carrying singletons land in the offices of regular ob-gyns. Difficult as this may be to believe, obstetricians and their staffs regard pregnancy as an entirely natural, commonplace, uneventful experience. While it may be a bit startling to encounter a calm, "nothing to worry about" welcome, this may be the beginning of you feeling like a "normal, pregnant woman." The words, *Everything looks fine, take your pre-natal vitamins and I will see you in a month"* mark a shift from the step by step crawl towards pregnancy that you've experienced over the past many months or even years.

Los Angeles Marriage and Family Therapist, Carole Lieber Wilkins, who has worked with many women pregnant after egg donation, observes that many of the women she meets with feel a sense of panic rather than relief when an obstetrician takes an "everything's normal" approach. She reports that some of her patients wish they could "have my own personal ultrasound machine" in order to continue to be closely monitored.

Not everyone is referred to a regular ob-gyn and not everyone's donor egg pregnancy is uneventful. If you find yourself carrying twins, you may decide that you are more comfortable with a high risk obstetrician, particularly someone affiliated with a hospital that has a level 3 neonatal unit (this is the highest level of infant care and important in multiple gestation when babies come early). If you have diabetes, an "incompetent" cervix, or any other condition that puts you at risk for complications during your pregnancy, you will probably be encouraged to work with a high risk ob.

Being in the care of a high risk obstetrician can be a mixed experience for women pregnant with a donated ova. On the one hand, it can be comforting and reassuring to feel that you are going to receive that extra measure of care. You don't really feel "just like everyone else" and so it can be helpful to know that you won't be treated "just like everyone else." On the other hand, there is something reassuring about the calm, "there is nothing different about your pregnancy" approach that many women with donor egg pregnancies receive.

Fear of Complications Due to Age

Although many women turn to donated ova in their 30s and some, in their 20s, a growing percentage of ovum donor moms are over 40. As part of the pre-ovum donation medical and psychological counseling, older would-be moms are advised of the added risks that come with age. Older women experience more gestational diabetes, pregnancy induced high blood pressure (which may lead to pre-eclampsia or toxemia) and preterm labor with their pregnancies. How people hear and process this information varies from one person to the next and may change during pregnancy.

We have found that women who are 42 or so when they become pregnant through egg donation seem to have far fewer concerns—and understandably so—than their fellow travelers who are past 45. Since many women are having babies in their early 40s and since spontaneous pregnancy can occur during this time, pregnancy at 41 or 42 or 43 has become almost routine. Women can easily spot women in their age group at birthing classes or wheeling a stroller in the park.

When a woman is pregnant in her late 40s through donated eggs, she has stepped outside of "normal reproduction." There may be compelling reasons to do this—a significantly younger husband, the desire to have a sibling for their two- or three-year-old—but it is still new reproductive territory. Understandably, women may be tempted to overlook known and imagined medical risks because they feel such a deep desire to have a baby. However, once pregnant, anxieties may set in.

> Suzette, who had her first child (spontaneously) at 41, turned to donor eggs at 45 and found herself worrying a lot about her age. Specifically, she was worried that she was simply too old to safely carry and deliver a baby. When she told her physician of her concerns, he repeatedly tried to reassure her, saying that she was in great shape and should be fine. Nonetheless, Suzette, who had not personally known anyone who had had a baby at 45, remained concerned that her "organs would shut down." In the end, she had a successful and medically uneventful pregnancy, but she remained filled with fear until she was holding her son.

Ambivalence

Therapist Peg Beck notes that there are several points along the oocyte donation journey when people experience bursts of ambivalence. These often come when people first look at/talk with prospective donors, when they make arrangements to move forward, when they undergo embryo transfer, and when they learn that the pregnancy test is positive. However, the most fertile ground for ambivalence is during the pregnancy. You may feel excited, relieved, optimistic, even elated and still experience times of uncertainty, of wondering if you have done the right thing, of wishing you could have your regular, non-pregnant body back.

We realize that we probably sound strange telling you that it is really okay—actually normal and healthy—to feel some ambivalence during pregnancy. After all, you worked so very hard to make this pregnancy happen, you knew you wanted it, you made all sorts of bargains with yourself, your partner, even God. *What's wrong with me*, you wonder, *that I'm not elated about this pregnancy 100% of the time?*

Ambivalence is a natural part of impending parenthood—through spontaneous pregnancy or donor gametes or adoption. Who wouldn't feel some ambivalence about having a little being take over one's body? Who wouldn't wonder about how the baby now surely on his/her/their way will change the family? Who wouldn't ask themselves—at least on occasion—whether this was the "right" decision?

Couples who become pregnant spontaneously generally feel entitled to their ambivalence. They can label the pregnancy an accident or they can protest, "We didn't know it would happen so quickly" (readers, we know how you feel about them!) or they can simply say, "We wanted to get pregnant, but now we're having a second thought or two."

Infertile couples rarely feel entitled to their ambivalence. Years ago, there was an ad for Toyota automobiles that said, "You wanted it, you got it, Toyota." In those days there were a fair number of people pregnant after infertility nicknaming their growing fetuses "Toyota." They wanted it, they got it…there was nothing to complain about.

Egg donation leaves even less room for ambivalence. Seeking and securing an egg donor and going through all that is involved in terms of time, energy, finances and, above all, emotional gymnastics leaves people little room to think *I'm not sure* or *Maybe I don't want to do this after all.*

Ambivalence is part of pregnancy. It is also part of parenthood. We expect that you will adore and cherish the child you give birth to, but there will be moments (maybe hours or even days) when you wonder, *Was it really worth it?* or think wistfully of the days when you had the freedom to do whatever you wanted without thinking about childcare, naps, school vacations schedules and the lot.

What to Tell People Now That You Are Pregnant

Finding out that you are pregnant is a very exciting and nervous time in your life, especially after you have struggled to conceive for so long. Once you've had that positive pregnancy test you are faced with many decisions, among which are when you should tell, whom you should tell, and how much you should tell. Some people believe in telling only their immediate family for fear of early pregnancy loss. Others believe that they will tell anyone and everyone, reasoning that if they did have an early pregnancy loss they would need the support of others. Most people fall into a middle ground.

Many people decide to wait to reveal their joyous news until after the first trimester, when the miscarriage rates drop drastically. Others open up only as their abdomens begin to grow. Sometimes it can be difficult not to tell for a variety of reasons. Severe nausea and vomiting may make it fairly obvious that something is going on, as will multiple visits to care providers. If you are intent on not telling everyone right away, then you need to be conscious of your actions. It's also very hard not to scream with delight when you are in an emotional high.

> "My husband and I couldn't wait to get home and start calling people. I realize that conventional wisdom is to wait until you are three months along to tell people, but when people know that you are going through this process, they also know that you are going to find out around a certain time frame whether treatments worked or not," says Jennifer, age 39, now mom of twins.

Finding Support

Often women who have become pregnant through egg donation say, "I don't feel part of the fertile world or the infertility world—I just feel different." You may actually find that relationships established with other infertile couples that you have met throughout your journey are threatened by the news of your pregnancy. It is important for couples to have discussions about the issues of pregnancy early within your friendships, addressing the need for honesty about conflicting feelings of joy and jealousy which may occur with pregnancy. The transition from the infertile to the fertile world can be scary. You should try to maintain as many support systems as possible.

One major transition from the infertile to fertile world involves the right of passage for nearly all first time parents—the childbirth class. Most obstetricians (as well as insurance companies) recommend that first time parents participate in some sort of childbirth education class. Typically, childbirth classes include several weeks of classes meant to prepare you for the impending delivery of the baby. Not only do you learn about the biology of labor and delivery and coping methods for the pain of childbirth, but also you are given the opportunity to meet and get to know other expectant parents with due dates similar to yours. As you introduce yourselves to one another, you will invariably hear the details of their pregnancy and often even stories about how their child was conceived. Consequently, you will find that most of these parents-to-be became pregnant without complications, the "old-fashioned" way. However, it is important to point out that ARTs, including egg donation, are becoming more and more common in our society. It is very likely that you will meet others in your group who also went to great lengths to have a baby. In fact, a few hospitals around the country are offering special childbirth classes specifically for couples who became pregnant with the assistance of infertility treatments and ARTs. Regardless, this issue may stir up feelings and emotions for you. It is important for you to think about your own pregnancy story and how you want to introduce it to others.

Making a Grand Entrance

For those women who have experienced prolonged infertility and successful treatment, natural childbirth may seem less important than for others. The decision to undertake a Caesarean section is usually reached by taking into account a combination of factors. A history of infertility, particularly when pregnancy has been achieved after many years and with high-tech treatment, is considered to be one factor in favor of operative delivery. For ARTs, maternal age tends to be higher and there may be concern about the function of the placenta even with pregnancies from donated eggs. Multiple pregnancy may be an additional reason for opting for Caesarean section.

There is some anecdotal evidence that suggests that the Caesarean section rate for women conceiving with ARTs is higher than for those that conceive spontaneously. However, the individual couple, together with their obstetrician, must ultimately decide on their preferred type of delivery—natural childbirth, vaginal delivery with pain medication (including epidural) or a c-section. Safety and patient satisfaction are the most important considerations when making this important decision. No matter what you decide, you may want to take a childbirth class and make sure you read several books and articles about labor and delivery so that you can make the most educated decision and be as prepared as possible.

As Ann, age 44, writes, "Nine days after his due date, my son, Ian, made his much anticipated entrance. I was tense and worried about his well-being throughout the delivery and consequently unable to rely on any of the relaxation techniques that had served me so well (before). When it finally came time to push, I didn't care if I ended up with a ten inch tear; I wanted him to have him safely in my arms. He took his first breath and made those precious newborn snuffling sounds. I thought I would cry, but I was strangely numb—exhausted not only from the delivery, but also from the nine months that preceded it. It wasn't until a few hours later when he and I were finally alone that I was able to celebrate his safe arrival with tears of joy."

Breastfeeding

There is no data that suggests that giving birth to a child concieved through egg donation negatively affects breastfeeding. If you desire, you should be able to successfully breastfeed. Because breastfeeding can sometimes be difficult or overwhelming for any new mother, it is best to talk to a lactation consultant for advice. Lactation consultants are health care providers that are specially trained and certified in breastfeeding education. They can be found in nearly any community and often work in doctors' offices, hospitals or in private practice. In addition, you may want to enroll in a breastfeeding class before the baby arrives so that you will know what to expect with breastfeeding.

Bringing Baby Home

Bringing home baby is the culmination of years of waiting and emotional and physical exhaustion. It can be difficult to balance your new life in healthy ways. Joan, age 43, hardly put her baby down for the first seven months of his life. She took him to her office and worked while he slept. She made calls with him on her lap. She carried him in a Snuggli as she attended important meetings. Joan held her baby so much she even needed cortisone treatments for arm pain.

For some parents, fears about their children's unusual conception still lingers in the back of the minds. One such mom, Anna, age 39, explained, "I used to fear at the end of the day when my twins were asleep, that their 'real' parents were going to show up at the front door to take them home any minute—I truly couldn't believe they belonged to me and my husband."

On of the most common characteristics of couples who struggled with infertility over a long period of time is overindulgence. Take the case of 39-year-old Gail, who adopted a baby girl from Russia after years of failed infertility treatments.

> Each day on her way to work, Gail stops at a children's clothing store. "If I see a pair of shoes for $80, I buy it for her. I spoil her completely," Gail says. For her child's second birthday, she and her husband rented a restaurant and invited 120 guests. "We cherish her," she says. "There's nothing we won't do for her."
>
> Gail indulges her daughter in time as well as material items. Since she works full time, she spends her weekends "sitting and playing with her, reading to her." She can't stand letting her daughter cry. "I'll always be overcompensating," she says. "I don't think I'll forget [the infertility] so easily."

A close cousin to overindulgence is over protectiveness. Infertile parents of babies and toddlers may baby-proof their houses to the hilt and install monitors in every crevice. The theme of loss—real, feared and imagined—runs through the experience of most infertile parents.

"I'll never lose the bond I had with the infertile community, but that doesn't mean I feel I can share my joys and frustrations of parenting with them," says Stephanie, age 43. Hopefully, you will have found new support systems that will help you as you enter this new stage of parenthood, such as through your birth preparation or breastfeeding class, new mom exercise class, or even new mom support groups.

Some Tips for When You Are Pregnant

You May Want To Keep a Journal

Making regular entries into a journal can be helpful in several ways. For one, it will give you a place to put thoughts and feelings. This will help you preserve memories you don't want to lose and to organize feelings that may seem scattered and intense. You can record them, read them over a day or week or month later and, perhaps, see them from a different perspective. Your journal can also serve as a repository of information that you might otherwise risk losing. For example, if you have a meeting with your donor, you can record specific information she gives you about her history and that of her family and you can preserve a description of your meeting—where you met, what you thought when you saw her, how you felt sitting there and talking with someone who was giving you such an incredible gift.

Save Your Child's Story

Remember that children love to hear stories about themselves and in particular, the story of how they were born. Photos make it even more fun. For parents concerned about how their child will make sense of it all, what could be better than having a visual diary of your journey to parenthood through donated oocytes. Take photos of the people at the program, meetings with the donor if you do this, a visit to the donor's city, etc. Keep copies of ultrasounds.

Before and during your pregnancy, obtain as much information as you can about your donor. Make sure that photos, a biography, letters and all else that you can gather are duplicated and kept in two places—a safe deposit box or something else that is completely secure—and someplace easily accessible in your home.

Psychologist Maggie Kirkman, PhD, a researcher at the Key Centre for Women's Health in Society at the University of Melbourne in Australia, advises parents to make a book about each of their donor-conceived children as a "contribution to explaining their origins and to developing their own stories." She recommends accompanying photographs, with a text that emphasizes how much the parents wanted a baby and how happy the birth has made them. "It can explain that all babies need an egg and sperm to grow and that Mum had no eggs. The story of finding the donor can be told, as well as the role of the doctor in putting the egg and sperm together. A book may serve several purposes: it allows parents to work on an acceptable story at their own pace, which may in turn play a role in clarifying their own understanding of what it means to them; it encourages children to take the initiative in talking about their own stories and to indulge in the repetition that children enjoy; it is a fixed point to which they can refer when matters become confused; it can give children pleasure and reassurance to see their own name and story in a book; and it has a status of legitimacy, like other books, that oral accounts may lack. This may not work for all parents or all children, but it is a technique that several families in my research found to be helpful."

Take Lots of Pictures of Yourself (or Your Wife) Pregnant

For moms through egg donation the profoundly intimate experience of pregnancy is of paramount importance, and photos of that experience can be validating and affirming. You and your child will be physically connected from the time the embryo(s) is transferred to you. The pictures taken of you with your child growing inside you will provide wonderful memories of your union.

Find Some Traveling Companions

It will be helpful for you to know other women who are pregnant, especially others who are pregnant through egg donation. You may have made some friends in a support group or from your physician's waiting room and be pregnant at the same time as some of them. If this isn't the case, we encourage you to reach out. There are on-line support groups (complete with "virtual showers!") and groups through RESOLVE and AFA and IAAC.

Do not feel that you need to limit yourself to groups made up only of others pregnant with donor eggs or pregnant after infertility. Although it may frustrate you to hear other women worrying about stretch marks or complaining about how much weight they've gained, this is normal pregnancy talk, and yours is a normal pregnancy. You may not always feel it, but you have finally joined the club.

Multiple Gestation

Whenever someone undergoes IVF (or other fertility treatments), multiple gestation is a possibility. Some intended parents feel so strongly about having one baby—or one at a time—that they restrict embryo transfer to one embryo. Yes, that one embryo could split and result in identical twins, but this is a long shot. When two (or more) embryos are transferred, twins are not a long shot.

Not me, you think. *Not us. We're so infertile, we could never have twins.* Indeed many women who become pregnant with donated eggs carry singleton pregnancies, but there are many twin pregnancies and some triplets as well. According to the the 2001 Centers for Disease Control and Prevention statistics about ARTs, about 42% of fresh embryos from donor eggs resulted in multiples, while frozen embryos from donor eggs resulted in multiples 28% of the time. The news that you are carrying more than one can baby generate an assortment of feelings, questions and concerns.

Disbelief

No one really believes they will be pregnant with twins, let alone a higher order multiple pregnancy. Remember Carla and Rob, whom we met in Chapter 1. In their words, "We weren't surprised to learn it was twins, we were shocked!" And that is how it is for many of you—you've had ample preparation for the possibility of multiples, but when it *really* happens, you're in shock.

Why is it that people are so startled when they've been so "well prepared" for the possibility of multiples? It seems that for many, it is nearly impossible to really hear a physician when he or she discusses this risk with them.

Carole Lieber Wilkins reports that some of the women she has worked with who have had triplet or higher pregnancies found themselves in very difficult positions on the morning of the embryo transfer. At a time of heightened anxiety and on medications that affected their mood, many had to make a decision about "that extra embryo that doesn't look good."

"The physician will suggest 'we put it in anyway' because it looks 'bad', and then that embryo ends up being the triplet or the quad," Lieber Wilkins says. She encourages her patients to be conservative and to consider hypothetical situations in advance. For example, one couple may decide that they will transfer no more than two embryos regardless of what the physician recommends. Another couple might decide to defer to the physician's recommendation up to three embryos, but no more.

Fear of Loss

When you began your cycle, you probably weren't thinking about twins. You knew you would be thrilled if you were able to take one baby home, and if you thought about twins at all, it was as a potential bonus—something, perhaps, to dream about but not to count on. Now, if you are pregnant with two or three babies, your expectations have changed. You went from hoping for one to counting on two (or three, if it is triplets). *How wonderful it will be if all goes well*, you think. *But what if it doesn't? What if we lose one of the babies along the way? What if we lose all? What if they are born too early and there are problems?*

Without a doubt, a multiple pregnancy brings with it certain risks. You may experience a partial loss, either early in the pregnancy or later on. This may feel like a disenfranchised grief—you wanted one, you're getting one, so what are you sad about? The answer is that you are sad because your perspective changed once you learned you were carrying more than one. It is entirely natural for expectant parents to attach to the idea of twins and to want to celebrate the specialness of this pregnancy, the advantages of "two for the price of one," and the excitement of "instant family."

Feelings about Multiples

Although many people are delighted to learn that they are pregnant with twins, not every expectant parent feels this way. There are a number of reasons why women pregnant after donor ova hope to learn they are carrying one baby and why some hope that a multiple gestation may reduce on its own early in the pregnancy.

If you are concerned about your ability to successfully carry a pregnancy to term, you may be particularly alarmed by the thought of carrying more than one baby. It is all well and good, you think, for people to celebrate "instant family," but your goal is a healthy baby, and that seems more likely with a singleton pregnancy. It is very scary to think that you may have gone through so much effort, anxiety, emotional and financial expense to find yourself with a high risk pregnancy.

Because transferring two embryos can result in a twin pregnancy (a triplet pregnancy in which an embryo splits is possible, though rare), couples going through ovum donation should think very carefully about how many embryos they want to have transferred. If you really want to avoid multiples, don't be afraid to ask your physician to limit the transfer to one embryo. He/she may caution you against this, telling you that you are reducing your chance of pregnancy, but it is ultimately your right to make a decision you can live with. Most physicians do not transfer more than two or three embryos.

Privacy Issues

To the extent that women pregnant with donated eggs wish to maintain some privacy, a multiple gestation challenges this. Twin pregnancies generate questions about the use of fertility drugs, and once the babies are born, all the more attention comes your way. Strangers on the street or in the supermarket have no qualms about asking you if you took fertility medications. And even those who refrain from such intrusive comments feel fully entitled to comment on the twins, to ask how old they are or where they were born or how you manage with two. Such questions have nothing to do with egg donation, but they are an intrusion on your privacy.

> Natalie, 42, was self-conscious about the fact that her twins did not look like her in any way. People often commented on this, and when they did, she often felt that they were "suspecting it was egg donation." Although it was difficult, the mom was able to handle these incidents. Then something happened which proved much more challenging. "I went to a store and a woman said, 'Are they yours?' I was used to that and had learned to simply smile and say a proud, 'Yes." But the woman went on and said, 'Your grandchildren are beautiful.' I felt like I wanted to fall off the face of the earth."

Another privacy concern comes for parents who have children through two different donors or who have a biological child and then a child through donated ova. Parents worry that if their children look different from one another and people take note of it (which they inevitably do), the family's privacy will keep being challenged. We remind people that even within "regular" biological families, siblings often look very different from one another. When people comment on these differences, they are simply making superficial observations, and there is no need to respond to them with anything of substance. It is really no different, we feel, than if they were to say, "Your baby looks young to already be walking," or "Your daughter has beautiful eyes," or "Your twins look so cute sleeping next to each other." You say "Yes" or "Okay." or "Thank you" and move on.

Pregnancy Loss

"It's nature's way; it wasn't meant to be." All too often women and men who lose a pregnancy hear this pronouncement. The words sting, especially when the pregnancy, so quickly dismissed, was long sought and deeply cherished.

Pregnancy loss after egg donation brings added dimensions of pain. In addition to the loss that any expectant parent feels when the baby who was beginning to make their heart sing is gone, parents through oocyte donation face an array of questions ranging from, "Did we force something to happen that really was not meant to be?" and "Was I diligent enough in taking care of myself?" to "Should we try again with a different donor?" to "Can we afford to try again?" to "How much more frustration and loss can we endure?" to "Maybe it really wasn't an egg problem after all?" and "Maybe there is something so wrong with me and my body that I can't carry a baby, even with 'good' eggs?" We will take a look at each of these questions, but before we do, we need to take a moment to briefly define the various forms of pregnancy loss.

Miscarriage

First Trimester Loss

Miscarriage, also known as spontaneous abortion, is usually defined as the loss of a pregnancy in its first twenty weeks. The vast majority of these losses occur within the first twelve weeks, making miscarriage after the first trimester much less common. In fact, most miscarriages occur before eight weeks of pregnancy, but since many women miscarry before they even know they are pregnant, the prevalence of early miscarriage is under reported. Although miscarriage can be caused by chromosomal problems in the embryo or by problems in the uterine environment, current understanding is that most of the very early losses are the result of chromosomal abnormalities. Problems in the uterine environment are less often a cause of first trimester losses. However, some uterine factors, such as Asherman's syndrome, a scarring of the uterus, can cause miscarriage by preventing an embryo from implanting properly.

Placental problems can also cause early miscarriages, but they are much more often implicated in later losses. Placenta previa is a condition in which the placenta attaches to part or all of the cervix. Abruptio placentae is a condition in which the placenta separates from the uterine wall. Losses can also occur when the placenta does not function properly and denies the fetus essential nutrients. Early losses can also be caused by systemic diseases such as thyroid disease, diabetes, and autoimmune conditions in the mother. However, as with placental problems, these illnesses are more likely to cause loss later in pregnancy.

Contrary to what women have been told their entire lives, you actually can be "a little bit pregnant." The "little bit pregnant" that no one ever heard of is known as chemical or biochemical pregnancy, an experience that appears to be a direct outgrowth of assisted reproduction. In biochemical pregnancy, the first pregnancy test comes back indicating a very low positive, yet subsequent pregnancy tests reveal that the pregnancy has not progressed. Physicians believe that a biochemical pregnancy occurs when an embryo stops growing and developing before it ever really implants in the uterine wall.

Second Trimester Loss

Late miscarriages, like early ones, can be caused by either maternal or fetal factors. The most common cause of late miscarriage is a maternal factor involving premature dilation of the cervix, sometimes as early as eighteen or nineteen weeks. If the problem is detected early enough, a miscarriage may be prevented by a cerclage—a suture that holds the cervix shut—which, if put in place early enough (usually around 12-14 weeks of pregnancy), is successful 80-90% of the time.

Fibroid tumors and uterine abnormalities are other maternal causes of late miscarriage. Physicians recommend a myomectomy (the surgical removal of a fibroid tumor) prior to attempting pregnancy in women whose fibroids may appear problematic. However, there are times when even a small and therefore seemingly non-problematic fibroid will grow so large and so rapidly that it causes the uterus to contract prematurely.

Although most chromosomally abnormal fetuses do not survive beyond twelve weeks, some do. A fetus may appear to be developing normally, but still have something inherently wrong with it which will cause it to abort. Worse still are those instances in which the pregnancy continues, but a routine ultrasound reveals devastating news. Expectant parents sometimes find themselves in the dreadful position of having to consider termination because the ultrasound reveals grave problems with the fetus.

Immunological problems, related to either parent, are another possible cause of second trimester losses.

Ectopic Pregnancy

Ectopic pregnancy, a pregnancy in which the embryo implants somewhere other than the uterus, is a relatively rare experience, occurring approximately 1% of the time in the general population and approximately 5% in women undergoing assisted reproduction. The vast majority of ectopic pregnancies occur in the fallopian tubes (probably 90-95% of the time), but it is possible to have an ectopic pregnancy in the cervix or in the abdominal cavity or on an ovary.

Ectopic pregnancy constitutes a medical emergency. If caught early, before it ruptures, it may be treated by medical or surgical intervention. After rupture, emergency surgery is required, often to resolve a life threatening situation. Either way, an ectopic pregnancy cannot be saved since even one that has not ruptured cannot be transferred to the woman's uterus. A pregnancy in which embryos are found both inside and outside the uterus is termed heteroectopic. If discovered early, it is possible to save the uterine pregnancy, since the ectopic pregnancy can be surgically removed before it ruptures and damages the uterine pregnancy.

Because IVF—whether with a woman's own eggs or with donor eggs—involves placing embryos in the uterus, one would assume that undergoing IVF would help prevent ectopic pregnancy. Unfortunately, this is not the case. Embryos are placed in the uterus, but they can migrate into the tubes and possibly become trapped. Although some women who experience ectopic pregnancies following ART treatment have known tubal blockages, which are most likely the cause of their ectopic pregnancies, others are thought to have clear tubes. This group includes women who turned to the ARTs because of unexplained infertility or a male factor. Some physicians feel that the fertility medications alter the hormonal environment of the fallopian tubes, making it more likely that an embryo will implant there.

Stillbirth

A pregnancy loss after twenty weeks gestation is often referred to as a stillbirth. However, we feel that loss at twenty weeks, before viability, is very different from a loss several weeks later, at a time when a baby could live outside the womb. We will focus our discussion on loss after viability.

There are many potential causes of stillbirth. One possible loss is a malfunction in the umbilical cord, resulting in a loss of oxygen to the fetus. If the umbilical cord is compressed during the delivery, or if it becomes wrapped around the baby's neck, it can cut off the oxygen supply and result in the death of the infant.

Placental problems can also lead to intrauterine death. If the placenta is implanted too low in the uterus (placenta previa), it can separate prematurely and cause the mother to hemorrhage. Alternatively, if the baby is post mature, the placenta may begin to malfunction, thereby depriving the baby of oxygen.

Other possible causes of stillbirth include conditions in the mother such as toxemia, diabetes or high blood pressure. Each can compromise the flow of nutrients to the baby. Or, if the mother's water breaks prematurely, the baby may contract a life threatening infection.

Loss in Multiple Pregnancy

Since pregnancy rates are higher when more than one embryo is transferred and since transferring more than two embryos raises the risk of a high level multiple gestation, most physicians recommend transferring two embryos during an egg donation cycle. Certainly there are many instances in which three—or even more—embryos are transferred and there continue to be triplet pregnancies after ovum donation. However, since the majority of multiple pregnancies after egg donation are twins, we will focus on the loss of one or both twins in this discussion.

Women who have had two or more embryos transferred are usually monitored closely early in pregnancy. Frequent blood tests and ultrasounds help determine how the pregnancy is progressing and how many embryos have implanted. The purpose of the early ultrasounds is not only to determine how many sacs are in the woman's uterus, but also to rule out the possibility of ectopic pregnancy.

Another form of partial loss early in a multiple pregnancy occurs when initial ultrasounds reveal two or more gestational sacs, but later ultrasounds fail to detect heartbeats in all of them. Often, the sac that has no heartbeat vanishes on its own. Sadly, "vanishing twins" and other partial losses are often dismissed by medical staff and others who seem to think, "You wanted one, you are getting one—so what is there to be sad about?"

Although others may still be inclined to minimize the impact, partial loss late in pregnancy is more often acknowledged as traumatic. By the second and third trimesters, expecting parents have formed bonds to each of their babies. When an ultrasound reveals that a fetus has died in utero or that it will not survive past birth because of congenital problems, this constitutes a real loss for the parents who had come to expect two babies, had begun to know two babies, and were looking forward to being parents of twins.

Multifetal reduction refers to the termination of one or more fetuses in a multiple gestation. This process is emotionally painful for parents who worked so hard to achieve a pregnancy, is generally recommended for anyone carrying four fetuses and often for triplet pregnancies. Only in unusual circumstances would multifetal reduction be recommended in a twin pregnancy. Although most women attempting pregnancy with donated ova have no more than three embryos transferred, there are instances in which one splits, resulting in a pregnancy composed of identical twins and a triplet. Sadly, these expectant parents, who so deeply want all their children, are forced to make the best decision they can for the future health of their babies and often, that decision seems to be to partially reduce the pregnancy.

Selective reduction refers to the termination of one or more fetuses in a multiple gestation when something has found to be "wrong" with that baby. In the event that pre-natal testing reveals some condition that the expectant parents do not feel prepared to handle, they may choose selective reduction.

Multifetal reduction and selective reduction are different in many ways, but the pain they bring to expectant parents is similar. In both instances, there was the initial excitement of carrying a multiple pregnancy and the anticipation, however brief, of what it would be like to be the parents of twins or triplets. Sadly, this joy ends in loss, a loss made all the more poignant by the fact that the couple worked so hard, even to the point of using donated eggs, to achieve the pregnancy.

Sadly, not all loss in multiple gestation is partial. There are couples who lose an entire pregnancy, often because of severe prematurity. As hard as moms-to-be work to try to delay labor, and as much as their physicians attempt to assist them in this, there are too many times when the babies simply come too early. Jean Kollantai, founder of The Center for Loss in Multiple Birth (CLIMB), a support network for parents throughout the United States and Canada who have experienced the loss of one or more fetuses during pregnancy, observes that parents who lose both their babies often feel angry at the technology that was successful in helping them conceive their children, but was unsuccessful in saving them. This loss is all the more painful when it follows a multifetal reduction, which attempted to create space for the healthy development of one or two fetuses, but which unintentionally resulted in the loss of all. Kollantai adds that some feel guilty for having wanted children so much that they turned to technology that put them at greater risk for multiple gestation.

Reconsiderations

Although we have provided some of the medical explanations for pregnancy loss, the reality is that in many instances, pregnancy loss is a mystery. All too often, grieving parents are left to wonder what they could have done differently. Sadly, many blame themselves, and perhaps to a lesser extent, their physicians. Some people blame God, wondering why they are being "punished" for wanting to be parents.

How does the fact that a pregnancy was achieved through egg donation impact upon people's feelings when they suffer a loss? As we have seen from the descriptions above, early miscarriage differs significantly from late miscarriage which differs from ectopic pregnancy in important ways and from stillbirth. Nonetheless, there are certain themes that apply to all forms of pregnancy loss after egg donation. We return now to the questions noted earlier, the first of which addresses the primary concern of many who lose a pregnancy after ovum donation.

Did We Force Something to Happen That Was not Meant to Be?

Pregnancy with donated oocytes is surely not a spontaneous, "natural" occurrence. Rather, it is the result of hard work and of advanced medical technology. While they are seeking an egg donor or attempting pregnancy after they have found her, many would-be parents wonder if what they are doing is morally right.

When all goes well, an on-going pregnancy and a healthy baby help confirm that parents have done the right thing—that sometimes hard work and determination help make something happen that was truly meant to be. On the other hand, when pregnancy fails, it is easy to reach the opposite conclusion—that it was not meant to be. This is what we meant in Chapter 1 when we spoke of "the blessing and the curse of the meant-to-be." "Meant-to-be" can provide great comfort or harsh condemnation.

Sadly, women who lose a donor-egg-assisted pregnancy may be plagued by the question of whether they tried to make something happen that was not meant to be. Although any grieving parent may ask this question, it is most likely to arise for those who had reservations about forcing nature to begin with. Included in this group will be older women, as well as older women and men who turned to egg donation with great reluctance, perhaps because their partners preferred this option to adoption (pregnancy loss can be especially painful for this group, who may now feel guilty for having lost their husband's child). Another vulnerable group are those with unexplained infertility, who chose egg donation because their physicians said, "It's worth a try."

Was I Diligent Enough in Taking Care of Myself?

Since it seems that any woman who loses a pregnancy looks back and scrutinizes her every action and reaction during pregnancy, it comes as no surprise that donor egg moms-to-be are experts at self doubt and recrimination. After all, you are the expectant moms who took self care most seriously, having promised yourselves that you would do all you could to grow your babies well. Unfortunately, nature has its way of making its own decisions, regardless of what you did and thought and ate. Even our brief summary of the causes of pregnancy loss reveals that many pregnancy losses, especially miscarriages early and late, are caused by problems in the fetus that have nothing to do with the maternal environment. Other losses are simply unexplained. And even those losses that can be attributed to a problem with the placenta or cervix or uterus are unrelated to your actions and reactions.

We know that when we say that it isn't your fault, the words are unconvincing. This seems to be the nature of pregnancy loss in general—it is hard for people going through the experience to really believe that it is simply something which happens and there is usually little, if anything, that a pregnant woman or her physician could have done to prevent it. And for women who have turned to ovum donation there is what psychologist Carole Lieber Wilkins calls a "double sense of failure." "They (patients) tell me that they failed once when their bodies and eggs could not make a baby, and now this loss makes them feel incompetent and according to some, 'worthless.'"

Should We Try Again with a Different Donor?

Following a few failed cycles or a pregnancy loss, people find themselves wondering if they should consider another donor. Depending upon who your donor is, how you came to enter into a donor pregnancy effort together, and what your other options are, you may be more or less reluctant to think about changing donors.

If your donor is your sister or your best friend and both of you feel great about this decision, you probably won't be thinking about changing donors. In fact, you and your donor may be grieving together and trying to see this as a step forward towards your shared goal. Similarly, if your donor is someone you found through a program, met, spent time with, and liked, you are probably reluctant to move on. On the other hand, if she is someone you have never met, you may feel that this pregnancy and perhaps, this match, "wasn't meant to be."

Decisions about choosing another donor will be shaped by the nature of your pregnancy loss as well. If you have suffered an ectopic pregnancy or a loss caused by an "incompetent cervix," you may feel certain that this loss had nothing to do with the donor. On the other hand, an early loss, which could be caused by chromosomal abnormalities, may prompt you to wonder about another donor.

Your donor's reproductive history will likely be a factor in your thinking about whether to continue with her. If your sister or friend has three young children, you and your doctor are likely to feel more confident about her egg quality than if she is 36 and had her last child ten years ago. Similarly, if your program-recruited donor has young children of her own *and* has donated successfully, she offers more reassurance than the childless, first time donor.

Whatever your thoughts and whatever you decide, this will not be an easy process. No one chooses a donor—whether family member or friend—without careful thought, exploration and discussion. By the time you start a cycle with a given donor, you will have already begun to bond with the idea of a baby conceived with this donor's egg. Having actually experienced a pregnancy through her eggs has only served to solidify your dream of a baby created with her egg, your partner's sperm and your love.

Can We Afford To Try Again?

As we see throughout this book, cost plays a huge role in some decision making about using donor eggs, and a negligible one in others. Differences are tied not only to family finances and to whether you have a volunteer donor or not, but also, to insurance coverage for egg donation. Hence, the question, "Can we afford to try again?" is irrelevant to some couples and central to others.

If you are self-paying for your medical treatment and for the donor, the costs of doing another cycle are high. You might have decided, prior to treatment, that you could only afford one cycle—that some financial resources had to be left in place for adoption if the cycle didn't work. However, now you have had a pregnancy, and if it was an early loss, you may feel, *We got one step closer to our goal; we can't quit now.* You may find yourselves in a real dilemma, not wanting to commit money you may later need for adoption, but reluctant to give up on egg donation when you now know that you can achieve pregnancy.

Fortunately, some couples are spared concerns about cost. In mandated states, most women under 40 have coverage for oocyte donation, and some in their early 40s are also covered. In non-mandated states, even women with sisters or friends willing to donate face significant medical costs in pursuing egg donation.

Cryopreserved embryos from a first donor cycle enable many couples to try a second time without worrying excessively about the cost of treatment. Yes, there is the cost of medications and monitoring which help prepare your body to receive an embryo, and there is the cost of transfer, but these costs are relatively small in comparison with the high costs of a full treatment cycle and of locating and paying a program-recruited donor.

How Much Frustration and Loss Can We Endure?

Here it is, the question that runs through all infertility treatment: "When is enough, enough?" Couples who have never conceived ask this question, and couples who have recurrent miscarriages ask it, as do those who don't conceive with donated gametes and those who have pregnancy loss after gamete donation. How do people know when they have reached their limit, when they are simply putting good money and good time and energy after bad?

In talking with countless couples facing the question "When is enough, enough?" I (Ellen) have developed a profound respect for people's ability to know when the time has come to move on. It may sound simplistic, but people have a way of knowing. Sometimes that "knowing" comes because one or both members of a couple realize that he/she simply has to stop—the person has run out of steam, of hope and belief. Other times, someone feels they have been given a sign. For example, I had a client, a physician who found herself treating a very sick woman who worked in adoption, specifically with China. My client, deep in the throes of IVF, remembers thinking, *now it has come together—I am going to save her life and she is going to help me get a baby*. Finally, there are those who reach an end point based on practical considerations. Their financial resources are drained and they want to keep some in reserve should they choose adoption.

After losing a donor egg pregnancy or simply having the procedure not work, you are likely to need some time to grieve and to "re-group" as a couple before you can make decisions about further cycles. The question, "How much frustration and loss can we endure?" is probably best answered after you have taken some time to mourn the baby you have lost and to return to being a couple, including some recreation and enjoyment, as well as mourning, in your time together.

Maybe It Wasn't an Egg Problem after All?

What a thorny question this is. Again, it is one of the questions that concern only some couples who suffer pregnancy loss after egg donation. Spared this question are those of you who know—for sure—that you need donated eggs in order to conceive, as well as those whose pregnancy loss appeared entirely unrelated to egg quality.

But what about those who turned to ovum donation because of unexplained infertility and have now had an early loss? More frustration. Sadly, you have no way of knowing whether your loss was simply a random event—which it probably was—or whether the real problem may be uterine or male factor. At this juncture, you will probably want to talk with your physician to see what he/she recommends about exploring uterine factors or possibly, introducing donor sperm with your ova, assuming you, as a couple, are comfortable with parenthood through sperm donation. Depending on your stamina and on the accessibility of other medical treatment, you may also want to seek a second opinion. We are not suggesting that you keep yourselves on an endless pursuit of pregnancy, but want you to avoid the painful regret that so often comes when people look back and question, "did we do all that we could?"

Maybe There Is Something So Wrong with Me and My Body That I Can't Carry a Baby even with Good Eggs?

How very, very sad that people sometimes get the impression or the message that "all you need are good eggs." And so we remind you, yet again, that reproduction is a mystery. This really isn't about there being something wrong with you, and most likely, it's not something wrong with your body. Even today, with all the recent advances in reproductive medicine, so much remains unanswered about conception and pregnancy.

Grief, Mourning and Moving On

Whatever form the loss takes—and we again acknowledge that there are enormous differences between early miscarriage and full term stillbirth—grieving parents need to mourn the loss of the child they were expecting before taking steps to bring another child into the family. This will be all the more true for those of you who decide to move on to adoption, since you will be grieving not only the child you have lost, but also, the opportunity to share pregnancy, childbirth and partial genetic connection. However, it is also true for those of you who suffered an early loss. Even if you are optimistically resuming efforts with the same donor, there has been a loss. You were expecting a particular baby, you were beginning to imagine him, to name her, to become excited about being pregnant.

Once again, we turn our attention to the particulars of egg donation. How does the fact that your pregnancy was donor-assisted impact
your loss and perhaps, help shape your grieving process?

Shared Grief

If your donor is your sister or your close friend, she is likely to be
part of your grief process. Although the magnitude of your loss is different, she, too, has lost something. She went through a great deal to help you
achieve pregnancy and she was invested in its outcome. Hopefully, the
camaraderie you feel with her softens your grief rather than intensifies it.

Complicated Mourning

Psychologists and others who offer counsel around grief and
mourning have long noted that grief becomes more complicated and
challenging when the mourner has had an ambivalent relationship with
the person or role that has been lost. Such may be the case with pregnancy loss after egg donation—the pregnancy was most often deeply
wanted, but it was also the source of some ambivalence. In addition to
the normal ambivalence that many pregnant women feel when a little
person "invades" their body, women pregnant with donated eggs arrive with a complicated history. There may have been earlier pregnancy
losses, perhaps with one's own eggs. There may have been much uncertainty about trying donor ova, There can be ambivalence about the
donor, especially if she is an eager family member or friend.

Grief and mourning after loss of a donor-assisted pregnancy may
include considerable anger (at oneself for turning to egg donation, at
physicians for promoting this option), regret (for forcing conception),
and deep sorrow (this may have been a last chance pregnancy).

Rituals

Few established rituals and ceremonies exist for early pregnancy
loss. Sadly, even late losses are sometimes dismissed as unworthy of a
funeral and burial. Hence many grieving parents, whether their pregnancy was conceived spontaneously, through their own gametes and
ART, or with donor gametes, feel that theirs is a disenfranchised grief.
All too often, the rest of the world, pours salt in their wounds by saying,
"At least you know you can get pregnant," or "It wasn't meant to be,"
or worse still, "Do you think you should quit your job next time and
just rest?"

The absence of rituals and public acknowledgement of loss is complicated for donor egg parents since many felt very private when they were pregnant. Hesitant to tell people about the pregnancy until it was well established, some of you may have suffered your loss before others even knew you were expecting. Others may have told people you were pregnant, but still handled the pregnancy with circumspection and ever a keen eye on privacy. Now you long for others to acknowledge your loss and to honor the memory of the child or children you were expecting. The distance you understandably maintained during weeks or months you were pregnant may make it all the more difficult for others to reach out to you now, especially in the absence of a memorial service or other observance of your loss.

We encourage you to create your own rituals. You may want to talk with clergyperson for some assistance or with a professional at a funeral home. Or you may feel comfortable creating your own ritual. Some grieving parents have planted trees, written good-bye letters to their lost child(ren), or donated children's books to a local library or goods to an orphanage. Some have stood at water's edge and recited a prayer or a poem. Others have created a gravestone to capture their feelings towards the child they lost. One especially moving stone had an etching of a small angel with the words, "If love had been enough to save you, you would have lived."

Remember that the means of conception is not necessarily something you need talk with others about. You have a right to treat conception as a private matter (and a right to tell others, if you prefer). What you are looking for, after all, is a means of remembering the child you had so looked forward to parenting. How he or she was created is not as important, by any means, as the fact that this young life touched yours in ways that will always be remembered, appreciated, missed and celebrated.

The Odds Are with You

Although loss is possible, it is not probable. If you conceive through ovum donation, the greatest likelihood is that you will deliver a healthy baby. You may have been told that you had a 50% chance or so of becoming pregnant, but once pregnancy is achieved, the odds shift dramatically in your favor. And they improve as time goes on—when you are six weeks pregnant you may be told that you have a 75% or so chance of taking a baby home, but by twelve weeks, the odds are probably in the high 90s. So when you are pregnant with your donor-egg-conceived child, we encourage you to look forward, not back, and to begin to anticipate the arrival of your much-wanted and long-sought-after child. You are pregnant. Life is growing inside you. This, as you know all too well, is a glorious achievement. Take some time to celebrate.

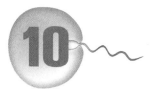

Parenthood after
Egg Donation

Parenthood is filled with a multitude of tasks, rewards and burdens, most of which have nothing to do with how a child joined a family. Being the kindergarten room parent or the tooth fairy or the one who plans a birthday party is unrelated to conception. Helping with homework, doing piles of camp laundry, driving carpool are the same for parents who adopt their children or conceive them spontaneously or create them with donor sperm or donor eggs.

The birth of every child is a miracle that leaves nearly all new parents overflowing with excitement and wonder. Imagine how over the top couples are when they finally deliver a child through oocyte donation. Many of you have traveled a difficult path to get here and although happy to be pregnant, you were probably anxious as well. You questioned everything…"Will the baby be o.k.?" "Will something more go wrong?" "Will we really love the child?" "Will we know how to care for a baby?" and of course, the ubiquitous, "Will we be good parents?"

As new parents of a child born through donated ova, you are likely to be thinking about how you will talk with your child and about how others will view your donor conception. You are probably also thinking about your donor and about how your child may be like her. But when your baby first arrives, there will be more immediate concerns. Diapers, car seats, nursing, announcements, maternity and paternity leave, religious ceremonies and more. We will touch on few of them here, because most of those issues are not colored by how your baby was conceived!

Since this is a book about egg donation and not about parenthood, we will not be talking about selecting a car seat or shopping for school supplies or taking your child to the dentist or convincing them to eat their vegetables. Rather, we turn our attention here to aspects of parenting that appear different, in some ways, when ovum donation is part of a family's story.

The Dynamics of the Parenting Partnership

In contemplating egg donation, some intended parents worry that they will experience an "inequality" in the family since the father will have a genetic connection to the child and the mother will not. We have found that this fear rarely materializes, since the gestational connection between mother and child is so powerful. Nonetheless, as the child matures and the pregnancy connection recedes more into the past, there is more room for feelings about the donor, especially if she is someone the parents have never met.

Many moms through egg donation say that having a child be genetically connected to their husbands is very reassuring. In particular, those with anonymous donors look to identify their husband's physical and personality traits in the child. They say that they feel comfortable when they can make the genetic connection from father to child. By contrast, they feel somewhat adrift when they see a particular trait that cannot be readily found in their husbands.

One mother through oocyte donation speaks of being tortured for years by a flip remark made by a friend of hers shortly after her son was born. The friend, probably having no idea of the impact of her words, said, "Well now you can never get divorced!" When the new mother asked why, her friend said, "Because your husband will surely get custody since he is the real parent." Sadly, these words stayed with this loving and otherwise content mother until she eventually sought counseling to try to exorcise them from her mind.

Just as moms through egg donation are proud and pleased to have a child that is genetically connected to their husbands, so, also, do the fathers feel appreciative of their wives' ability to carry a baby and to go through labor and delivery. Although there are probably some new fathers through egg donation who feel some anxiety about the fact that they have the genetic connection with their child and their wives do not, this is not something that new fathers have expressed to us. Rather, they seem to feel that they and their wives are very much on "equal footing." After all, these dads have just watched their wives go through the different stages of pregnancy as well as the pain and triumph of child-birth. Nonetheless, like all new parents, they must adjust to the arrival of this new person who has invaded their space, their time and, in many ways, their relationship.

If you and your husband are feeling some stress in your marriage following the arrival of your child, remember that you have lots of company. Like all new parents, you must negotiate who will do what and when and how you will do it. Sometimes this can feel like a "tug of war" or a "scorecard." What may make it more challenging for parents through oocyte donation is the history that brought you to this point. A new dad may be thinking, *But she wanted a baby so much, doesn't she remember all those tearful nights when we faced disappointment? Why, then is she grumpy when she has to get up at 2:00 a.m. to nurse the baby?* At the same time, as an exhausted new mom, you may have your own set of troubling thoughts: *He's the lucky one. He gets to sleep through the night, to go to work in the morning and he gets to be genetically connected to our baby. I shouldn't be complaining but it doesn't seem fair.* Parenthood should not be a balance sheet, but it is sometimes difficult, especially in the first few days and weeks after your child arrives, to avoid keeping score. If you find yourself feeling shortchanged for free time or under appreciated, you need to talk with your partner. The years of infertility taught you that the two of you can pull together in stressful times, but that doesn't mean they prepared you for parenthood.

For most couples it gets easier. Round about four months or so, your child will start to be a lot of fun. The little crying-pooping-sleeping machine of the early days and weeks will grow into a smiling, cooing, playful baby. We expect that it will feel easier to share parenting respon-sibilities when you are also sharing smiles and when you are really able to play with the your baby. But remember that everyone is different, that it takes longer for some than for others to adjust to parenthood, and that even strong, loving couples can have a hard time. Don't let stress between you mount. If you aren't feeling good about how things are unfolding in your newly expanded family, ask for help. Those of us who counsel infertile couples welcome the opportunity to help you with the new challenges that parenthood brings.

Talking with Others about Donor Conception

Remember all the times that you were reluctant to open the mail for fear there would be a baby announcement? Now, perhaps at long last, it is your turn. One of the many joys of new parenthood is sending out announcements.

Baby announcements come in all shapes and sizes and flavors, from email announcements, to cards bought at a Hallmark store, to handmade announcements or true artistic creations. We encourage you to take your time and enjoy the process of figuring out what you will say and how you will say it. We're not suggesting that the card read, "Tom and Sally welcome their new egg donor baby," but you may want to say something that acknowledges how much you wanted a baby or how long you waited. One announcement read, "Arrived...at long last...." Another said, "Our dreams finally came true." And many parents after infertility say something like, "Our little miracle has finally arrived." You may take this route—the route of acknowledging your efforts—or you may do what Steve and Pam did. "We're going for 'regular'. We've had enough of being different. The announcement is simply going to have our son's name, date of birth and weight. That's it. They can figure out the rest."

When you think about who you will talk with about how your child joined your family, please remember that there are really very few people who need to know about donor conception. We include in those who need to know this select few:

- Other children impacted by this donation (a known donor's other children and your other children)

- Your obstetrician

- Your child's pediatrician and other medical providers when a history of donor assisted conception might impact care.

- Family members and close friends who may later hear this from the child anyway.

So how do you make decisions about talking with others? Remember that you can always add information, but you cannot subtract it. If you feel that you want to maintain privacy, it is probably best to think carefully about with whom you talk about having used donated ova. Friends and family can know you are having difficulty conceiving without knowing specifics about the options you are considering. Similarly, upon learning of your pregnancy or hearing that you have had a baby, people can know that this didn't come easily without knowing exactly how you found resolution.

We are *not* suggesting that this be a secret. We've just finished encouraging you to be confident and proud, and we're not trying to turn that recommendation on its head. Rather, we want you to feel that you have choices, and that being honest and open with your children does not automatically mandate being open and honest with others. Every family should have comfortable privacy boundaries.

Rebecca Gordon, the 11-year-old whose family was introduced in Chapter 1, has known her entire life that she was conceived through DI and she was an active participant when it came time for her parents to select an egg donor. Still, Rebecca chooses not to tell her friends nor her teachers about her donor origins.

If you believe, as many adoptive parents do, that your child's story is his or her private information, then there is a lot to be said for telling as few people outside your close circle of family and friends as possible before you tell your child. Family should know so that they never see donor conception as a secret.

"What will happen," you might ask, "if our child later tells people and they don't believe him? Or they get angry or feel hurt by us because they weren't privy to this information sooner?"

Social worker Judy Calica, reminds us that children generally develop a clear sense of what is private in a family. Calica notes that children become attuned to social cues and advises parents to trust that their children will only talk about donor conception if and when it is appropriate. On the other hand, we have all known instances where a child blurts something out and then does not know how to handle questions or comments that may follow. For the most part, these questions pass quickly and the curious inquirers move on to other topics. Still, as a parent, you may face times when your child talks about egg donation publicly and then is at a loss to respond to the reactions of others. Again, we return to our mantra: be confident, honest, direct with your child. The process that the two of you go through in addressing the issue will be more important than the actual words you come up with. Consider it yet another opportunity for you to show your child how comfortable you are with the truth. We like to think that people will not only understand why you have maintained your child's privacy, but that they will also respect you for it. Adoptive parents have reported this experience again and again—people may be surprised, at first, when an adoptive parent declines to answer a question about the child's birthparents, stating that it is his or her information to share or not share. However, upon brief reflection, people seem to get it. We hope that with ovum donation, something even more private because it involves the physical act of conception, privacy will be all the more respected and accepted.

Do you tell other people? Teachers? Your child's dentist? Your clergy? In each instance, we encourage you to ask yourself, "Is there any reason that this person should know that our child was conceived through egg donation?" Keeping in mind that there will probably be other people you think about telling, let's look at three examples, just to provide a little practice for you about how you might think through other situations.

Medical Specialists. We advised earlier that your child's pediatrician will need to know about donor conception. Although much of pediatric care has nothing to do with family history, certain conditions, illnesses and traits have hereditary components. You will want your child's physician to be basing his/her care of your child on an accurate family history, but what about other medical specialists? We suppose that if your child breaks his arm, the orthopedic surgeon doesn't really need to know about donor egg. However, when anesthesia and medications are involved, it seems safest to provide all physicians with as much information as possible.

Teachers. Is there any reason that a teacher would need to know that your child was conceived through oocyte donation? We can think of only one: elementary school units on the family. In the early school years there are often class discussions of family formation. Adoptive parents have worked hard to sensitize teachers and other educators to the fact that there are many ways to form a family, a message that has been further communicated by single parents and gay and lesbian parents. Adoptive parents have also succeeded, in many school systems, in eliminating the often troublesome "Family Tree" assignment and having it replaced with something more akin to a "Family Orchard." Nonetheless, your child may be in a first or second grade class in which the teacher asks, "Did anyone join their family through adoption?" or "Does anyone here have a step-father or a half-sister?" Since it is possible that your confident little son or daughter may proudly raise a hand to say, "My Aunt Pat gave my mommy and daddy an egg," you might want to talk with a primary grade teacher about egg donation.

Dentists. Does your child's dentist need to know that he/she was created through egg donation? It may become a good idea. Although brushing and flossing habits are not hereditary, family history can be relevant in other aspects of dental medicine. These can include use of medications and anesthesia which are needed for dental surgery.

Clergy. Does your priest, minister or rabbi have reason to know that your child was conceived with donated oocytes? Your response to this question has a lot to do with your relationship with your clergyperson. If you don't have a religious connection or are only an occasional participant in your congregation, you won't be thinking about talking with clergy about egg donation. However, if your clergy is someone you are close with, and especially, if you are planning some religious celebration such as a baby naming or a christening, you may (or may not) want your clergy to know the special way you became a family.

If your child grows up in a religious community, he/she may someday want to talk with clergy about his origins. Donor conception may feel very relevant, for example, to an eleven- or twelve-year-old preparing to become a bar or bat mitzvah, since this service often makes reference to ancestry. However, this event comes at a time when it should be your child's decision—not yours— whether to talk.

Meet Corey…

Corey, 39, had her daughter, Lindsey, last year through anonymous egg donation. She offers some interesting observations about talking with people. Corey says that she often tells strangers about Lindsey's conception. "They're safe. I feel I can tell them and it won't matter. Also, it gives me the opportunity to delight in her without feeling like I sound boastful. When people say, 'Your daughter is beautiful,' I can say, "Yes she is, but please don't think I'm bragging—she was born with the help of an egg donor.'"

Corey goes on to say that with friends and acquaintances she will see again, she is often more circumspect. She remembers one incident during her pregnancy. She was with a close friend, also pregnant, who commented that she had been a big baby and expected her baby would be big. She turned to Corey and asked about her weight at birth. Corey answered her but did not say, "I'm not sure it matters, since my child was conceived with a donated egg."

Corey tells us that her daughter's donor conception has be-come easier and easier for her over time. She remembers feel-ing very tentative early in the pregnancy, but reports that she felt much more confident and optimistic once she felt the baby move. When Lindsey was born and came out looking just like her father, Corey felt relieved. "She was familiar. I was relieved to see the familiar look." Then Corey smiles and tells the story of a conversation she had with a lifelong friend when Lindsey was four months old. She and her friend, whom she had told about Lindsey's donor conception, were looking at their babies and commenting on the fact that both girls had big ears. Her friend said, "Remember, we each had big ears when we were little." Corey said, "With moms like Biz and Bombo (the nick-names they had given each other as kids) of course our girls will have big ears." It was not until later that day that Corey realized what she had said and how her friend had respond-ed—neither had "remembered" or noted that Lindsey probably didn't inherit her mom's big ears.

Talking with Children about Reproduction and about How They Entered Their Family

Remember that every child has questions about where babies come from. Our goal is to help you feel confident in your ability to talk with your child in an open, honest, helpful way that will promote trust in your relationship and self-confidence in the child.

"How will I tell my child?" All too often this question torments people considering egg donation. In fact, some are so troubled by it that they either postpone talking openly with their child or, worse still, contemplate lying to their children. In the past many well-intentioned, deeply loving parents were ill-advised by medical and even some men-tal health professionals, who took the approach that "what he doesn't know, won't hurt him." Oddly, these professionals relabeled *speaking the truth* and called it *disclosure*. The idea, it seems, was that there was a deep, dark secret that needed to be kept hidden, but some parents might choose to "disclose" it.

We don't get it. We don't understand why anyone would advise parents to intentionally deceive their children. What makes it all the more baffling is that the parents involved are people who deeply love their children and who created them with great happiness and anticipa-tion. The story of how their children joined their families is a joyful one that we would think people would want to celebrate again and again. Instead, it has often been transformed into a dark, hidden secret.

Fortunately, there is wise and informed guidance about the importance of speaking truthfully to children. This guidance comes from children of donated oocytes and from donor sperm offspring who are old enough to talk about their experience.

> Daniel, 16, was conceived through egg donation. His parents have always been fully open with him and so Daniel doesn't get why people are so worried about talking with their kids. Daniel says, "It's not a big part of my life. I think it would be hard for me if I learned now that I came from a donor, but I've always known it. I'm not interested in meeting the donor, but I know that if I was, my mom would put me in the car and take me there."

Contrast Daniel's relaxed, candid approach with that of donor sperm offspring who were not told the truth when they were young. Now adults, some men and women who joined their families through the help of an anonymous sperm donor are speaking loud and clear about their need to know the truth about their origins. Many have likened themselves to adoptees, explaining that they are not looking for new or better parents, but rather, for information which will help them better understand who they are. In addition, they seek medical information as well as knowledge about others to whom they may be genetically related. Guidance has also come from their parents, many of whom learned the hard way the consequences of secrecy. And, at long last, the Ethics Committee of the American Society for Reproductive Medicine, (www.asrm.org) came out with a position paper in 2004 advocating truth telling with children.

The voices of donor offspring have recently been captured in writing and on film. In Caroline Lorbach's book *Experiences of Donor Conception,* she chronicles the history of secrecy in donor insemination and then tells about the pain that secrecy wrought on donor families. Lorbach offers the voices of several donor offspring, including Bill, Christine, Barry, Nicky, Lynne and Lauren. They cover the most of the concerns of DI offspring—the value of truth telling, the avoidance of shame, the need for accurate medical information and the longing for information about the donor.

> Bill tells us, "DI parents have raised us, but, because of the shame they feel about their infertility, they are reluctant to discuss our origins with us, fearful we would reject them for their

decision....They do not understand that we are undergoing genetic bewilderment."

Christine, who learned the truth about her origins as an adult, says, "I no longer have to be vigilant about the onset of the diabetes which killed my legal father and other members of his family, and I am heartily glad that I hadn't volunteered to take part in ground-breaking medical research in our locality involving people with a family history of diabetes. My involvement could have given false results and impaired the success of the whole research program."

And from Barry, "Things have changed, but secrecy is a legacy of that period. Secrecy is isolating; when you have a secret in the family, it is a barrier. When you have a secret, you have power over the person who does not know the secret. Many women feel the need to tell someone, and kids tend to pick up on secrets...and medically, you have to lie to a doctor when you are asked your family history."

And from Nicky, a more positive report, "In my case, I have a very loving family who have done the best they could with the little they knew about donor insemination. I have always felt loved and treasured by both my mother and (social) father. They answered my questions when I sensed that Dad wasn't my biological father, and they have never resented me for or prevented me from exploring the possibility of finding out information relating to my history. I respect and thank them for that."

And of course we agree with Lauren, who tells us, "The rights of the children must be made paramount in assisted reproductive technologies. We didn't have any choices in the beginning—we were simply created and I think people forgot we would grow into intelligent adults. I believe we should have the choice to access our birth information, if that is what we desire. I wish I was given that choice."

Janice, who learned of her origins when she was 22, says, "Our mother carefully and lovingly told us the truth of our origin. Though originally loyal to our father's desire we should never know of his infertility and of the choice of DI, she felt that we should know the truth after all. It was an immense surprise and shock. I remember examining my hands and face in the mirror, seeking physical evidence of this 'new' biological father's presence, being fascinated by the prospect that half of me was 'unknown.' I also felt sadness and frustration that I would never be able to talk about this new revelation about my identity with the man whom I had now discovered was my 'social' father; but he was still my 'father.' I wanted to tell him how I admired him and my mother for the courage that it took to choose DI."

Barry Stevens, also a DI offspring, has written and produced the exquisite film, *Offspring* (produced by Barna Alper Productions, 366 Adelaine St. West. Suite 700, Toronto, M5V 1RG Canada in 2001 and first aired on CBC, then on BBC, then in the US on Sundance). In it, Stevens chronicles the search that he and his sister undertook following the death of their father, and the news, from their mother, that they were both conceived through donor sperm. As he searches for information about his genetic father, Stevens poignantly and powerfully captures the longing of DI (and we assume, DE) offspring to know the truth about where they came from.

> Karen, a donor offspring, wrote in a personal email to me (Ellen), "I am not adopted in the traditional sense. I know my mother, but was raised 'as if' my father was actually my biological father. I wasn't told the truth until I was 16. I challenged my mother with the knowledge, and she confessed. To this day she insists that someone must have told me. No one had. It was just knowledge I had in my inner being that I blurted out one day.
>
> "Anyway, to get to the point. I just attended a family reunion this weekend on my father's side of the family. I've been in a funk ever since. It is a four-and-a-half hour drive home, and I hardly spoke the entire way and the crying started as soon as I hit home (I am a well-adjusted, functioning, member of society, 47 years old).
>
> "I can only describe what I am going through as grieving. My issues seem to come in waves. First at 16, again at around 32, and now here it comes again apparently. Just when I think I have come to terms with everything, I've been blind-sided with another surge of emotions."

"But isn't donor egg different from donor sperm?" you may ask. Yes. There are some fundamental differences. In each instance, the child is genetically related to only one of his/her parents. However, with donor egg the child has the very significant gestational connection to his/her mother. We feel it is this connection that fully authenticates both parents and should make donor egg a much more comfortable topic of family conversation.

What is it, then, that makes people uncomfortable about speaking truthfully to their children? When asked this, some prospective parents offer a vague, "I don't want to confuse my child" or "We're afraid we'll upset him." We don't understand what they feel is upsetting or confusing about the story of two people lovingly and with great care and excitement and joy deciding to create a baby. Does the fact that a third person helped them create this cherished child diminish the story? We think not.

> Patrice, 42, and mother of twins through donated ova, told us that she fears her children will reject her. This is something that has been on her mind since she first learned she was pregnant. The children, now five, adore her, but sadly, this loving and capable mother continues to worry, We find her worry so sad and so very unnecessary and blame those who talk in terms of "disclosure" for creating and fostering her sense of shame. Why would two children, created in love, cherished from the moment their parents learned of the pregnancy, raised in a nurturing and supportive home reject their parents? They wouldn't, they won't, but tell this to their mother. We tried, but it is difficult for Patrice to hear this. It is our hope that she will seek counseling, or perhaps better yet, a support group for mothers through egg donation.

Boston-area therapist Peg Beck notes that talking with a child about donor conception offers parents the opportunity to teach their children two valuable lessons: that it is okay to ask for help when you need it, and that there are often kind people who are willing to help those in need. Isn't this a much more sensible approach to egg donation than one that attempts to cloak it in shame and secrecy?

Chicago therapist Judy Calica lends further support to this perspective by reminding us that all parents, including donor parents, want their children to have a full and authentic sense of themselves. Open, honest conversations with their parents that include full and accurate information can only help reinforce a child's sense of authenticity and wholeness.

Young children are egocentric. They see themselves as the center of the world. How wonderful it is for them to have their parents tell them the joyous story of how they were born. Remember that the central message of this story is one that applies to most children: "Mommy and Daddy (or Mommy and Mommy or Daddy and Daddy) wanted to have a baby and were so happy to be able to have you."

We encourage parents to feel confident about talking with their children and, hopefully, to enjoy the experience. We know that may sound idealistic to those of you who are not yet parents and who are anxious about talking with children, but please think about what you will be doing. How often in life does someone have the chance to let someone you love know how much you wanted to be with them and how overjoyed you were when they came into your life? How nice, also, to be able to express gratitude, respect and admiration for the person who helped make it possible.

"But what exactly do we say and when and how do we say it?" Los Angeles marriage and family therapist Carole Lieber Wilkins advises the parents she works with to tell their children by the time they are 3 years old. "The reason for telling a child about a third party reproduction is not because they need to know the technical details of how in vitro fertilization or inseminations were performed; it is because children need to begin the process of acknowledging that there is another person or people in the world to whom they are connected in a significant and lasting way." Lieber Wilkins goes on to say that it is normal for children to "fantasize about the pieces of the puzzle that may not be filled in for many years" but adds that this is not a reason to delay talking with them when they are very young. She cautions people against waiting, saying that to tell a child of 9 or 10 that they are not genetically connected to their mother or father in the way their friends or other family members are related to their parents "would be a tremendous shock, indeed perhaps perceived as a betrayal."

We turn to developmental psychologist, Anne Bernstein, for her guidance. Bernstein, who feels "What you don't know *can* hurt you," has written a remarkable book about talking with young children about sex and reproduction. In *Flight of the Stork: What Children Think (and When) about Sex and Family Building* (Perspectives Press, Inc., 1994) she advises that when a child asks, "Where do babies come from?" a parent should first respond, "Where do you think?" This lets parent know what the child knows or guesses (pg. 44).

Bernstein's book guides parents through a series of six levels of cognitive development at which children understand more and more about reproduction and family connectedness. Bernstein reminds parents, again and again, that children have a great deal of curiosity about where babies come from and that talking with them at a level they can understand not only strengthens bonds between parent and child, but enhances a child's growth and development. "A child's questions about procreation are an early foray into their search for knowledge," Bernstein writes. "Encouraging the child's unguarded questions and answering responsively also encourages the child as an active, inquisitive explorer of the world." (pg. 29)

In *Flight of the Stork*, Bernstein's six levels of understanding offer parents practical information about what children can understand and when they can understand it. Throughout her discussion, Bernstein emphasizes the importance of parents listening very carefully to what their children are saying, reminding themselves that children really do see the world through a different lens than do adults. Bernstein also urges parents to use correct terminology about body parts. For example, it is crucial that children be told that a baby grows in a mommy's uterus or womb—not tummy—so that a child does not confuse eating or becoming full with pregnancy. Children need to know that babies have a place to grow in women—womb or uterus. Teaching about anatomy using real names increases self esteem and reduces confusion. And of particular significance to parents through ovum donation is the need to use the word *ovum* not *egg*. Otherwise, children will be envisioning an egg like the one that was boiled for their breakfast being a central player in their lives.

The following are brief summaries of each of Bernstein's levels. What becomes quickly apparent when reading them is that you will not be having one conversation with your children. Like all other parents, you will be telling and re-telling and telling again the wonderful story about how you became a family. Your child will understand this story in one way when she is 3 and comprehend it in a very different way when she is 8 or 15. You may think he "gets it" at 7 and later be totally surprised by a comment he makes or a question that sounds like it comes from a much younger child. Remember that the following levels are only guidelines, that each includes children of a rather broad age span and that the most important thing always is that you speak with confidence in your relationship with your child regardless of his or her level of comprehension.

Level One children are described by Bernstein as "The Geographers." Between ages 3 and 7, Level One children believe that babies always existed and it is just a question of where they were before they joined their families. They learn that babies grow in their mother's bodies, but they assume that they always existed.

Understanding level one thinking helps parents through ovum donation remember that young children are not thinking about *who* created them and *how* it happened—they assume they always existed.

Level Two children are described by Bernstein as "The Manufacturers." Children reach level two between ages 4 and 8, and when they do, they realize that babies did not always exist; they had to be created. These "manufacturers" also know that a man and a woman are needed to create a baby, but they are not clear of the role each plays.

Understanding level two helps parents through egg donation introduce their role as "manufacturers" to their young children. They have the opportunity to let their child know that *they* created him/her together, but that others (donor, doctor) *assisted* them in their creation.

Level Three children are described by Bernstein as "The In-Betweens." During this transitional time, usually arrived at between ages 5 and 10, children explain procreation as a mixture of physiology and technology. They know Mommy and Daddy can't open and close their tummies, but they may assume that conception is impossible without marriage. At this level they know there are three major ingredients to making babies—social relationships such as love and marriage, sexual intercourse, and the union of sperm and ovum—but they can't combine these factors into a coherent whole. They can be aware that their explanations don't add up.

Understanding level three assists donor egg parents as they begin to explain assisted reproduction to children. Their task is to convey to young children that sometimes love and science need to work together to create a much wanted child.

Level Four children are described by Bernstein as "The Reporters." These diligent little people, ages 7 to 12, feel the most important thing is to report accurately. The world is full of laws, and they limit explanations of reproduction to the facts. They understand that paternity is not just a social relationship—it is tied to biology.

Understanding level four assists parents as they help their children grapple with the fact that someone can have a genetic connection to a child and not be a parent, and that someone can be a parent without having a genetic connection to their child.

Level Five children are identified by Bernstein as "The Theoreticians." Children arrive at this level between ages 10 and 13 and in some cases may remain there for the rest of their lives. "Theoreticians" see both sperm and ovum as necessary, but believe that a baby really begins in one or the other.

Bernstein reminds her readers that the idea that a life began in either egg or sperm—but not both—was accepted for much of history.

Only since the 1870s, she reports, have scientists realized that genetic material comes from both egg and sperm. Level Five children (and adults) feel that embryos are preformed and that sexual intercourse provides conditions for it to grow.

Understanding level five can help parents of pre-teens as they put complicated pieces together, beginning to comprehend that life is created through a union of one sperm and one egg and cannot exist without both essential ingredients *and* the equally essential ingredient of a gestational environment.

Level Six is the point at which someone "puts it all together." According to Bernstein, level six can begin as early as 11 or 12 or it may not occur at all. Those who do reach level six "can assimilate the concept that two distinct entities, sperm and ovum, can become one qualitatively different and unique entity, the embryo. Level six requires an appreciation that the genetic materials are transformed in the process of uniting." She goes on to add that Level Six thinkers are ready to consider the moral and social aspects of reproduction and they "can integrate physiology with emotion, religious teaching and social convention."

Understanding level six helps prepare parents of donor offspring for adolescence and for the "Who am I?" questions that inevitably arise. As they watch their children grapple with the relative influences of genetics, gestation, family environment, friends, community, faith etc, parents can feel confident in their roles and respectful of the complex questions their children are asking.

"O.K." you say, "We know we should feel confident talking with our children. We know we should use correct terminology and should pay attention to levels of understanding. We know we should be prepared to tell the story many times and for there to be questions that remind us that our children don't really understand what we are saying. We know all these things, but we still don't know how to get started. What should we say and when should we say it?"

We subscribe to the "always knew" school of talking with children. Generations of adoption-expanded families have demonstrated that this approach works better for children in the long run than does "sudden disclosure" in late childhood or adulthood. Whether the topic be egg donation or sperm donation or adoption or surrogacy, it seems that everything is simpler for both parent and child if there is no single moment of telling. Instead, parents begin using words and concepts when their children are very young, before the children have any idea what it all means.

So, for a starter, you should begin talking about how your family was formed when your child is very young, perhaps three or four. Bernstein (and we urge you to read *Flight of the Stork*) reminds us that at this age, most children should know the correct names for body parts and the socially shared words for elimination. They should understand that babies grow in a woman's body, and if they want to know, or ask about it, they should know that babies are made by mothers and fathers together. Remember, also, that as Caroline Lorbach puts it, "Things trickle down in a family." If you have more than one child, your younger child will hear you talking with your older child and will learn important information this way, though because he is less cognitively mature, he may not process this trickled down information accurately. This is why you will, of course, have to provide each of your children with specific information that relates to their personal story.

Marriage and family therapist Carole Lieber Wilkins advises the parents she works with to practice. Talking to themselves and to one another, before their child can possibly understand, helps parents become comfortable with language which might otherwise feel awkward. Lieber Wilkins feels this also enables parents to deal with the feelings that arise at a time and in a context that feels safe.

Social worker Peg Beck offers the following suggestion for talking with a very young child, "I begin by saying that all babies are made the same way—with an egg and a sperm—and they all grow in a uterus. Then I go on to say that some parents who want a baby very much need help in creating a baby. I emphasize that it is a good thing to ask for help when you need it and that many times in life, there is a kind person who will offer the help that is needed. That is what happened when this couple created this child—they wanted a baby, they needed help with an egg, and a kind, generous woman offered to help. I explain that all three people worked together to make this baby so that he/she could grow in this Mommy's uterus and become these parents' child."

Nurse Mary Fusillo offers some tender stories of parents talking with their children. We found one, in particular, especially moving. Fusillo tells of one mom who did all the right things. She brought up egg donation from time to time. Her children ignored her. She showed them pictures of her when she was pregnant with each of them. They seemed to have no interest. Then everything changed. The mother of one of her daughter's friends had a baby. Suddenly both girls, then 3 and 5, had questions. They wanted to know how they got in her womb. Fusillo says that her client told the girls that she "didn't have any ova, but another woman offered to give her some of her ova so that she and the girls' father could have babies." Fusillo's client then added, "So you each grew in my uterus and we were attached by our belly buttons. There was a cord that connected us and our belly buttons will always be a reminder of that connection."

Marriage and family therapist Shelley Smith shares this story— her own. "My twins have always known they were created through oocyte donation. But when they were 3 or 4 years old, we did a family project that really brought it home to them. We planted seeds for tomato plants in our garden. Then we went next door and asked our neighbor if we could add a few of their seeds to our garden. They happily obliged, and we added their seeds to our plantings. Then we spent the spring and summer watering the plants and watching them grow. My children saw that all the plants were our plants because we were the ones who tended to them and helped them grow. They saw that without water and attention and love the seeds would not have grown into sturdy plants."

Carole Lieber Wilkins has worked with parents who have little or no information about their donors and who worry about how they will talk with their children without information. She reminds these clients that our job, as parents, is not to keep our children from all pain, but to be there for them when they do hurt. She adds that we can't control how they will feel about our decisions but we need to be there for them if they long for more information or express other feelings about the way they joined our families.

Surely you can vary your story, depending upon whether your child asks a lot of questions or you are offering this story in the absence of questions. The important messages, as we repeat them yet again, are the following:

- Be confident—this should be an opportunity, not a burden.

- Remember that your child thinks and understands in ways very different from the way you, as an adult, think and understand.

- Be prepared to tell the story many times. You won't make a mistake. You will have many opportunities to share the details.

Relationships with Donors

Known Donors

When people decide to have a family member or friend as a donor, they usually give at great deal of thought to questions of how the donation will affect their relationship. A common concern among those beginning to contemplate known donation is that the donor will feel some parental authority and will interfere with the way the child is being raised. Fortunately, pre-donor egg counseling and lengthy discussions between donors and recipients seem to do a good job of minimizing the times that the relationship turns out to be problematic. Our experience is that people who donate—whether they are sisters or friends or volunteer donors—really *do not see themselves in a parental role.* Indeed, it is the ability to see an egg as "extra body material" rather than "a future child," that enables people to donate.

Uninvited parental advice is but one fear that people have when thinking about using a known donor. Another is the fear that they will feel forever indebted to the donor. After all, how can you thank someone for giving you the gift of life? As much as payment to egg donors can be troubling, it serves an important purpose: it reduces the "lop-sidedness" of the donor-recipient relationship. For this reason, we feel that it can be helpful for recipients in known donation to give something of substance to their donors at the time of donation. As we suggested before, this might be a contribution to the donor's child's college fund or something else that relates to the donor's family.

Whatever feelings you have towards your donor, it will be important to accept and respect that your child will have his/her own feelings towards this person. For some offspring, an aunt who donated is the same aunt that she would have been had she not donated. For other offspring, the relationship may feel more special because of the unique relationship that now exists between aunt and niece or nephew.

....

Meet Bev...

"Day to day, you totally forget. I hadn't realized it would go away. But I'm a mom now and she is my child and that is all there is to it."

These words capture much of Bev Marshall's approach to motherhood through egg donation. They speak to the part of her that is open, at ease, natural and fully content with the decision to pursue motherhood using donated oocytes. They speak to the part of her that has been comfortable telling friends, family, even some colleagues about the way she and her husband, Todd, built their family. They are content, proud, grateful.

Another part of Bev is more cautious. Yes, egg donation went well for them. Theirs was a very special situation since it was Todd's brother Hank's wife, Toby, who offered to donate for them. Toby, mother of three and age 34 at the time of donation, was a perfect candidate. Even though the families lived several hundred miles apart, things went smoothly and Bev became pregnant on the first cycle. However, the pregnancy was not an easy one and it led to another set of feelings: gratitude and caution.

"My pregnancy actually began as two, but one was ectopic. We went through a difficult time—getting rid of the ectopic and then taking extra special care that nothing happened to the surviving fetus. I remember being very frightened during the remainder of the pregnancy and then, very relieved when Jenna emerged—a big, strapping healthy baby. I thought, *We've been really really lucky. We've been really, really blessed. We'd better not be greedy and push our luck.* And that is how we ended up as a one child family. Todd is one of three. I am, too. We would have loved more children, but I was 40 when Jenna was born and didn't want to push our luck."

When asked her feelings about having a child through egg donation, Bev expands on her gratitude. She adds that she is not only grateful to have become a mother after going through an early menopause, but she is also very grateful that Jenna was able to inherit certain characteristics from Toby's family, and to be spared the depression and early menopause that run through Bev's family.

"Toby did an amazing thing for us and I'm hoping that will make her special to Jenna, as she is certainly very special to us. We live far from each other but I think of her all the time, of what she did for us and of how much I want her to be close with Jenna. Toby only has boys and I think it would be special to her to be close with Jenna."

When asked if she has any other thoughts about becoming a mother through egg donation, Bev adds the following, "Family is very important to me and it always has been. Living far from family members makes it difficult for people to be close. Our family's experience is different. We live a few hours from Toby and Hank and their children, but we're close, very close. I don't know that we see each other more often than we would if Toby hadn't donated, but I do think there is something different in the closeness we feel. I'm not sure I can find better words to express it."

Feelings and Fantasies about Anonymous Donors—and Their Families

Among the many lessons adult donor sperm offspring have offered all of us is that children conceived through donor gametes have a deep and often abiding curiosity about their donor. Their feelings are very similar to those reported by generations of adult adoptees, their parents and birthparents—feelings which have greatly influenced the growing trend toward more openness in adoption. This curiosity is one of the reasons why it is critical that recipients of anonymous donation obtain as much information as possible about their donor and, if at all possible, arrange an in person meeting with her. Although this may feel awkward or unwelcome at the time, think of how much easier it will be when your child asks questions about the donor.

While you are raising your child, you are likely to find that the donor comes and goes from your mind and from your child's. There will be some times when you think of her and other times when she is completely forgotten. We expect that she will be on your mind when your child accomplishes something remarkable or displays an unusual talent or, on the dark side, when a serious medical question arises. We assume she will vanish temporarily at those moments when you are busy chasing your toddler around the house to make sure he doesn't accidentally destroy himself. Then she'll be back at a quieter moment.

In the absence of information, your child is likely to have fantasies. Hopefully, you will have met your donor or have substantial information about her so you can answer your child's questions. A photo will help your daughter who may be imagining that the donor is someone she saw at the mall or on TV. Information about the donor's family and about the other families she donated to will help your son who wonders if his new girl friend could be genetically related to him. Adoptees and donor sperm offspring have taught us that children have these fantasies and questions, that they somehow cope with them and that the most important thing for parents to do is to continue to talk openly and honestly with their children. Remember that your children can accept the fact that you have limited information as long as they know that they can count on you to speak with them with sincerity and compassion. If they become angry with you, try not to become defensive or apologetic. You did the best you could when you chose ovum donation, and now you are doing the best you can to raise your child with the information that is available to you.

Feelings Common to Many Parents after Infertility

Parents through ovum donation, like nearly all parents after infertility, carry with them some special expectations. And they face some unanticipated challenges. The following are but a few of the "after infertility" issues that confront donor egg parents.

The Need to Be Eternally Grateful

When they are going through infertility treatment and oocyte donation, people make "bargains." Among them is the pledge, "If only I am able to have a baby, I will be eternally grateful." When a real live child comes along, parents are grateful—*very grateful*—but they are also tired, stressed, ambivalent and inexperienced. It is difficult to maintain a consistently high level of gratitude, but that is what they feel they have pledged to do. Many become angry with themselves and remorseful when they feel the normal feelings of new parents—fatigued, trapped and wondering, *what have I gotten myself into?*

Parents who feel committed to eternal gratitude may find it more difficult to discipline their children. You know that your child needs limits, but you may feel like you are being cruel and ungrateful if you say "no" to him. Logically this makes no sense but there is a lot of "magical thinking" connected to infertility and parenting after infertility. Having endured so much disappointment and loss, parents sometimes associate leniency with gratitude (e.g., "If I love him so much and am so grateful to have him, then how can I punish him?").

Questions of Authenticity

"What do you know about her real mother?" This question has plagued adoptive mothers for years and now it can undermine moms through ovum donation as well. Once they have changed hundreds of diapers and tended to scrapes and bruises and been the tooth fairy and the kindergarten room mother and... moms become more convinced that they are "the real thing." But certainly in the beginning, feelings of being a fake or a fraud or "found out" are torturous. Again, we blame those who suggest that there is something to keep a secret about and who talk about "disclosure."

Feelings about Being Older Parents

Parents through ovum donation are often older parents, either because they first attempted parenthood at advanced age or because they spent years pursuing pregnancy on their own or years considering and pursuing egg donation.

Whatever got them to advanced age, all older parents (we're thinking over 40) face certain issues. One is the fact that their own parents are older, or, perhaps, they have died along the way. There is a loss of grandparenting, or, for some, the experience of being in "the sandwich generation"—having to meet the needs of young children and aging parents at the same time.

There are also worries about their own age and health. Many illnesses and medical conditions become more common when people are in their 40s. New parents may be surprised by how tired they are taking care of a baby and begin to worry about what it will be like in a few years, let alone when their child reaches adolescence.

And there may be questions about having a second child. Many donor egg parents would like to have more than one child, but is it fair to bring another child into the world when you are in your mid-40s? One mom through egg donation, who had twins at 40 and is now 45, said, "I would love to have another baby, but I can't. It's simply not the right thing to do."

Which brings us to…

Questions of Family Planning

Among the many legacies of infertility is the inability to plan your family. While your fertile friends are busy talking about timing and ideal spacing, you may be wondering whether you will be able to afford another donor cycle. Or perhaps you are worrying about your cryopreserved embryos or thinking a lot about whether you can ask your sister or close friend to donate again. You may also be focusing on your age, feeling that you cannot delay adding to your family because you don't want to be any older when your next child is born.

How nice it would be to enjoy your long awaited first child and wait a year or two or three before adding to your family. Unfortunately, the concerns we just listed and the inevitable fear that it will take a long time to achieve another pregnancy prevent many parents though ovum donation from postponing decisions about adding to their family. Those who want to remain a one child family and those who have twins and feel their family is complete are spared family planning worries, but most others are not.

Feeling Caught between the Fertile and Infertile Worlds

In the fertile world women can talk endlessly about pregnancy, labor and delivery. They can moan about stretch marks or groan that they had a c-section. Now you are among them, but your experience may seem vastly different. You may have labored for years to have a baby and a few extra hours in labor are of little consequence. Yes, you are having some trouble taking off the weight you gained, but you don't mind it all that much—it's a temporary souvenir of your pregnancy.

So one way that you are caught between the fertile and infertile worlds is that you are with fertile moms and you feel different. Another place you feel different is with infertile women—you may feel that you are still one of them, but sometimes they don't see it that way. You have had a baby and that puts you in a new place.

Although it is important for you to be with other moms—"regular" other moms—you will probably also find it helpful to connect with other moms through egg donation. You should be able to access them through your local RESOLVE chapter or AFA or through the web. In the Boston area, for example, there is a donor egg network that meets for lunch each month.

Our Real versus Our Fantasy Children

When contemplating parenthood, everyone fantasizes about what their child will be like. Inevitably, partners focus on the traits they like best in themselves and in each other and they imagine a child who combines the best of both of them. In anticipating parenthood, it is much easier and more natural to picture a child with her beautiful eyes and his great hair or her athletic ability and his musical talent than it is to imagine a child who has her anxiety and his stubbornness, her Uncle Fred's schizophrenia genes and his Aunt Sally's paranoia. You get the picture.

Our *real* children are not the children of our fantasies. They are not exactly who we expected, but as parents, we realize that our task is to love them for who they are and not for who they are not. This can be a challenge for all parents, but perhaps all the more so for donor egg (and donor sperm and adoptive) parents. While other parents can celebrate differences with a sense of curiosity and wonder, you may be more inclined to experience disappointment. If you had an anonymous donor, you may be wondering whether your child has inherited some of his/her less appealing traits from the donor. You may feel added sadness that some qualities you'd hoped to see in your child seem to be missing.

We encourage parents through ovum donation to realize that all parents deal with disappointment. As much as we love our children, they are always different in some way from what we wanted and hoped they would be. And that, in many ways, is the magic of parenthood. Philosophy professor, Michael J. Sandel (*Atlantic Monthly*, April, 2004) concludes his article, "The Case against Perfection," with these words about those who seek to "design" children, "But that promise of mastery is flawed. It threatens to banish our appreciation of life as a gift and to leave us with nothing to affirm or behold outside our own will."

Extraordinary Joy

Lest we end on a down note, we turn now to the most prominent feature of parenting after infertility: Joy! Ecstasy! Exuberance!

How often have we seen people who struggled and struggled to build their family be transformed into content and happy parents. Yes, they are tired. Sure they feel ambivalence. But what we notice most of all is their happiness. They look younger, they look more relaxed, their cars and their homes and their very selves are permanently altered.

In her wise and comforting essay, "Entitled to All That Parenting Has to Offer," psychologist Carole Lieber Wilkins, herself a mom through egg donation and adoption, concludes with theses words, "We get it all. Whether infertile or not, genetically related or not, whether we gave birth to them or not, we are entitled to all the title of Mom and Dad confers upon us—the blessing and the curse—with our eyes open and fully cognizant of the blessing which we have finally received."

....

Meet Debby and Stephen...

Debby and Stephen have created their family through adoption and donor egg. Asked how she feels about building a family this way, Debby smiles and says, "I'm very positive about our experience." Then she pauses for a moment and adds, "But that's because I got my kids. I wasn't feeling so positive when we were in the middle of things!"

"The middle of things" proved an incredible challenge for this spirited, open, communicative couple who knew they wanted two children. Debby and Stephen suffered several years of infertility including four miscarriages before they began thinking about both donor egg and adoption. "We knew we would make something work. Maybe it wouldn't be our first choice but it would be a way to have a family."

Debby and Stephen went through an anonymous egg donation cycle when Debby was in her late 30s. She did not become pregnant, and the couple, feeling parenthood was long overdue, chose to move on to adoption. They had cryopreserved embryos, but, at that point, adoption—a sure thing—was looking more attractive than another attempt at pregnancy. And so Debby and Stephen, frayed by all their losses, set out to adopt a baby.

"We went to an adoption agency which was placing kids pretty quickly. There were people there who submitted their applications one month and were parents two or three months later. And so it was hard not to assume that the same thing would happen to us. Well, it didn't. We ended up waiting ten months for Bobby. Ten months may not sound like a long time but Stephen and I had been waiting years to be parents."

As much as Debby and Stephen hated waiting for "The Call," they admit that when it finally came, it was incredibly special. Debby, a clinical social worker, was leading a therapy group when she noticed that her beeper was repeatedly signaling her to call the adoption agency. She remembers thinking to herself, *Oh them, what could they want? They're probably bothering me about a bill or something.*

The call wasn't about a bill; it was about a baby. Not a pregnant woman. Not a baby soon to be born, but their real, live Bobby, a baby waiting for them. When she finally called the agency to learn this news, Debby tried her best to stay calm and to reach Stephen. Her calm turned to frenzy when she couldn't find him. Eventually they connected and by the end of the day, they were parents.

And so the couple that woke up one morning assuming it would be a work day no different from any other work day, ended the most eventful day of their lives as parents. "Bobby was our dream child from the moment we saw him—and he still is." In addition to being crazy about Bobby, Debby and Stephen were crazy about adoption. They had learned that pregnancy can't be counted on and that adoption really works. So how is it that they ended up having their second son, Jeffrey, through donor egg?

"We had frozen embryos that we wanted to use. If I hadn't become pregnant, we would have certainly adopted again, but we had the embryos and this time one worked." Debby goes on to say that the pregnancy she'd waited so long for was anything but the nirvana she'd anticipated. "I was hospitalized several times, warned that the baby would never make it, sick as can be." It was extraordinarily difficult for Stephen as well, since he had to take care of Bobby, as well as watch his wife suffer and worry.

Despite several close calls, Debby did give birth to a healthy baby. Like his older brother, Bobby, 4 1/2, Jeffrey, now 2, has been a delight to his parents. Debby and Stephen are busy and tired these days, but also jubilant. "We realized, along the way, that the important thing was to get our kids, we knew we would love them and we felt that the love we would have for them would be bigger than anything."

Debby and Stephen, mental health professionals who are active in the infertile community, both speak publicly about their blended family. Do they have any advice to readers? we asked. To this, the couple responds, "Yes, you make it work. If you want to be parents, you figure out a way to have that happen and then you make it work."

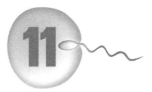

Ethics, Faith and Egg Donation

Entire books have been written on the ethical and religious concerns raised by assisted reproduction. Included in them are lengthy discussions of ovum donation. Because the focus of this book is on your journey to parenthood through egg donation and because we have addressed many ethical questions in other chapters, we are limiting our discussion here to an overview. Because there is so much to explore and consider, we will refer you to articles we found especially helpful and which we encourage you to read.

Ethical Considerations

As someone who is considering using donated oocytes, you probably feel that you are being bombarded with overwhelming life-altering decisions, beginning with whether you even want to try egg donation. Ethical perspective may play a role in your decision making.

Ovum donation, for all it has to offer, raises many ethical questions. We have briefly introduced several of these questions in other chapters, but we have waited until now, after you as a reader have had considerable time to get to know us through our writing and should have, we hope, come to see us as your advocates, to deal with these issues in depth. We feel, though, that we would not be serving you well if we did not suggest that you think seriously about the ethical reservations that have been raised by others about the process of family building through egg donation. Some of these opinions and concerns may be difficult to think about, but we believe that you must think about them before making a final decision to pursue this family building option.

We would like to take the opportunity and the challenge now, then, to seriously explore with you some of the central ethical dilemmas raised by egg donation.

Ethics are a set of principles that motivate us to engage in "right" behavior. Each of us has our own unique personal code of ethics and specific definitions of behaviors we feel are right and wrong. Our personal code of ethics has been developed and influenced by many factors in our lives—our family culture, our religious training, our schooling, etc. We draw upon this code of ethics when we need to make difficult decisions. For most of us, it is our ethics that we rely upon to guide us and keep us from crossing ethical lines in situations which may tempt us. The use of donated oocytes to form families is complex ethically because it raises many questions that we never thought we would have to think about, and it forces us to carefully consider new ways of creating families.

Ethics related to medical and health issues are governed by four major principles. The first is *autonomy,* or the obligation to respect the decision making rights of individual people. This allows each individual patient to decide which course of treatment to pursue or refuse. Regardless of how strong your views are, however, it is difficult to predict what you will do in a situation until you are actually faced with it. It is the responsibility of medical professionals to ensure that each patient is accurately informed about his or her medical condition and all of the treatment possibilities that are available and then to respect that each patient has the autonomy to make his decision on his own. As long as it does not infringe on the welfare and safety of others, autonomy encourages us to assume that everyone is making the best decision possible for themselves and their families.

The next two principles, *non-maleficence* and *beneficence,* go hand-in-hand. Non-maleficence emphasizes the obligation to "do no harm," while beneficence encourages not only the obligation to actually provide benefits, but also to balance these benefits against risks. With egg donation, it is easy to see that a benefit would be that a couple gets a new baby, and who could argue with that? Well, someone could, based on the idea that harm could be done. It is important to examine the risks involved or the harm that could be produced as a result of ovum donation. We are not talking only about physical harm here, but rather "hidden" risks, such as emotional harm possibly affecting you and your partner, the lives of the donor and her family, as well as the child conceived through donated ova. We do not think any of us would purposely wish harm on someone, but the bottom line is that we do not know the long term effects of egg donation. Consequently, these unknown factors must be carefully weighed when deciding if oocyte donation is the best choice for you and your family.

The final medical health ethical principle is *justice*. Justice obligates fairness in the distribution of benefits and risks. In other words, everyone should be treated fairly and have access to what they need, including the most advanced forms of reproductive technology. While most of us would agree with this concept in theory, the reality is much more complicated. Since reproductive technologies are not typically covered by insurance nor are they available in every small town, there are limits as to who has access to these technologies and who does not. This raises the question of who should control these limits and ultimately decide who should be able to attempt certain ARTs and collaborative reproductive options, including egg donation. Often, it is money that speaks the loudest. Is it fair to assume that just because you have enough money to spend, you have the right to attempt to conceive with donated oocytes regardless of the circumstances?

As you can see, when any of these principles clash, an ethical dilemma results, and we are forced to ask the age old question: just because we can do it, should we? Since autonomy is the cornerstone of medical ethics, in most instances, medical professionals are inclined to accept a patient's autonomy and respect their right to make any decisions that they feel are in their best interests. However, is it always acceptable to allow someone to do this, especially when it may cause possible harm in the future, as perhaps may be the case with egg donation? Moreover, who should have the power to make these "gate keeping" decisions

In this chapter, we will provide an overview of issues related to the ethics of ovum donation. As with most ethical questions, there are very few definite right or wrong answers here. As we have said before, you will encounter many different opinions and point of views over the course of your journey, from family and friends, as well as respected professionals such as clergy and physicians. They will all claim that they are in indeed right regarding their views on ova donation. Consequently, this experience will challenge you to rely on your own ethical and moral frameworks to navigate through these gray areas. Our goal for this chapter is to better prepare you to face these difficult issues with knowledge and confidence as you travel down the road toward using donated eggs. We sincerely hope that you take from this book as much information as possible and decide what is best for *you* and *your family* while taking into careful consideration all the risks and benefits and the overall justice of your final decision.

Is Ovum Donation Ethical?

Since its inception, assisted reproductive technology has been plagued by ethical concerns. In the early 1900s, society in general had difficulty even accepting the relatively simple procedure of artificial insemination with a husband's own sperm. Some groups quickly condemned the practice altogether, citing that it was un-natural and sacrilegious. However, it was not long before this practice was not only common, but for the most part, supported by many. However, it seems as though once one issue is resolved, it is time to tackle a new one. For instance, once public opinion moved towards accepting artificial insemination with a husband's own sperm in order to achieve the desired pregnancy, donor sperm became an option. People were forced to ponder yet again what this all meant and to reflect on whether it should be done. It is no surprise, that as technology has grown more complicated over the years so have the ethical issues.

A little more than thirty years ago, when IVF was in its infancy, it was almost immediately met with worldwide public outcry. Most of Western civilization felt that assisted reproductive technology was "against God's will" and feared that it would destroy traditional family values that had long been established and actively promoted within society. Physicians and scientists throughout the world argued about the ethics of IVF and its implications. With one in seven couples unable to conceive on their own, supporters of IVF thought it a valid means to help many couples realize their dream of becoming pregnant. How could they deny couples this chance, most likely their only chance, to have a baby? On the other hand, there were many who thought IVF was just one step further down a slippery slope. What is so slippery about giving people the chance to have babies, you may ask yourself? It is important to remember that IVF is the first step towards genetic engineering, creating "designer" babies and perhaps new species, as well as stem cell research and cloning, all of which remain political hotbeds even as we speak. As Eunice Kennedy Shriver explains, even beneficial developments can be the first step on a slope that might lead to great harm.

Even though IVF was allowed to continue, the debate over the ethics of ARTs was never fully resolved. In fact, concerns were amplified when oocyte donation became available in the early 1980s. Egg donation was believed to be just another step down that slippery slope. Just how far should man go in manipulating the creation of life?

Where are we today? Some counties, such as Austria, Norway, Sweden and Switzerland have completely banned the use of donated oocytes, mainly due to the slippery slope philosophy—having decided that the benefits do not outweigh the risks involved. Other counties, such as the United Kingdom, Australia and Canada, have put in place specific regulations concerning use of donated ova in hopes of mitigating these risks. In the United States, thousands of babies have been born through the use of egg donation. Even though there will always be some who oppose assisted reproduction in almost all cases or more specifically gamete donation or other third party reproduction, oocyte donation, generally speaking, has come to be accepted by American society as an appropriate means to build a family.

However, we still have not found the answers to so many of the major ethical questions raised by egg donation, such as at what point do we cross the line of potentially causing harm? It seems as though the obvious benefits of reproductive technology are surpassing our ability to fully comprehend and reconcile concerns we might have. To make matters worse, no one can decide who should further explore these issues. Many governments, including the United States government, have been reluctant to take a stance on ovum donation—specifically, about what should be allowed and what should not. This puts anyone who is considering using donated eggs in a difficult place. How can you be expected to make important life-altering decisions about egg donation, when so many others, including prominent leaders across various disciplines such as medicine, science, theology and law, who deal with similar tough ethical issues every day, have not been able to do so?

Now back to the original question, is egg donation and conception using donated eggs ethical? We wish we had the definitive answer, but ovum donation is one of those gray areas through which you must navigate. You must understand that this is a decision that is entirely yours to make based on your own sense of personal ethics. What is right for someone else, may not be right for you, and vice versa. It is our hope that this chapter will provide you with the knowledge and tools to guide you and help you feel good about making vital decisions that will affect you and your family and a potential donor and her family for the rest of your lives.

In Whose Best Interest?

In order for ovum donation to be ethically sound, all participants should enjoy some benefit or beneficence. Their autonomy should be respected and they should be treated with justice. By "all" we refer to the donors, the recipients, the offspring, members of their extended families and the society at large. Let's take a look at what might be in the best interests of each group.

The Children

We begin with the question of the best interests of the children since, unlike the donors and recipients, the offspring of donated ova cannot speak for themselves—at least not at the time of key decision making. Who, then, looks after their best interests and what might these interests involve?

On the positive side, children created through egg donation are given the gift of life, something they would not otherwise have and the value of which may trump any negatives associated with egg donation. Add to the gift of life the fact that these are children who are wanted, planned for and who will be raised by those who intended, from the start, to parent them. Those who are created with the help of family donors also have the gift of being born into two families with which one shares a genetic history and heritage,

If children created using donated oocytes are given gifts of life, love and family, then surely, it can be argued that egg donation is ethically sound. However, that does not negate the losses experienced by some of the offspring of donated eggs . There are those who are permanently cut off from one side of their genetic families. This occurs not only because some donors remain anonymous, but also, because some donors donate multiple times, offering their offspring no way of finding or identifying one another.

Even those whose program-recruited donors met with the parents in the course of the donation process may face questions about the payment the donor received. Although egg donation is fundamentally different than sperm donation, since egg donors undergo significant inconvenience, discomfort and even risk to donate, it is possible that some offspring will react in much the same way as those sperm donor offspring who accuse their donor fathers of "doing it for the money."

Some donor offspring will be born to much older than average parents, and this raises further questions about what is in their best interests. Although it was always possible for a child to be born to a 60-year-old man, prior to the availability of oocyte donation, the mother was almost always under 45. It is now possible for a child to be born to two people over 45 or even significantly older. Is it in a child's best interests to have parents who are over 60 when raising an adolescent? Is oocyte donation creating children who will need to take care of elderly parents before they, themselves, really reach adulthood? Does it create children whose parents are likely to die before they themselves have gotten through an increasingly lengthening adolescence (now presumed to include not just the teen years, but also a significant portion of the twenties)?

And so we see, in reviewing ethical principles, that when it comes to donor offspring, some fundamental questions arise. Surely the gifts of life, love and family are evidence of beneficence, but when we look at the potential suffering associated with being cut off from genetic relatives and history and being born to older parents, we see that for *some* egg donation offspring, there are questions of justice and non-malificence.

The Donors

Does egg donation offer benefit to donors? Where do the other central ethical principles of autonomy and justice fit in? From a positive perspective, ova donation respects a donor's autonomy. A woman can decide to donate her eggs to her sister in need, to a close friend, or she can become an altruistic donor. Researcher Judith Bernstein documented in Seibel and Crockin's book *Family Building Through Egg and Sperm Donation,: Medical, Legal and Ethical Issues* (1996) and others have observed that egg donation offers donors "gratification through altruism, increased self-esteem or fulfillment of a desire to rework a negative past experience with a better outcome." At the same time, however, Judith Bernstein and others address the question of non-maleficence— the potential for a donor to be vulnerable to harm, either psychological or physical, as a result of the donation. Harm could occur if a family member feels coerced into donating, if a volunteer donor is enticed by payment, or if a medical or donor-recruitment program does not go to great lengths to help donors achieve informed consent.

With true informed consent, women donating eggs would be likely to recognize their need to know the outcome of their donation. They would understand that if their efforts to help a family have a child, that child may want to know more about the person who helped give him/her life. The truly informed donor would be prepared for a future in which questions might arise coming either from the offspring, or the recipient or they may arise within the donor herself. Unfortunately, true informed consent does not always occur. There are donors who are left wondering what happened with their ova and if there "is a piece of me out there," who are, indeed, harmed by the process. According to one study conducted by The Bioethics Institute at the Johns Hopkins University (Kalfoglou and Geller, 2000), most egg donors interviewed after their donations would, in retrospect, like to have known what happened to their donated eggs. The most common reason for this was that it would make them feel good to know that their donation was successful.

With egg donation there is also the potential for medical complications for the donor. Although egg donation is considered by the medical community as safe, there are risks. First, powerful fertility medications are used, as well as complicated surgical procedures. This raises the potential for physical risks, both short- and long-term. For example, there are risks to the donor of ovarian hyperstimulation, infection during ova retrieval, the potential for future infertility issues of her own, and the possibility of increased risks for certain types of cancers, including ovarian cancer. The question arises as to whether it is beneficent to encourage healthy women to undergo ovarian hyper-stimulation and ova retrieval in order to assist others to create a baby.

The subject of payment to donors has been the subject of extensive ethical debate. On the one hand, payment for time and effort and the inclusion of a broad range of women as donors meets the ethical standard of justice. The process is time consuming, intrusive, invasive and carries with it risks, so why shouldn't women receive compensation for their effort? However, some wonder whether payments of $5000— the "going rate" as of this writing—do not serve to entice women who might not otherwise donate eggs. In her essay, "What is Wrong with Commodification?" Ruth Macklin, Professor of Bioethics at Albert Einstein Medical College examines in Cohen's book (pp. 106-121) the question of payment to donors from a variety of ethical perspectives. She concludes that it all comes down to a "disagreement over commodification." Macklin explains that those who favor payment argue that to prohibit payment would be "moralistic and symbolic" while those who oppose it say that it treats reproductive capacity as "just another market force and leads to 'an inferior conception of human flourishing'." Macklin herself concludes that "although commodification is not immoral, it is nonetheless 'unsavory.'"

So what does this mean for women who volunteer to be egg donors and receive payment for doing so? For some, not much at all: they work hard to donate their eggs and are grateful to have some financial compensation for time loss of work, social and leisure time. For others, however, there may be the potential for future regret. Should these women face infertility or pregnancy loss in the future, we hope that they will not look back with regret, a regret that could be intensified if the payment was at all a factor in their decision making.

Unfortunately, there are no guidelines currently in place regarding the level of payment that should go to the donors. The ethics committee of the American Society for Reproductive Medicine (ASRM) has tried to draw a line between the selling and donating of ova. Due to both the physical and psychological burdens donors must endure, ASRM does not come out against compensation for these women. Instead, it says that "compensation based in a reasonable assessment of the time, inconvenience and discomfort associated with oocyte retrieval can be distinguished from payment for the oocytes themselves. This compensation should not be based on particular human traits. Furthermore, it concludes that sums of $5,000 or more require justification and those above $10,000 go beyond what is appropriate. In addition, ARSM further emphasizes the need for physicians to treat egg donors as they would other patients and suggests that programs should note the burdens and risks as well as the financial or other benefits in their advertisements for ovum donors.

A related question that many grapple with is whether it is ethical to "buy and sell" human eggs if it is illegal to sell human organs? As we have said many times, those involved in egg donation are always careful to identify the payment as being one for time effort, rather than for ova. Still, the debate continues as to how like and different eggs are from human organs. Jeffery Kahn, Ph.D., M.P.H, Director of the University of Minnesota Center for Bioethics, explains that historically, blood, bone marrow and sperm have been donated for money. Unlike egg donation, blood, bone marrow and sperm are all replenishable, have low or no risk with their donation; and therefore, they bring relatively low payments. Macklin, in her article "What Is Wrong with Commodification?" points out that, "even the sale of blood, like other human bodily materials, is a form of commodification." Macklin quotes the "Glover Report to the European Commission" by Jonathan Glover and others (DeKalb, Northern Illinois Univ. Press, 1989), which observes that payment "deprives donors of the chance of doing something purely for others."

Protecting donors from risks is more complicated than it seems. In their article, "Navigating Conflict of Interest in Oocyte Donation: An Analysis of Donors' Experiences," Andrea Kalfoglou, Ph.D. and Gail Geller, Sc.D., both of the Bioethics Institute at the Johns Hopkins

University, explore the issue that egg donation places oocyte donors in a unique situation. Egg donors are not truly patients. They are not seeking medical attention in order to achieve better health. Instead, they are perfectly healthy individuals who are volunteering to undergo medical procedures that are being paid privately by someone else to help the recipient (often someone they do not even know in the case of anonymous donation) have a baby.

Kalfoglou and Geller raise many questions. First, what exactly is role of the egg donor and what are the recipients' and the medical community's expectations of and responsibilities towards her? For example, when she undergoes psychological screening to be an egg donor, whose interest is the mental health professional looking out for—the donor's or the recipient couple's? In their study about donors' experiences, Kalfaglou and Geller illustrate this point through a quote by egg donor Claire, age unknown, who commented without any prompting, "I was sort of curious to see how (the mental health counselor) handled her position in terms of disclosure and that sort of thing—about what her purpose was. And I expected her to say, 'I am being paid by the recipient couple. I am not your advocate.' Nothing. She did not even have me sign a release, which I thought was a little tacky."

Kalfoglou and Geller point out that mental health professionals' ability to provide appropriate care may be clouded by the fact that it is the recipient who is paying the entire bill and it is the recipient who wants to find an egg donor. Hence, the mental health professional may feel pressure, whether overt or more subtle, to secure a good egg donor candidate for this couple. Similarly, because the donor knows the mental health professionals wants to find a good donor, she might be reluctant to provide any information, such as abuse, rape or abortion, that might put her in a bad light or hurt her chances of becoming a donor.

Likewise, conflict of interest and poorly defined roles may affect the donor's treatment by medical and legal professionals as well. Again, it is the recipient couple, not her, who pays the bills for the medical treatment and any legal representation. Consequently, donors may be unclear about their own rights and responsibilities when they agree to treatment or sign contracts. Because people are taught to trust people in authority positions, including doctors and lawyers, donors may be more hesitant to ask questions and voice concerns. Whose interest is actually being protected during the egg donation process, that of the recipient couple who is paying the clinic, lawyers and psychologists for services, or the donor who is being "evaluated" and "screened?"

We turn now to what we call "involuntary donors"—infertile women who donate ova through what is called "egg sharing." Egg sharing asks a woman who is undergoing infertility treatments to donate some of her ova in exchange for a reduction in the costs of her treatment. Egg sharing can mean that patients only have to pay half of their treatment fees or may even receive free infertility treatment. Some clinics actively promote the egg sharing concept because there is such a shortage of voluntarily donated eggs.

Although this practice is popular in some places, we feel that it raises significant ethical issues. It strikes us as coercive to ask an infertile woman (or couple), so eager to have a child, to relinquish some piece of her own fertility in order to secure treatment. Ethical questions around beneficence, justice and autonomy all arise if someone's only access to assisted reproduction comes at the cost of her own eggs.

While it is difficult to predict how involuntary donors will feel later on, it is important for these women to discuss potential issues that may become evident at sometime later in life with a trained counselor before beginning the egg donation journey. Donors need to carefully explore what they want to get out of this oocyte donation process and how these expectations may change over time as their lives continue to change.

The Recipients

For the recipients of donated oocytes there appear to be many advantages to receiving donated eggs. The process seems to meet ethical measures of autonomy in that people who seek parenthood have an opportunity to make decisions for themselves; justice in that egg donation is available to a vast range of would-be parents; non-maleficence since as long as donors have informed consent; there appears to be no harm; and beneficence, because as we have said, many times, the child created through ovum donation is planned for, wanted and deeply loved. All of this is true, but there are other perspectives that can be applied to the question: Is ovum donation in the best interests of recipients?

Some people feel a need to try to conceive using donated ova, despite its emotional and physical risks, "because it is there." Some say that their medical programs promote egg donation as a form of "treatment, "rather than correctly identifying it as an alternative path to parenthood. These patients say that adoption is presented as much more challenging, risky and unfamiliar. In addition, there are instances in states with insurance mandates where ovum donation is presented as much more affordable. This occurs often in Massachusetts, where there has been an insurance mandate to cover ARTs since 1987. As a result, I (Ellen) have seen a vast number of couples who have said that without the mandate, they would have adopted, but adoption often costs close to $30,000 (now reduced by the tax credit and other adoption benefits) while ovum donation often costs as little as $4000 (if the donor is a family member and medical costs are covered, there are only legal and counseling fees remaining).

Those who pursue egg donation "because it is there" and who become successfully pregnant, may suffer some harm because they have a child they may not be fully prepared to welcome into their families. Those who do not conceive are likely to suffer greater maleficence—egg donation becomes another failure, another set back, and for those who would otherwise chose adoption, it costs them valuable time and money.

Another aspect of the "just because it is there," perspective on egg donation is that there will be recipients who pursue conception through oocyte donation at advanced age. At one time women past their early 40s, made peace with the fact that they could not bear children and faced big challenges adopting (challenges which have diminished greatly as some are adopting even into their 50s). Now this cohort of women has the opportunity to become pregnant, and some feel that if the opportunity is there, they should seize it. I (Ellen) recently met with a 47-year-old, newly married woman who raised serious concerns about whether it was "right for me to have a baby at this age," but who felt she should try it because "I would love to be pregnant and the doctors say it can happen."

It can happen, but is it in the best interests of recipient couples to enter into parenthood if both are of advanced age? We realize, of course, that there are 43-year-old women with 33-year- old husbands now becoming families through egg donation, but what of the couple in which both are past 45? As one medical program I (Ellen) worked in determined it, "It does not seem right to us to work with couples whose combined age is over 90." At some clinics, however, such combined-age-of-90 couples are becoming parents and their advanced age may not only put a burden on their children, but on the couple as well. A friend who is an elementary school principal observed, "People in their 50s with kids in elementary school are out of the loop of the parent network. They stand out as different and receive limited support from the community at a time when they could use it most." Another friend, a radiologist specializing in breast disease, said, "Every day I have to talk with women in their 40s and 50s about a new breast cancer diagnosis. It seems unfair to me to think of these women facing breast cancer treatment at the same time as having young children at home. Yes, younger women can become ill, but diseases like breast cancer become more common in the 40s and certainly, when a woman passes 50." And we might add, so do heart disease and other age-related health problems in both men and women.

Women who decide to attempt pregnancy with donated eggs and who do not succeed in becoming pregnant often report a sense of failure. They say that their bodies let them down and speak of diminished self-esteem. For those who tried other ARTs before ovum donation, there can be a more profound sense of failure. "Nothing seems to work. Even when there are great eggs, I still cannot become pregnant." It can be argued that these women received benefit from egg donation in that it gave them another chance at pregnancy, but harm also can be seen, since they ended the process feeling an increased sense of failure.

Another ethical consideration regarding recipients is one of justice—should everyone have the opportunity to obtain donated eggs? If so, then we are likely to see more 60-year-old women deciding to pursue pregnancy and we have already acknowledged some of the ways in which this may not be non-maleficent. Furthermore, recipients from certain groups, for example, lesbians, single women, low-income women, and older women may find it more difficult to access egg donation technology. What choices should they be allotted as far as family building? Exactly which characteristics should be used to evaluate potential egg donors? Should criteria beyond medial and reproductive health considered? Is it appropriate to select oocyte donation recipients based on certain subjective criteria such as lifestyle, social status and ability fit someone's definition of a "good" parent?

However, if certain groups are excluded as egg donor recipients, questions of justice arise. What if a particular program decides to deny access to lesbians or to single women or perhaps to people who already have children? We can easily see how access to oocyte donation and restricting that access create some ethical quandaries.

The Extended Families

The families of recipients of egg donation enjoy many benefits and so it can well be argued that ovum donation is in their best interests. Grandparents get new grandchildren, cousins get cousins, aunts and uncles get nieces and nephews. The family expands and this brings happiness to many, all the more so when the new parents are known to have endured much suffering in order to become parents. On the other hand, the feelings of the donor's extended family are rarely addressed. At a recent meeting of mental health professionals involved in egg donation, one group member said that she "cringed" when her step-daughter said she wanted to donate eggs. Others in the group all said they could identify with her reactions. Although they help others become parents through egg donation, none of them—the potential grandparents—would want their daughters donating eggs to strangers.

The ethical question that arises for extended families is "who am I related to?" While this is unlikely to be a problem in intrafamily donation or even friend-to-friend donation, questions do arise when a program-recruited donor provides ova to several families. The children in those families, as well as all members of the donor's genetic family, may not know who one another are and may be cut off from contact. This may take an emotional toll and, possibly, a medical one as well, since there are instances in which genetic relatives may be able to donate life saving bone marrow or become live organ donors for one another.

The Society at Large

The greatest ethical questions posed by oocyte donation are those that relate to our society at large. Is there benefit to society as a result of egg donation?

Surely, there are positive societal outcomes from ovum donation. Egg donation brings new children into the world, some of whom may make major contributions to humankind through their work in medicine, the arts, education and more. Egg donation also enables cancer survivors and others who have suffered significant loss early in life to bear children. It offers couples in which the woman is significantly older than her husband the opportunity to share a pregnancy and raise a child together, something which has long been afforded older men and their younger wives. The world expands in many ways through the use of donated ova, and with this expansion, come many potential benefits.

What are the drawbacks? We have already addressed some of them—payment to donors raises concerns about people and body parts becoming commodities and whole segments of the population being cut off from their genetic relatives and heritage. Prospective parents can now extend their childbearing years, bringing children into the world who may be caring for aged parents before the children, themselves, reach adulthood or who may be in need of care should their parents die before the children are independent.

In addition, the different approaches to egg donation worldwide have led to "fertility tourism"— people traveling from one country to another seeking eggs. Although this travel could be defended in terms of autonomy (people have an opportunity to create the families they want) and justice (people worldwide can access egg donation), ethical questions arise. Ruth Deech, author of "Reproductive Tourism in Europe: Infertility and Human Rights," (*Global Governance*, Oct/Dec. 2003;9[4]:425-33), explains that the rapid development of health-related technologies and the mobility and knowledge of people have led to the globalization of assisted reproductive technologies. Gametes and embryos may be passed from country to country in search of one that permits the desired treatment or allows the chosen gametes to be used. This is becoming more and more popular with oocyte donation, as women are becoming "fertility tourists" and paying high sums of money to travel abroad in their desperate search to find egg donors and programs that will allow them to become parents at any cost.

In London, waiting lists at clinics can range from six months to eight years. Because of much more lenient guidelines for egg donors, other countries, such as Spain, Crete, and Romania seem to have a higher volume of egg donors. Couples with money may regard this situation as inviting, simply traveling abroad in search of eggs. In its October 25, 2004 article, "EU faces fertility tourism threat," the BBC write about the Bridge Centre in London which reportedly "sends frozen British sperm to Bucharest to fertilize eggs provided by Romanian women." The article goes on to explain that the frozen embryos are then shipped back to London and transferred to British women. The motivation for going to Eastern Europe is that an IVF procedure in the UK typically costs between $4000 and $7500 while the same procedure in Slovenia or Hungary is about $3000. (Interestingly, the article reports that success rates are 36% and 31.9% in Slovenia and Hungary and 28.4% in UK.) The article also notes that women in Romania are paid a couple hundred dollars for an egg, a fee that is a good portion of the average Romanian yearly income, while donors in the UK are permitted to receive about $25. Fertility tourism raises the possibility of one group "exploiting" another, something that. concerns Professor Macklin (Cohen, 1996) when she looks at the issue of payment to donors and questions whether the availability of ovum donation will result in wealthier couples "paying money to poorer women for the use of their bodies." Macklin responds to this question by concluding that "All things considered, it is implausible to conclude that paying egg donors is exploitive. The facts surrounding the socioeconomic status of ovum donors show that they do not come from the poorest class of society." Still, if people are encouraged to travel from one country to another for donated eggs, there may be more opportunity for egg brokers to entice poorer women to donate eggs.

In her article, "Toward a Feminist Perspective on Gamete Donation and Reception Policies," (Cohen, 1996) Dr. Rosemarie Tong, Thatcher Professor in Philosophy and Medical Humanities at Davidson College in North Carolina offers another perspective on the societal impact of egg donation. Tong observes that "cultural feminists" see in oocyte donation (as well as in sperm donation), "possibilities for increased human connection—the kind of collaborative reproduction that, in the 1960s, was supposed to defeat the view that children are 'genetic possessions.'" Having noted this way in which egg donation contributes to a fabric of society, Tong emphasizes that feminists who hold this position insist, as we do, that donation be open and, they add, "non commercial." She adds, "If gamete donors are interested, they should at least be kept posted on their genetic child's development, and at some point in time, perhaps when the child has reached the age of majority, at least be introduced to him or her."

Another societal question involves the use of medical and societal resources. Although there have been some who have argued that infertility is "not a disease," RESOLVE and other organizations have worked hard to educate the public and the health insurance industry so that infertility is, indeed, recognized as a serious medical condition. Nonetheless, with children worldwide needing homes, many argue that the pursuit of treatment for infertility should have its limits and that some infertile couples should be encouraged to consider adoption, not because it is their obligation, but because familiarity with adoption often makes it more attractive to infertile couples..

Where does oocyte donation fit into the debate over the use of medical and social resources? Again, some would argue that egg donor recipients should be offering homes to children who need them rather than "creating children who will be 'half-adopted' anyway." Others counter and ask why shouldn't a 32-year-old woman who lost her ovarian function during chemotherapy not be able to become pregnant, carry and deliver a child that is her husband's genetic offspring? Isn't egg donation, which enables a woman to use half of her reproductive capacity, something beneficent, just and respectful of people's autonomy.

In Massachusetts, where there has been mandated coverage for infertility for many years, health insurance companies have found ways—some just and others, less so— to address the question of when medical resources should be allocated for ovum donation. In general, insurance will cover egg donation for any woman whose ovarian failure is premature. By contrast, insurance plans find ways of distinguishing peri-menopause and menopause from early ovarian failure and do not offer coverage in these instances. Although this leads to frustration and disappointment for some couples, it appears to adhere to medical ethics in that all those with ovarian failure that is truly premature and hence, a medical problem, receive the benefits of coverage. As we have seen, egg donation brings with it complex ethical questions. Who should decide what is right and what is wrong? Currently, much is left to individuals, at least in the U.S. Because infertility falls outside government regulations in the United States, George Annas, Professor of Health Law at Boston University's School of Public Health, calls the world of assisted reproduction the "Wild West." And indeed it is in many instances. Worldwide, it remains the "Wild West" in some countries and has been severely restricted in others. Both situations seem problematic.

One of the darkest sides of egg donation is that it has unleashed the possibility of "designer breeding" and thereby raises disturbing questions about eugenics. Currently, few couples have sought specific traits in selecting egg donors; thus there is not an abnormally large proportion of, say, tall, blonde, athletic, Ivy League-bound children running around. But as egg donation becomes more widespread, these questions will become increasingly real.

It is one thing for people to select *out* for medical conditions, for people to decide they don't want a donor with a family history of mental retardation, depression or alcoholism. That's one of the benefits of current medicical technology—to identify what's a disease, and what we can do to prevent it. But it's quite another thing for people to choose specific enhancements and improvements. That's a question society will have to answer. What kind of people do we want to create? Smarter? Taller? More athletic? Those kinds of decisions are more or less inevitable if we go down this road of selecting specific egg donors.

And yet—while realizing that question must be asked for the sake of society, individuals must still make decisions. Whether one particular potential mother accepts the social stereotypes associated with education, IQ, or physical appearance, and whether she pays more money to a college-educated donor than to a working-class donor, will have little impact on general patterns of social stereotyping and class division. Each individual's decision is limited in scope, and her responsibility for overall social patterns—even ones she has contributed to—is likewise limited. However, this does not mean the issues are not significant and can be ignored. Like other broad social issues—conservation, racism, and so forth—each single person's actions are of little consequence, but each person's contributions are necessary to creating a solution to the problem on the large scale. Egg recipients who object to "social engineering" on the basis of education, IQ, physical appearance, and the like can be true to their values by seeking egg donors on the basis of socially neutral criteria like overall health alone. While their contribution to the trend in general may be small, they can feel good about adhering to their own ethical and moral code.

As you can see, there remain many unanswered questions with egg donation. It is our sincere hope that people will continue to raise, explore and attempt to respond to the ethical questions raised by assisted reproduction. We hope, also, that world-wide there will be increased cooperation and collaboration, as people from all nations face many of the same questions and quandaries regarding egg donation's ethics. However, these controversies should not necessarily provide a reason to avoid participation in egg donation if this is where you journey has led you. In most cases, we generally do not think that because some social practices are imperfect, this means that no one may benefit from those practices at all.

Questions of Faith

"Be fruitful and multiply."

Whether you are a Christian or a Jew, a Muslim or a member of the Buddhist or Hindu faiths, you have most likely been raised in a religion that values family and encourages its members to bring children into this world. Regardless of your faith, you probably read in your *Bible* or *Torah* or *Qu'ran* about the pain of infertility and the quest for children. Indeed, the pain of infertility dates back to earliest Biblical times and to the recorded suffering of Sarah, Leah, Hannah, Rachel and so many others. Rachel's plaintive cry, "Give me children, or I die," has been echoed and re-echoed throughout recorded history with people of all religions and all degrees of faith struggling with infertility.

When an individual or couple is struggling to have a child, they often find that their struggle precipitates a crisis of faith. It is not unusual to question your beliefs, your faith in God, your relationship with God, and your participation in your religion. Since organized religion celebrates the arrival of children, you may find yourself avoiding your place of worship at a time when you may most need the solace of prayer. After all, who wants to enter a sanctuary, seeking comfort, only to encounter a baptism or a naming ceremony?

Similarly, you may be tempted to avoid religious holidays and celebrations. Take Easter and Passover, for example, two profoundly significant religious holidays. Each is a time when families gather together for prayer, food *and* a celebration of children. These holidays are made all the more poignant for their infertile participants by their central symbol: the egg. It is easy to understand why many struggling with infertility feel that they must distance themselves from religious practice, if not also from faith.

Again, volumes have been written about religion and infertility, and in his article, "Religious Views Regarding Gamete Donation," Dr. Joseph Schenker (*Family Building through Egg and Sperm Donation*, Siebel and Crockin), narrows the focus to egg and sperm donation. Schenker examines the specific religious doctrine applicable to egg donation in the Christian (with special sections on Roman Catholicism, Eastern Orthodox, Anglican and Protestant perspectives), Jewish, Islamic, Hindu and Buddhist faiths. Such an examination is beyond the focus of our book, though we encourage you to read Schenker's article and others. Instead, we address here some of the central questions of faith that arise when people are enduring infertility and considering using donated ova.

Is God Punishing Me/Us, and If So, for What?

One of the first questions raised by people of faith is about punishment. Since infertility is a terrible affliction, people who are suffering and who have little or no control over the outcome of their efforts, wonder why they are being punished. Rather than regard infertility as a random misfortune, many are apt to assume that God has decided to punish them. But for what?

Since many of us live with regret, often around reproductive or family building decisions, it can be easy to identify something we "did wrong" that generated this dreadful punishment. Some go directly to an abortion or the decision to place a child for adoption, two of the most painful histories for those experiencing infertility. Others, who have secondary infertility, quickly conclude that they are being punished for not being good enough parents, for not fully appreciating the child or children they have, "for wanting more when we should be grateful."

For others, explanations for punishment are less clear. "Maybe it was because I focused too much on my career?" "Maybe I should have stayed with my first husband, when I was young enough to have a child, and somehow worked it out?" "Perhaps God is punishing us for inter-marriage." And the list goes on.

Why Is God Doing This to Me/Us When I/We Have Been So Good?

While some people of faith conclude that God is punishing them for some transgression, large or small, that warrants punishment, others are left baffled. They examine their behavior, past and present, and feel that they have conducted themselves in ways for which they are proud. They know that they would be good parents or are good parents deserving of another child. Unlike those who become angry at themselves for inviting this punishment, these people of faith become angry at God. In many ways, this is far more painful.

Feeling betrayed by God is extraordinarily difficult for people of faith. For one thing, it shakes their faith: "How can we continue to believe in a good and just God when this happens?" For another, it estranges them from family and friends, especially those who do not seem to lead their lives so virtuously but who are still rewarded with children. And as we said earlier, it is tempting to stay away from church, synagogue, temple or mosque when you are going through infertility. This aversion to religious services becomes all the more prominent when someone feels betrayed. After all, who wants to attend a service that praises God when you are feeling let down, alone, cheated and unfairly punished?

Is This God's Plan?

A question directly related to the egg donor decision is one regarding "God's plan." Although many people of faith do not regard God as all-knowing, all-giving and all-planning, some do. For them, there is a sense that God has a Plan.

The idea of a plan may be comforting. Maybe God intends you to adopt a child? That perspective may offer some solace and some guidance in your decision making or it can feel like you are in a bind. What do you do if you are interested in egg donation but you *believe* God intends you to adopt?

For some people of faith, God's plan is something that can be flexible. You may conclude that God has a plan for you to take an alternative path to parenthood, but it is left for you to determine that plan. For example, Nina, who had just about concluded that she should adopt because that "seemed to be God's plan," reversed direction when she renewed contact with an old friend who then offered to donate eggs. From Nina's perspective, "God brought her back into my life for a reason."

At other points in this book, we have talked about "the blessing and the curse of the meant-to-be." Surely, it is in the area of faith that we see both sides of this perspective. It can feel like a burden to "have to conform to God's plan" or a blessing to believe that God has guided you in your decision and freed you from having to make decisions for yourself.

What If My Religion Does Not Support Ovum Donation or Places Significant Restrictions on Our Participation?

Religious faiths offer varying perspectives on egg donation. Although individual members of the clergy accept and support the availability of donated ova, many faiths do attempt to limit, if not ban, the practice. According to Dr. Schenker, an expert on religious faith and professor at Hadassah University Medical Center in Jerusalem, Islam prohibits gamete donation as well as adoption. Roman Catholicism prohibits all gamete donation. The Eastern Orthodox churches regard gamete donation as an adulterous act. Hinduism accepts both egg and sperm donation, as does Buddhism, as long as the child has the right to know his or her genetic "mother or father." The Reform, Conservative and Reconstructionist movements in Judaism accept egg donation, as do several, but not all, Protestant denominations. Orthodox Judaism accepts egg donation but places severe restrictions on the timing and protocol for medical diagnostic and treatment procedures. Jewish law states that "a child is related to the one who finished its formation, that is, the one who gave birth." Christian Scientists are instructed by their faith not to pursue assisted reproductive technology, including egg donation.

And so we see that there will be many people of faith who find themselves in a quandary: "How do we follow the commandments of our religious tradition—to bring children into our faith—when our religion is telling us that we cannot use donated eggs?" Some conclude that they cannot turn to egg donation if their faith instructs them otherwise. However, others feel that religious doctrine can be interpreted in various ways and that the important thing is that a child will be born into a faith and raised to respect and honor it. Some are comforted in this approach by clergy or by physicians who are members of their faith and who encourage and support their actions.

Does Prayer Help, and If So, How?

Prayer is comforting. Prayer offers solace. Prayer is communal. But does prayer work and if so, how? Some people pray, seeking only one response from God. If the desired response is the birth of a child, anything else that happens feels as though one's prayers have not been answered. However, others approach prayer in a different way, feeling that the experience of praying is, in its own way, healing. In addition, they may feel that "God works in strange ways" and that this may include a different response to their prayers. Other traditions teach that prayer should ask from God only the strength to accept whatever is His will.

Some people of faith derive enormous comfort from repeating prayers that come from their tradition and that have been spoken for generations before them. Others seek to develop their own prayers, either by writing them or by combining existing prayers into something that seems to fit with their particular circumstances. In her book, *Tears of Sorrow, Seeds of Hope,* (Jewish Lights Press, 1999) Rabbi Nina Cardin includes some prayers written by women and men struggling with infertility and pregnancy loss. Although some are clearly rooted in Jewish tradition, others offer words that apply to people of many faiths, regardless of their religious affiliation. Among them is this one we felt our readers might find meaningful...

> Choose from Your sacred treasury of souls and give us a child who is wise and caring, healthy and secure. May we be blessed with a pregnancy that lasts, with a birth that yields life and a child who gives us joy.
>
> May our family grow through the years and through your kindness, may we be a blessing to all who know us.
>
> May the words of our mouths and the desires of our hearts please You, our Strength and our Deliverer.

Creating Ceremonies

In their book, *Creating Ceremonies: Innovative Ways to Meet Adoption Challenges*, (Zeig, Tucker and Co., 1999) authors Rhea Bufferd and Cheryl Lieberman talk about the value of creating ceremonies for adoptive families, a concept that has been borrowed by many who have built their families through other alternative means, including egg donation. Included in the ceremonies Lieberman and Bufferd refer to are ceremonies of celebration. Although Lieberman and Bufferd's ceremonies are not religious in nature, the idea of creating rituals and ceremonies is one familiar and comforting to people of faith.

If you bring a child into your family through donated ova, you will surely want to participate in your faith's rituals and ceremonies around birth and infancy. Baptisms, Christenings, Bris' and Naming Ceremonies are all sacred events that confirm that a child is authentically a member of your family and your faith. In addition to celebrating these long awaited occasions, you may want to create some of your own ceremonies. For example, adoptive families sometimes bring home some soil from the place they adopted their child and mix that soil with the soil in their yard, planting in it a tree or flowers. You may want to find some way to similarly honor and celebrate your egg donor and your experience with her.

For many couples, the crisis of faith that arises during their infertility experience and their egg donor journey actually serves to strengthen their religious connections. Just as infertility will challenge, but usually not destroy, strong relationships, so also can it shake, but not destroy, religious faith. Some find that they are comforted, fortified and renewed by prayer. Others receive enormous support and guidance from clergy or from other members of their faith. And many draw strength from knowing that the birth of a child will bring delight to their families, who will join them in welcoming that child into their faith.

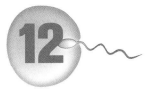

Families with Special Circumstances

For most of this book, we may have seemed to limit our primary focus to traditional couples. However, the ranks of people seeking donated eggs are not confined to this group. Four other groups may seek ovum donation. In fact, one of the groups—gay men—requires oocyte donation and a surrogate in order to achieve parenthood. Two others—single women and lesbian couples—may travel through various fertility treatments before coming to a fork in the road where the choices include donated oocytes. The fourth group—families of color—may face "supply issues" in their journey.

Single Women

In today's society, more and more single women are choosing to become parents without the involvement of a male. Some assume that as long as a single woman has a sperm donor, she can get pregnant whenever she wishes. Readers of this book would of course know that this is not always the case, since problems in the female reproductive system create at least half of all infertility problems.

We have found that most women who choose to become mothers without partners are older—usually in their late 30s or early 40s—when they attempt pregnancy. Although there are women who truly *choose* single motherhood, many of the single moms by choice that we meet had hoped and expected to find partners before parenting. Most have kept a keen eye on their biological clocks, and when they didn't have a partner for parenting by their late 30s, they tackled the complicated question of whether they should pursue pregnancy on their own. For most, this decision was made with much soul searching and many discussions with close friends and family about social, financial and logistical issues. Although many of these women do go on to successfully have children through donor insemination, there are those who have aged out of using their own eggs. It is from this group that most of the single women who consider using donated eggs come.

There are other single women who turn to donated ova. They include women like Jenny, whom we introduced in Chapter 3.

> Jenny and her late husband were going through fertility treatments when he was diagnosed with what proved to be a terminal illness. As a couple they put their efforts to conceive aside, but Jenny's husband, Pierre, cryopreserved sperm in the hope that he would recover and they would have a child together. Pierre also told Jenny that if he did not survive and if she chose to have a child with his sperm, she had his permission and his blessing.

> Sadly, Pierre did not survive. Jenny took some time to grieve and then examined whether, as a busy physician, she could embark on parenthood on her own. When she concluded that this was indeed something she could do, she learned that her eggs were no longer viable. Jenny turned to ovum donation, an option which enabled her to have Pierre's child. This decision not only brought her much joy, but was especially meaningful for Pierre's elderly parents, who had no other grandchildren and who were so happy to have their son "live on in our beautiful, beloved granddaughter."

Although Jenny's story is unusual, it illustrates that there are a variety of circumstances that might bring a single woman to egg donation.

> One of Jenny's friends from her "Single Mother's By Choice" group is Sandra, a single woman who began trying to conceive when she was 37. Sandra had always wanted to be a mom, and when her own mother died, she decided to attempt pregnancy "before it was too late." Four years of fertility treatments later, Sandra did give birth to her first child, Abigail. When Abigail was 2 and Sandra was 43, this exuberant single mom tried for a second child. Like Jenny, she learned that she'd "aged out of good eggs" and turned to ovum donation. When asked why she made this choice rather than adoption, Sandra replied that she now felt a connection to the sperm donor—Abigail's biological father—and she wanted to have a second child with whom her daughter had a genetic link. "Although we don't know him, our donor is now part of the family."

Mary is another single mom who struggled with many questions before pursuing parenthood through both egg and sperm donation. Mary knew that she would love any child she gave birth to, but she was troubled by what combined egg and sperm donation would mean to the child. After considering many possibilities, including exploring adoption, Mary decided that she would take a risk and ask her brother, Alex, to be her sperm donor. It felt like a risk because she didn't want to put him in a difficult spot, but she knew she would be deeply disappointed if he said no.

Fortunately for Mary, Alex said yes. As it turned out, he liked the idea of being able to help bring another child into the world. He is the happy father of two teenagers and he was tickled to be able to help give them another cousin. And so he said yes, making Mary's path ever so much easier for her. "With Alex's o.k., I realized I could accept having an egg donor, even if she wanted to remain anonymous. It felt like an extra bonus when I learned that the donor I chose was willing—actually very willing—to meet me."

Mary's son, Matthew, is now 3 years old. His mom, who didn't know if she could handle one on her own, has recently spoken with Alex, as well as with her donor, Stephanie, about donating again. "This time I'm asking my doctor to transfer just one embryo. I'm pretty sure I can be a mom to two children, but I'm not risking twins."

Jenny, Sandra and Mary chose to use donor oocytes in their family building. Nancy Docktor, RN, MSCS, program counselor for the Fertility Center of New England in Reading, Massachusetts, comments, "Many of the single women I see prefer ovum donation to adoption. Yes, they are disappointed, because they set out to have a child that was genetically connected to them, but they see ovum donation as an opportunity to have a child without 'being scrutinized.' As single women, they fear that adoption agencies will treat them as 'second best' and force them to prove that they can parent on their own. Ovum donation presents them with no such hurdles."

Such fears may or may not be accurate reflections of adoption practice, but they are what some single would-be mothers believe. Other single women choose adoption, concluding that, for them, it is more ethically correct since the child already exists and is not being created by both donated eggs and donated sperm. Women who choose adoption, especially adoption from China and South or Central America, options which have attracted many single women, feel this choice brings with it an easily identifiable peer group.

However, for some women, the pregnancy experience, the chance to influence their child prenatally, and, with intrafamily egg or sperm donation (if a non-family donated ovum is being used, the sperm donor can be a family member), the chance to have a genetic connection to a child, all make using donated eggs attractive.

For single women, the oocyte donation process is very much the same as outlined in this book, however it offers some additional challenges. First, it must be mentioned that some egg donation programs do not accept single women as recipient clients. Among those that do, there are programs which will not agree to both ova and sperm donation, or if they agree to it, will require that at least one of the two donors be a family member so the child will have some genetic connection. Furthermore, in cases where donors have some input into who receives their oocytes, there will be women who want their eggs to help only married couples become pregnant.

If you are a single woman interested in pursuing pregnancy with donated eggs, it is important that you find a clinic that is sensitive to the issues faced by single women. You should expect more intensive counseling and screening sessions in order to fully assess your ability to parent a child alone. Specifically, a counselor will attempt to confirm that you have support systems in place, including people who can help if you are ill, and a guardian who can take over in the event of severe illness or death and that financial planning takes into consideration your child's possible future without you. Counselors will also want to confirm that you have spoken with other single mothers and with at least some family members and friends about your plan.

As we indicated earlier, some single women seeking ovum donation look to family members as either egg or sperm donors. Assuming that a sister or brother or cousin offers to help, you will then need to locate the "other donor." If it is an egg donor you seek, most of what we have written in other chapters about identifying an ovum donor will hold true. If it is an anonymous sperm donor you need, you will want to contact a sperm bank.

There are currently approximately 150 sperm banks in the United States. With so many to choose from, you should be able to find one that meets your needs and is both ethical and effective. Depending upon your race and ethnicity, you may prefer one sperm bank over another because it offers more donors who will feel like good matches. Beyond race and ethnicity, you will want to work with a cryobank that offers extensive medical and social information about the donor (most do) and that can confirm with you that they maintain long term record keeping. Ideally, the bank you choose will also identify itself as one that includes "yes donors"—men who have agreed to be contacted in the future, if, by mutual agreement, offspring, donors and parents all agree to contact or to a meeting.

In contacting a cryobank, the following are some things you should be able to get and some things you should be cautious about:

You Should Be Able to Receive:

- A lengthy questionnaire, often completed in the donor's own handwriting (to make the document more personal), that includes extensive medical, family and personal history and which captures something of the donor's personality, outlook on life, values. This questionnaire will probably include a statement from the donor about why he chose to donate and hopefully, there will be a message to a potential offspring.

- Confirmation that the program conducts a thorough medical and psychological evaluation of the donor. The importance of careful medical assessment was highlighted in recent years when a donor checked out "family history of kidney disease," and the cryobank did not investigate this further. When the recipient couple had a child with significant kidney disease, they brought a law suit against the cryobank.

- Prompt, efficient service. As one woman said, "It feels weird enough charging sperm to my VISA over the phone. I want to talk with a real person." Selecting a sperm donor is a deeply personal decision and one that can feel daunting. As a single woman, you should not feel alone in the process. Hopefully, family and friends will be there to help, if you ask, but the cryobank also, should be available to respond to questions.

- The opportunity to purchase and bank extra sperm so that you can have a second child, with the same donor, should you make that choice in the future.

You Should Be Cautious about:

- Programs that are hard to reach or in any other way inefficient. Using donated eggs is a very expensive undertaking, and you will want to feel complete confidence that the cryobank will send you healthy sperm on time.

- Programs that do not offer access to records. In recent years, most sperm banks have come to appreciate the importance of record keeping and of access to those records by the recipient couple and their child. This proves especially important for those families in which a medical question or problem arises. Be cautious about a program that cannot or will not provide you with access to donor medical records. Ideally, the program should agree to help you access the donor, himself, should a medical problem arise.

Lesbian Couples

As more gay and lesbian couples are being accepted and supported by our society, their abilities to seek family building options are increasing. For lesbian couples, this often means having one or both partners become pregnant and give birth to children whom the other partner adopts. Although many lesbian couples will be able to achieve pregnancies on their own, with home inseminations or low tech inseminations in physicians' offices, some find that they need more assistance in achieving pregnancy. They need ova as well as sperm.

Not all infertility clinics are supportive of lesbian couples, but most will not exclude lesbians from their practice, and a growing number are welcoming lesbian couples. In seeking a program, you should explore their approach to lesbian couples and work only with a program that is enthusiastic about working with you. It is important for you to know that many programs are enthusiastic. They recognize the hurdles you have had to overcome to get to where you are, and they genuinely want to help you. If you don't get the sense that this is their approach, go elsewhere.

Lesbian couples seeking fertility treatment and considering oocyte donation face many of the questions that heterosexual couples face but there are some added issues.

Two Potential Genetic Mothers

You and your partner may have decided that only one of you wants to become pregnant and bear a child. If this is the case, what happens if the intended genetic and gestational mom proves to have high FSH or some other significant problem? Do you turn to your partner for a donated egg or, in the reverse situation, to carry the child?

....

Meet Martha and Lynette…

Martha and Lynette met in college seventeen years ago and have been together ever since. When they were in their early thirties, Lynette told Martha that she wanted to become pregnant and hoped Martha would "be up for parenting with me." Martha, who loves children, but didn't particularly want to be pregnant, was supportive of Lynette's plans. However, as things turned out, Lynette was unable to become pregnant. Although only 33 at the time, her physician told her that it was an egg quality problem.

"It was at that point that I asked Martha if she would be willing to donate her eggs to me." According to Martha, this was hardly a question—she loved the idea of having a genetic connection to her child without having to go through pregnancy. The partners agreed to move forward and five months later, Lynette was pregnant. She gave birth to a baby boy, Owen, who is now nearly 3.

Time passes. Things change. Martha, who had never wanted to be pregnant, has loved being a mom with Lynette, and, she acknowledges, she has loved having a genetic connection to her child. To her surprise and surely Lynette's, Martha recently decided that she would like to become pregnant and to give birth to the couple's second child. The women have contacted their sperm donor and plan to begin inseminations soon. If their efforts succeed, their children will be full biological siblings.

Counselor Nancy Docktor describes Martha's ability to donate to Lynette, as "nice back-up" and observes that many lesbian couples have this added benefit as they go through IVF. "They know," says Docktor, "that if IVF doesn't work, they have a very attractive alternative."

For some lesbian couples the prospect of having one partner carry the child and the other be the genetic mother is not simply a Plan B. Some make it their first choice. In fact, it not only offers a certain parity—each woman makes a major contribution to bringing their child into the world, but it also opens up the option of their having a full genetic child. This becomes possible if a brother of the woman who carries the child offers to donate sperm.

Some lesbian couples choose to have one intended mother carry the baby and the other donate eggs for legal protection. They feel that dividing genetic and gestational motherhood between them ensures each her parental rights.

This sort of arrangement can occur whether initially chosen or as a "second choice," when the woman who intended to become pregnant is found to have a problem. However, many lesbian couples prefer, for a variety of reasons, to keep things simpler. The above arrangement may feel "too complicated," "too weird" or "too costly." Or it may ask the partner who did not seek pregnancy to become involved in a way she does not want. For all these reasons, as well as the possibility that neither partner has viable eggs, there will be lesbian couples who seek egg donation from a third woman. We are told that when there is a need for an egg donor, lesbian women often find that friends in the lesbian community offer to donate to them. Kathy, 32, said, "We have a rich, supportive network of women friends and so we weren't surprised when a few of our friends offered to donate."

Needing Two Donors—Egg and Sperm

If you are a lesbian couple seeking donated eggs, you will face many of the same questions that heterosexual couples face in selecting an egg donor. She can be a family member, a friend or an anonymous donor. What complicates your situation is that you also need a sperm donor, and he, too, can be a family member, friend or anonymous donor. So there are many combinations and permutations to consider. Since many of you will want your child or children to have a genetic connection to at least one of your families, you may find yourselves having complicated discussions about who you might want to ask and how you will ask him or her.

The Need for Social Support

Although lesbian, as well as gay, couples have come a long, long way in terms of gaining social support and recognition, lesbian parenting is still non-traditional. Add in egg donation and you have departed further from traditional family building. Needless to say, it will be very helpful if you have family and community support for your endeavor.

You may want to secure this support in stages—first letting people close to you know that you plan to become parents together and waiting until after a pregnancy is established to let them know that you have chosen pregnancy and parenting with donated ova.

When One or Both Already Have a Child or Children

It is not unusual for one or both members of a lesbian couple to have been married and to come into the new relationship with a child or children. Your existing family may influence your decisions about your future family building. For example, if one partner has never been pregnant, wants this experience and she proves to be infertile, you may then turn to egg donation rather than have the partner who is already a mother attempt pregnancy. This may feel more "fair" or more "equal" or you may conclude that the infertility prompts you to change your plans and consider another option—either having the presumably fertile partner attempt conception or perhaps, you will choose adoption.

If you need the sperm of an anonymous donor, please read the section for single women (above) for our advice on selecting a sperm bank.

Gay Couples

When two men want to have a baby together, they clearly need help from at least one woman. In the past, gay men faced many barriers to parenthood, both social and logistical. Then, when surrogacy became available in the late 1970s, those gay couples who had the financial resources and the stamina were able to choose this option as a way of having a child. This option was attractive to them, not only because they could have a child who was related genetically to one of them, but also, because until recently, it has been extremely difficult for gay men to adopt.

With the arrival of gestational care/gestational surrogacy, gay men had another option, and it is one that many gay couples are choosing: using donated eggs with a gestational carrier. Although this option is more expensive than traditional surrogacy, in that it requires ART and fees to two women collaborating with them in building a family, couples generally prefer it. In addition to avoiding the issues that arise with traditional surrogacy—a woman agrees to place her full bio-genetic child pre conception—ovum donation with a gestational carrier offers the intended parents the option for two genetic connections or, a genetic and gestational connection. How? If the egg donor is a family member (of the non-genetic father) or if the gestational carrier is a family member, the couple—sometimes both of them—has the opportunity to have more physical connection with their child.

In our experience, most gay couples choosing oocyte donation with a gestational carrier end up working with two women who were either previously unknown to them or who are unrelated to them. We recall Stan and Alan, whose carrier was a former colleague of Alan's and whose ovum donor was someone they found through a program that encouraged openness in using donated eggs.

If you are a gay couple considering donated ova with a gestational carrier, you face many challenges and decisions. We will list some of them below, but we want to begin with some words of encouragement. The path that lies ahead may seem incredibly complicated, but *it can and does work*. It is important for you to know that many medical programs, ovum donation programs and gestational care programs are very welcoming to gay couples. The men who have been trail blazers ahead of you have helped physicians, nurses and mental health counselors appreciate the obstacles you have faced in becoming parents and, for the most part, they want to help. Now for your challenges…

Familiarizing Yourselves with Both Ovum Donation and Gestational Care Programs

This is a brave new world of making babies, and unlike some couples, who need learn about either oocyte donation *or* gestational care, you need to educate yourselves about both.

We encourage you to see this as two tasks and to focus on each, preferably sequentially. Assuming that you will not be working with a family member for either process, you will need to think about what is important to you in an egg donor and what is important in a gestational carrier. You will quickly see that the characteristics you identify will likely be found in two very different women, whom you will be choosing for very different reasons.

I (Ellen) recall meeting first with Mark and Larry, hearing about their path to parenthood and then meeting with their gestational carrier, Christine.

> Christine is a strong willed, free thinking mother of three children. Married for nearly fifteen years, Christine sees motherhood as the ultimate profession. She devotes her life to her children and to making the family home a wonderful environ-

ment in which to grow. Christine completed high school, and although intelligent, never had additional education.

Two days after meeting Christine, I sat down with Mark, Larry and Bianca, their ovum donor. Bianca is a graduate student in art history who is single and unclear about whether she ever wants to marry and have children. While Christine came to gestational care because she loves being pregnant, Bianca decided to donate her eggs because her roommate from college went through three years of infertility before conceiving. This inspired Bianca to want to help a couple who could not have children, and with many gay friends, she was especially drawn to helping gay couples.

After meeting each of the women, I had a chance to talk with Larry and Mark. We spoke about how well they got along with each woman and how much they like them. We spoke also of the qualities they value in Christine and of those they value in Bianca and of how different those qualities are. Then we all laughed a bit, trying to imagine what Christine and Bianca would have to say together if they were seated next to each other on a train.

"Very little," quipped Larry. "But that is the beauty of this—each one is well suited to be doing what she is doing for us but they could never exchange places."

Becoming Patients in a Practice That Expects Its Patients to Be Women

Fertility clinics have a way of identifying the couples who come to them by the female partners. All too often, men tell us that they felt that they were ignored in meetings with physicians, that people knew only their wife's name, that they were called by her last name even if theirs was different.

Enter into this female-focused world, two men. Until recently, a strange experience. Fortunately, things are changing. Many fertility centers are welcoming gay couples; and adjusting their office practice so that their male patients feel included. Surrogacy programs, similarly, are gaining experience working with gay couples. Amy Zaslow, Director of A-Z Consulting in Lexington, Massachusetts, comments, "In some ways, this is an easier road for gay couples. I find that unlike the heterosexual couples I see, who come with a history of infertility defeats, gay couples come with optimism. They have thought about this decision for a long time and because they can choose their egg donor and their gestational carrier, they are optimistic things will go well for them."

Finances

This is going to be costly. As two men, you don't qualify for insurance coverage for egg donation, even in a state with a full insurance mandate. While this appears discriminatory to us, it is unlikely to change in the near future. So, whether you are insured or not, you are left having to pay medical costs out of pocket for both the donor and the gestational carrier (other than the pregnancy and delivery, which your program or your attorney will have confirmed is covered by her health insurance, if she has insurance). These costs, together with costs to a donor program, to a gestational carrier program, and to lawyers and counselors will add up. We can't say what the total will be, but it's a costly undertaking. For this reason, it will be important to select a donor who has a good chance of producing several eggs and a gestational carrier who is willing to undergo a second transfer if the first doesn't work or results in miscarriage.

Two Potential Fathers

Gay couples have to decide who will become the genetic father of their child. Although there are instances, as with lesbians, where one man already has children and the couple decides the other should get to become a genetic father—if he is able—there are many couples who hope to have children from each of them. Most approach this sequentially—"The first child will be 'mine' and the second, 'yours.'" Others attempt to have a twin pregnancy with an embryo from each of them and attempt pregnancy with both.

Larry and Mark, for example, split Bianca's eggs, inseminated half with Larry's sperm and half with Mark's, and had the "best" embryo from each transferred. In their case, they learned that Christine was carrying a singleton, though occasionally this can result in gestational twins who have the same mother and different fathers. When their son was born, they underwent DNA testing to determine which of them was his biological father. Both men felt that it was important to have the testing immediately so that they would be able to provide accurate family medical history to their son's pediatrician. However, because both families were so excited about their grandson's arrival and so convinced he was their genetic heir, the fathers decided to postpone telling anyone—other than Christine and Bianca—the news of who was the genetic father. "There will be time down the road," said the man who is the genetic dad.

Larry and Mark's decision to "mix embryos" is not accepted by some medical programs. When we asked people in such programs what they objected to, physicians and psychologists commented, "It doesn't feel right. The man who is not the genetic father needs to face this right away." Some added that it seems "wrong" to them to have a woman carry two children who are not full biological siblings. We are somewhat puzzled by these reactions, since we feel that Larry and Mark's arrangement is ethically sound: their child will know the truth about his origins and the dads, by making the choice they did, feel that they were able to exercise their autonomy and to experience a process that was fair and just.

Families of Color and Multi-Ethnic families

People of all races and ethnic groups seek egg donation, and in most instances, they feel it is important for the egg donor to match them racially. In addition, mixed race couples want to have children who represent the same racial mix. Boston area therapist Peg Beck explains this desire in the following way, "Biracial couples want to carry forward the wonderful mix that is their relationship. When they dream of making a baby together, they picture a child that is the racial and ethnic combination of their union."

Because the majority of donors are Caucasian, families of color and multi-ethnic families often face more challenges in finding a donor. If you are a family of color, or if you and your partner are of different racial groups, the following are some of the things you should know:

Ethnic Availability of Donors Varies from Program to Program

We have found that the availability of African American, Asian, Latino, and mixed-race donors varies from one program to the next. Some of this is regional—there are areas of the country, such as California, that have large Asian populations and hence, are more likely to have more Asian donors. Similarly, there are urban areas with larger African American populations and hence, more African American donors. Some of this is also an issue of recruitment. It just may be that oocyte donation services, most of which are run by Caucasian professionals, are not yet culturally competent enough to successfully recruit among minority populations. In general, however, there tend to be a limited number of Latino and Asian and African American women offering to donate their ova.

This is the case, also, with Jewish donors. Some Jewish couples feel that it is important to have a Jewish donor so that their child will truly be born into the "Jewish people." These couples are focusing on being Jewish not so much as a religion, which can be converted to or from, but as a historical people. Jewish donors, like African American and Latino donors, are not plentiful. We understand that some Jewish couples have turned to an Israeli "broker," who finds Israeli donors for couples seeking Jewish donors.

Nancy Docktor observes that couples seeking a donor from their cultural and ethnic group sometimes have to "settle for something akin to their ethnic group." Docktor remembers a Vietnamese woman who went with a Chinese donor when the program she was working with was unable to offer her a Vietnamese donor. Docktor also recalls a dark skinned couple from the Caribbean who, unable to find a donor from either of their islands, accepted a Swedish donor "because, on the island we live on, there is a racial spectrum. Some of our nieces and nephews are very fair." And Docktor counseled a couple from Nigeria who, unable to find an African donor, went with an African American. "It was this couple," Docktor says, "that helped me understand some of the cultural differences that influence what people tell their children. The Nigerian couple told me that they would not tell anyone—even the child—about egg donation because it would not be accepted in their culture."

Multi-Ethnicity

If you are a multi-ethnic or multi-racial couple, your quest for a donor may feel even more complicated. We assume that you will seek a donor who matches the female partner in terms of race and ethnicity (though this is not the choice made by all couples in your situation.) Some conclude that other factors, such as family medical history, motivation for donation or intelligence, etc. are more important to them than are race or ethnicity, They go with a donor who is of the husband's race or ethnicity but who offers some of the other features that they feel are important.

Whatever the "special circumstances" are which bring you to ovum donation, we remind you that you are not alone. Each of the four groups we mentioned includes many people considering and/or pursuing egg donation. If you are single, or if you are a gay or lesbian couple, we encourage you to find others who are in a similar situation. And if you are a multi-ethnic family, we remind you that while one program may have no donors that match you racially, another program will have several.

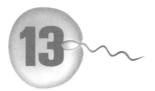

Looking to the Future

Change. One of the biggest challenges, and perhaps the greatest pleasure, in writing this book has been to participate in—and to try to keep pace with—change. News about developments in reproductive medicine and family building comes almost on a daily basis. No sooner did we write that "egg freezing is not available" than the news came that "100 babies worldwide are known to have been born using frozen eggs." And it was round about the time that we were writing about "special circumstances," that gay marriage became legal in Massachusetts. As we go to press, we have little doubt that readers will read this book a year or two or three from now and note that much of what we say is dated.

Much changes. Some things remain the same. As we look to the future, we hope for certain changes—donor registries, guaranteed access to genetic family information for recipients, widespread acceptance of donors' rights to know the outcome of their donations. We hope that secrecy will vanish and that the shame it generated will be replaced by pride, satisfaction and gratitude.

And so we come to the end of this book, knowing that our readers will be traveling down different paths to parenthood and to life after infertility. Some of our readers will choose adoption or perhaps living without children or may remain a one child family. We hope that this book has helped you feel clearer and more secure in those decisions.

We know, also, that many of our readers will choose egg donation, and for you, we are grateful to be able to offer some advice from one who truly knows and understands ovum donation. Daniel, who is 16 as of this writing, was asked several years ago to write about what it meant to be conceived through donated eggs. He generously shares his thoughts with you.

There is no such thing as a perfect child, so not matter what you do, they will screw up a few times. What you should do early is to have the child develop self-esteem. That was one of the most important things I have ever been taught to be. To feel good about yourself means that you will have a brighter look on life. Self-esteem will become important when you feel nervous about people finding out how you were born. But that is not in most times true. DE in my life has really not been a big deal. I am going to live the same and die the same no matter what the heck I was born with. I just want all mothers to know that their child is no different. When I told one of my friends that I was one of the first eleven children ever conceived through DE, he said, "Um...Huh?" So tell your child that he/she doesn't have to worry about fitting in.

Start early and start little by little telling the kids how they were conceived. If you disagree, I might be wrong because I can only say what worked for me. I think it would be worth a try though. I think one of the best ways to explain it is to put it in words they can easily understand and then, as they mature, tell them more finite details.

DE is just the way I got here, but now I'm just me. I hope moms and dads who used DE will feel good about the way they have their kids and good about their kids.

Thank you, Daniel, you have said it all.

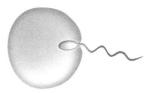

Acknowledgments

We end this book by acknowledging the contributions of the many mothers and fathers through egg donation who have shared their personal stories with us. Out of respect for their privacy, we have not used their real names in the book. But we have used their words, and we have done our best to convey their messages—messages of hope, joy, challenge and opportunity.

We were also fortunate to have several professionals in the field of reproductive medicine and law who have given generously to this project of their time, experience and expertise. Special thanks go to Carol Lesser, NP; Susan L. Crockin, JD; Judy Calica, MSW; Elaine Gordon, PhD.; Carole Lieber Wilkins, MA; Peg Beck, LICSW; Shelley Smith, LMFT; and Katrina Twomey, RN; all of whom spent time with us or reviewed chapters and offered us their comments. Others who made significant contributions include Mary Fusillo, RN; Amy Zaslow; Deb Fenn LICSW; Adele Kauffman, PhD.; Sharon Steinberg, RN; Robert Nichols, JD; Patty Mahlstedt, PhD; Nancy Docktor, RN, Olivia Montuschi, and Mark Johnson, Esq. We also thank Steven Bayer, MD and especially Eric Scott Sills, MD for responding to our medical questions in such a timely and generous manner.

I (Ellen) give a special thanks to my husband, Dan Manning, without whose patience, support and computer literacy this book would not exist. I also thank my Friday group—mental health colleagues in the field of reproductive science—with whom I have shared lively conversations and good food one Friday a month for the past sixteen years. The Friday Group is Ellen Feldman, Judith Bernstein, Geri Ferber, Jeanie Ungerleider, Susan Lynn, Susan Levin, Adele Kauffman, Deborah Silverstein and Sharon Steinberg. I thank my parents, Shirlee, Ira and

Helen Sarasohn, who continue to teach me how to live. And as the dedication of this book reflects, I am most grateful to my late co author, colleague and above all, dear friend, Dr. Susan Cooper, whose wise perspective on family building is hopefully reflected throughout this book

I (Evelina) would like to thank first and foremost my family—Dan, Ben and Ellie—for all of their patience and support throughout this project. Also, I thank Angie Best-Boss and Dr. Sam Thatcher for their tremendous help in formulating the initial concept for a much needed book on this topic. Finally, I am forever grateful to my parents, Donna and Steve Weidman, for instilling in me a lifelong passion for learning.

We are deeply grateful to Pat Johnston, Publisher, Advocate and Visionary Extraordinaire. Without her push and her faith in us, this book would not exist.

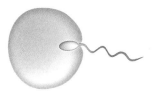

Bibliography

The following is a list of academic and consumer books as well as peer-reviewed journal articles that we consulted and read as part of our research for this book. In addition, we conducted many interviews with clinical professionals and experts in the field (see Acknowledgments) which also contributed significantly to the research base. Although you will not see quotations from all of these materials, this body of work informed our thinking. We offer it to those professionals who would like to explore more deeply any of the issues which we have raised in *Having Your Baby through Egg Donation*.

Achilles, R. (1989). "Donor Insemination: The Future of a Public Secret" in *The Future of Human Reproduction* edited by Christine Overall, Women's Press, Toronto, pp. 105-19.

Andrews, L. (1985). "When Baby's Mother is Also Grandma—and Sister: Commentary" *Hastings Center Report* 15: 29-30.

American Society for Reproductive Medicine (November 2003), "Family Members as Gamete Donors nod Surrogates, *Fertility and Sterility*, 80(51).

Annas, George. "Fathers Anonymous: Beyond the Best Interests of the Sperm Donor," *Child Welfare* 60 (1) pp. 161-174.

Baran, A and Pannor, R. (1993). *Lethal Secrets,* Amistad Books, NY.

Becker, Gay, (2000) *The Elusive Embryo: How Women and Men Approach New Reproductive Technologies.* University of California Press, Berkeley, CA.

Bennett SJ, Waterstone JJ, Cheng WC and Parsons J. (1993). "Complications of Transvaginal Ultrasound-Directed Follicle Aspirations: A Review of 2670 Consecutive Procedures," *Journal of Assisted Reproductive Genetics*, 10:72-77.

Bernstein, Anne. (1994). *The Flight of the Stork: What Children Think (and When) about Sex and Family Building*, Perspectives Press, Indianapolis, IN.

Blickstein, I (2003). "Motherhood At or Beyond the Edge of Reproductive Age," *International Journal of Fertility,* 48(1):17-24.

Boldt, Jeffrey, (Summer 2004). "Oocyte Preservation," *Family Building.*

Braff, A, (1977) "Telling Children about Adoption." *American J Maternal and Child Nursing* 2: 254-259.

Braverman, Andrea, (Summer 2004). "Agency Vs. Clinic: Choosing the Best Fit," *Family Building.*

Braverman, A and Corson, S. (March 1995). "Factors Related to Preferences in Gamete Donor Sources," *Fertility and Sterility* 63 (3):543-549.

Braverman, A (1993). "Survey Results on the Current Practice of Ovum Donation," *Fertility and Sterility*, 59:1216-20.

Brodzinsky, D.M, Singer, L.M. and Braff, A. M. (1984). "Children's Understanding of Adoption" *Child Development* 55: 869-878.

Burstyn, Barbara Sumner. (February 23, 2004). "The New Underclass," *New Zealand Herald.*

Centers for Disease Control and Prevention. (2001). "Assisted Reproductive Technology Success Rates and ART Surveillance in the United States," www.cdc.gov/reproductivehealth/art.hrm.

Cohen, Cynthia. (1996). *New Ways of Making Babies*, Indiana University Press, Bloomington, IN.

Craft, I, "(May 10, 1997). An Inconvenience Allowance Would Solve the Egg Shortage," *British Medical Journal*, 1400-1.

Curie-Cohen, M. (1980). "The Frequency of Consanguineous Mating due to Multiple Use of Donors in Artificial Insemination," *American Journal of Human Genetics,* 32:589-600.

Daniels, K. (September 1996). "Successful Donor Insemination and its Impact on Recipients," *Journal of Psychosomatic Obstetrics and Gynecology*, pp. 129-134.

Deech, R. (2003). "Reproductive Tourism in Europe: Infertility and Human Rights," *Global Governance*: 9(4):425-33.

Diamond, R. (Sept/Oct 1995). "Secrecy vs. Privacy," *Adoptive Families*, pp. 8-11.

Edelman, S. (February 7, 1993). "Egg-donor Programs Raise Questions," *The Record*, Hackensack, NJ, pp. A1 and A12-13.

Fielding, D. (1998). "Motivation, Attitudes, and Experience of Donation: A Follow-up of Women Donating Eggs in Assisted Conception Treatment," *Journal of Community and Applied Social Psychology*, 8:273-87.

Gloger-Tippelt, G. (1988). "The Development of the Mother's Conceptions for the Child before Birth." Paper presented at the Sixth Biennial International Conference on Infant studies, Washington, DC.

Golombok, S and Rust, J. (1986). "The Warnock Report and Single Women: What about the Children?" *Journal of Medical Ethics* 12: 185-88.

Gordon, Elaine and Kathy Clo (1992). *Mommy, Did I Grow in Your Tummy?: Where Some Babies Come From*, E.M. Greenberg Press.

Gurmankin, AD. (2001). "Risk Information Provided to Prospective Oocyte Donors in a Preliminary Phone Call," *The American Journal of Bioethics*; 1(4):3-13.

Hancock, M, (February 28, 1993). "When Dad's only Name is 'Anonymous donor,'" *The Brockton Enterprise* pp. 1-17.

Henig, Robin Marantz, (2004). *Pandora's Baby: How the First Test Tube Babies Sparked the Reproductive Revolution*, Houghton Mifflin Company, New York.

Humphrey, M and Humphrey, H (1986). "A Fresh Look at Genealogical Bewilderment," *British Journal of Medical Psychology* (59) 133-40.

Imber-Black, E, (1993) *Secrets in Families and Family Therapy*, WW. Norton and Company, NY.

Indichova, Julia (2001). *Inconceivable: A Woman's Triumph over Despair and Statistics*, Broadway, New York.

Inhorn, Marcia C. and Frank van Balen. (2002). Infertility Around the Globe: New Thinking on Childlessness, Gender, and Reproductive Technologies. University of California Press, Berkeley, CA.

Johnson, MH. (May 10, 1997). "The Culture of Unpaid and Voluntary Egg Donation Should Be Strengthened," *British Medical Journal*, 1401-2.

Kahn, J, "The Ethics of Egg Donation," *Minnesota Medicine*, October 1998;81.

Kalfoglou AL and G Geller. (2000). "A Follow-up Study with Oocyte Donors Exploring Their Experiences, Knowledge, and Attitudes about the Use of Their Oocytes and the Outcome of the Donation," *Fertility and Sterility*, 74(4):660-7.

Kalfoglou AL and G Geller (2002). "Navigating Conflict of Interest in Oocyte Donation: An Analysis of Donor's Experiences," Johns Hopkins University Bioethics Institute; not yet published.

Kaye, K and Warren, S. (1988). "Discourse about Adoption in Adoptive Families" *J. Family Psych,* 1 (4): 406-433.

Kellam S.G., Ensminger, M.E. and Turner, R.J. (1977). "Family Structure and the Mental Health of Children," *Arch. Gen. Psychiatry*: 34 1012-1022.

Kirkland, A, Power, M and Burton, G et. Al (1992) "Comparison of Attitudes of Donors and Recipients to Oocyte Donation." *Human Reproduction* 7: 355-357.

Kirkman, (2003). "Egg and Embryo Donation and the Meaning of Motherhood," *Women and Health,* 38 (2).

Klock, S. et al. (1998). "Predicting Anonymous Egg Donor Satisfaction: A Preliminary Study," *Journal of Women's Health,* 7:229-237.

Klock, S. and Greenfeld, D. (June 2000). "Psychological Status of in Vitro Fertilization Patients During Pregnancy: a Longitudinal Study," *Fertility and Sterility* 73 (6): 1159-64.

Klock, S. Jacob, M and Maier, D. (1994). "A Prospective Study of Donor Insemination Recipients: Secrecy, Privacy and Disclosure," *Fertility and Sterility*, 62 (3): 477-484.

Lauritzen, P. (1991). " Pursuing Parenthood: Reflections on Donor Insemination," *Second Opinion* (17):57-76.

Leiblum, S., Hamins, S. (1992). "To Tell or not to tell: Attitudes of Reproductive Endocrinologists concerning Disclosure to Offspring of Conception Via Assisted Insemination by Donor," *J. Psychosomatic Obstetrics and Gynecology* 13: 267-275.

Lessor, R. et al.. (1995). "All in the family: Social Processes in Ovarian Egg Donation between Sisters" *Sociology of Health and Illness,* 15, 393-413.

Lessor, R, et al. (1993). "An analysis of Social and Psychological Characteristics of Women Volunteering to Become Oocyte Donors," *Fertility and Sterility*, 59:65-71.

Lewis, G and Gillent, W. (1995). "Telling Donor Insemination Offspring about Their Conception: The Nature of Couples' Decision-Making," *Social Science and Medicine,* 40 (9): 1213-20.

Lieber-Wilkins, Carole. (October 1, 1994). "Sperm and Egg Donations: What you Need to Know" Audiotape of talk given at RESOLVE/ Serono Symposium in Los Angeles.

Lieber-Wilkins. (Summer 2002). "To Tell the Truth: Issues of Donor Disclosure" in *Family Building*, pp. 7-10.

Lorbach, Caroline. (2003). *Experiences in Donor Conception, Parents, Offspring and Donors Through the Years*, Jessica Kingley, Philadelphia.

Mahlstedt, P, Greenfeld, D. (1989). "Assisted Reproductive Technology with Donor Gametes: The Need for Patient Preparation, *Fertility and Sterility* 52: 908-14.

Marsh, Margaret and Wanda Ronner. (1996). *Empty Cradle: Infertility in America from Colonial Times to the Present*. The Johns Hopkins University Press, Baltimore.

Meyer, Cheryl. (1997). *The Wandering Uterus: Politics and the Reproductive Rights of Women*, New York University Press, New York.

Nachtigall, R. (1993). "Secrecy: An Unresolved Issue in the Practice of Donor Insemination," *American Journal of Obstetrics and Gynecology* 168: 1846-51.

New South Wales Infertility Social Workers Group. 1988). *How I Began: The Story of Donor Insemination* Ed. Julia Paul, Carlton, Victoria. The Fertility Society of Australia.

Perloe, Mark. (January 2004). "Determining Ovarian Reserve: A Review of the Tools, Tests and Techniques," www.obgyn.net..

Power, M, et al. (1990). " A Comparison of the Attitudes of Volunteer Donors and Infertile Patient Donors on an Ovum Donation Programme," *Human Reproduction* 5: 352-55

Raoul-Duval, A, Letur-Konirsch H and Frydman, R. (1992). "Anonymous Oocyte Donation: A Psychological Study of Recipients, Donors and Children," *Human Reproduction* 7:51-54.

Riegler, J and Weikert, A (1988). "Product Egg: Egg Selling in an Austrian IVF Clinic," *Reproductive and Genetic Engineering* 1: 221-23.

Robertson, John, (1989). "Ethical and Legal Issues in Human Egg Donation," *Fertility and Sterility* 52:355.

Rowland, R. (1988). "The Social and Psychological Consequences of Secrecy in Artificial Insemination by Donor Programmes," *Social Science and Medicine* 21: 395.

Rosenwaks, Zev (1987). "Donor Eggs: Their Application in Modern Reproductive Technologies, *Fertility and Sterility* 47: 895-909.

Sauer, M and Paulson, R. (1994). "Mishaps and Misfortunes: Complications that Occur in Oocyte Donation," *Fertility and Sterility* 61: 963-65.

Sauer, M, Paulson, R, and Lobo, R. (1992). "Reversing the Natural Decline in Human Fertility: An Extended Clinical Trial of Oocyte Donation to Women of Advanced Reproductive Age, *JAMA* 260:1275-79.

Sauer, M and Paulson, R. (1990). "Human Oocyte and Pre-Embryo Donation: An Evolving Method for the Treatment of Female Infertility," *Amer. Jr. Obstetrics and Gynecology,* 163: 1421-24.

Schover, L. Collins, R and Richards, S. (1992). "Psychological Aspects of Donor Insemination: Evaluation and Follow-up of Recipient Couples," *Fertility and Sterility* 57: 584-589.

Schover, L.R, et al. (1991). "Psychological Follow-up of Women Evaluated as Oocyte Donors, " *Human Reproduction,* 6: 1487-91.

Seibel, Machelle and Susan Crockin (1996). *Family Building through Egg and Sperm Donation* Jones and Bartlett Publishers, Sudbury, MA.

Seifer D, J Grifo and D Battaglia. (2000). "The Aging Ovarian Follicle: Can We Turn Back the Clock?," *Contemporary Obstetrics and Gynecology,* 3:76-101.

Seligson, S. (March 1995). "Seeds of Doubt" *The Atlantic Monthly,* pp. 28, 30 and 38-39.

Smith, Meyer et al. (2001). "Anonymous Oocyte Donation: A Follow-up Questionnaire," *Fertility and Sterility,* 75:1034-6.

Snowden, R and E, (1998) "Families Created Through Donor Insemination," in *Donor Insemination International Social Science Perspectives,* Cambridge University Press.

Spirtas, SC, et al. (1993). "Fertility Drugs and Ovarian Cancer: Red Alert or Red Herring?" *Fertility and Sterility* 59: 291-93.

Topp, Karen. (1993). "Positive Reflections Growing Up as a DI Child" *The Canadian Journal of Human Sexuality* 2 (3): 149-151.

Whittemore, A.S., Harris, R. and Halpern, J. (1992). "Characteristics Relating to Ovarian Cancer Risk: Collaborative Analysis of 12 U.S. Case-control Studies," *American Journal of Epidemiology,* 136: 1175-83.

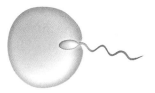

Resources

The list of resources for egg donation is ever expanding. We offer here a brief list of books, organizations and websites that may be of help to consumers. We expect that many of them will lead you to other valuable resources.

Recommended Reading

And Hannah Wept: Infertility, Adoption and the Jewish Couple by Michael Gold (Jewish Publication Society of America, 1988).

Building Your Family Through Egg Donation: What You Will Want to Know About the Emotional Aspects and What to Tell Your Children by Joyce S. Friedman and Celeste H. Friedman (Erlanger, KY:Jolance Press, 1996).

Choosing Assisted Reproduction: Social, Emotional and Ethical Considerations by Susan Lewis Cooper and Ellen Sarasohn Glazer (Indiana: Perspectives Press, 1998).

Confessions of a Serial Egg Donor by Julia Dereck (New York: Adrenaline Books, 2004).

Conquering Infertility: Dr. Alice Domar's Mind/Body Guide Enhancing Fertility and Coping with Infertility by Alice D. Domar and Alice Lesch Kelly (New York: Viking, 2002).

Experiences of Donor Conception: Parents, Offspring and Donors Through the Years by Caroline Lorbach (Philadelphia: Jessica Kingsley Publishers, 2003).

Family Building Through Egg and Sperm Donation: Medical, Legal and Ethical Issues Edited by Machelle M. Seibel and Susan L. Crockin (Jones and Bartlett Publishers, 1996).

The Fertility Sourcebook by M. Sara Rosenthal (Chicago: Contemporary Books, 1996).

Flight of the Stork: What Children Think (and When) about Sex and Family Building by Anne C. Bernstein (Indiana: Perspectives Press,1994).

Getting Pregnant When You Thought You Couldn't by Helane S. Rosenberg and Yakov M. Epstein (New York: Warner Books, 2001).

Helping the Stork: The Choices and Challenges of Donor Insemination by Carol Frost Vercollone, Heidi Moss and Robert Moss (New York: Macmillan, 1997).

Let Me Explain (A Story about Donor Insemination) by Jane Schnitter (Indiana: Perspectives Press).

Mommy, Did I Grow in Your Tummy? Where Some Babies Come From by Elaine Gordon and Kathy Clo (EM Greenberg Press, 1992).

New Ways of Making Babies: The Case for Egg Donation (Medical Ethics Series) Edited by: Cynthia Cohen, National Advisory Board on Ethics in Reproduction (Bloomington, IN: Indiana University Press, 1999).

Phoebe's Family by Linda Stamm. A story about egg donation for ages 5 to 10.

Rewinding Your Biological Clock: Mothering Late in Life, Options, Issues and Emotions by Richard J. Paulson and Judith Sachs (New York: WH Freeman and Company, 1998).

Six Steps to Increased Fertility: An Integrated Medical and Mind/Body Program to Promote Conception by Robert Barbieri, Kevin Loughlin and Alice Domar (Simon and Schuster/Fireside, 2001)

Tears of Sorrow, Seeds of Hope: A Jewish Spiritual Companion for Infertility and Pregnancy Loss by Rabbi Nina Beth Cardin (Jewish Lights Publishing, 1999)

What to Expect When You're Expecting by Arlene Eisenberg, Heidi Murkoff, and Sandee Hathaway (New York: Workman Publishing, 1996).

Organizations and On-line Resources

ACeBabes
A membership organization that provides education and support for families who have conceived through assisted conception.
www.acebabes.co.uk
email: eng@acebabes.co.uk

American Association for Marriage and Family Therapy (AAMFT)
The professional organization representing marriage and family therapists, believes that therapists with specific and rigorous training in marriage and family therapy provide the most effective mental health care to individuals, couples, and families.
1133 15th Street, N.W. Suite 300
Washington, DC 20005-2710
Tel. 202-452-0109
www.aamft.org

American Fertility Association
A national organization dedicated to educating, supporting and advocating for men and women concerned with reproductive health, fertility preservation, infertility and all forms of family building.
666 Fifth Ave. Suite 278
New York, NY 10103
www.theafa.org

American Society for Reproductive Medicine (ASRM)
A non-profit organization that is devoted to advancing the knowledge and expertise in reproductive medicine.
1209 Montgomery Highway
Birmingham, Alabama 35216-2809
Tel. (205) 978-5000
www.asrm.org

American Surrogacy Center
E-mail discussion and on-line support groups for those interested in surrogacy and egg donation. Hear from surrogate mothers, intended parents, egg donors, and leading experts in the field. Offers legal, medical, psychological, information, message boards, and e-mail Discussions.
Kennesaw, Georgia
www.surrogacy.com

Centers for Disease Control (CDC)
Offers a comprehensive listing of all infertility clinics registered with the federal government as well as ART success rate reports and other statistics on infertility.
Atlanta, Georgia
Tel. 770- 488-5372
www.cdc.gov/nccdphp/drh/art96

Childfree Network
A national organization for men, women, singles, and couples who are childless by choice or by chance.
6966 Sunrise Blvd. Suite 111
Citrus Heights, CA 95610
Tel. 916-773-7178
www.hometown.aol.com/cfnspm

Conceiving Concepts
An online community of support and education for those experiencing infertility
Tel. 877-487-9474
www.conceivingconcepts.com

DC (Donor Conception) Network
Organization offers information and support for anyone interested in donor conception
Box 265
Sheffield, S3 7YX
England
Tel. 020 8245 4369
www.dcnetwork.org

Donor Conception Support Group
Organization that supports, educates, and advocates for families created by donor conception
PO Box 53
Georges Hall, NSW 2198
Australia
Tel. 02-9724-1366
www.dcsg.org.au

Donor Offspring
Offers support to adults conceived by donor insemination
c/o Bill Corday

1415 Romona Ave.
Salt Lake City, UT 84105-3707
www.donoroffspring.com

Donor Sibling Registry
Helps donor offspring locate biological half siblings.
www.DonorSiblingRegistry.com

European Infertility Network
Aims to provide quality information on ARTs and infertility.
www.ein.org
email: webmaster@ein.org

Family Pride Coalition
National organization offering support, education, and advocacy for gay
and lesbian parents and their children
PO Box 65327
Washington, DC 20035-5327
Tel. 202-331-5015
www.familypride.org

Fertile Thoughts
A large community of information, forums and chats. Forums cover
specialized topics such as infertility over 35, secondary infertility, PCO,
and high tech treatments.
www.fertilethoughts.net

The Genetics and Public Policy Center—Johns Hopkins University
The Genetics and Public Policy Center has been established to be an independent and objective source of credible information on genetic technologies and genetic policies for the public, media and policymakers..
The goal of the Center is to create the environment and tools needed by
key decision makers in both the private and public sectors to carefully
consider and respond to the challenges and opportunities that arise
from scientific advances in genetics.
1717 Massachusetts Avenue, NW, Suite 530
Washington, DC 20036
Tel. 202-663-5971
www.dnapolicy.org

Hannah's Prayer
International Christian resource and support network for couples fac-

ing infertility, miscarriage or neonatal loss. Newsletter, support chapters, chat room.
www.hannah.org

Human Fertilisation and Embryology Authority (HFEA)
HFEA desires to safeguard the interests of patients, children, the general public, doctors, service providers, the scientific community, and also future generations. The HFEA ensures that all UK treatment clinics offering IVF or DI, or storage of eggs, sperm or embryos, conform to high medical and professional standards and are also inspected regularly.
21 Bloomsbury St.
London WC1B3HF
Tel. 02072918200
www.hfea.gov.uk

Jewish Infertility
Support for those of the Orthodox Jewish faith who are limited by their religion as to means of treatments. Contains a message forum and weekly chats.
www.atime.org

Journal of Assisted Reproductive Law
www.surrogatelaw.org/jarl.htm

Infertility Awareness Association of Canada (IACC)
National organization offering information, support and advocacy about infertility issues
201-396 Cooper ST.
Ottawa, Ontario K2P 2H7, Canada
Tel. 613-234-8585
email: iaac@fox.nstn.ca

The Infertility Network
160 Pikering ST.
Toronto, Canada
www.infertilitynetwork.org
email: info@inferitliynetwork.org

International Council on Infertility Information Dissemination (INCIID)
An on-line resource of comprehensive consumer-targeted information about cutting-edge infertility treatments.
P.O. Box 6836,

Arlington, VA 22206
Tel. (520) 544-9548 or (703) 379-9178
E-Mail: INCIIDinfo@inciid.org
www.inciid.org

International Federation of Infertility Patient Associations (IFIPA)
An organization that helps those affected by infertility.
www.child.org.uk
email: office@email2.child.org.uk

IVF Connections
Connects people going through IVF to information and support. Features
bulletin boards, email lists, chat rooms, questions and answers, stories,
links and an IVF in Canada section.
www.ivfconnections.com

Mind/Body Programs
Mind/body medicine integrates modern scientific medicine, psychology,
nursing, nutrition, exercise physiology and spirituality to enhance the
natural healing capacities of body and mind, including issues with infertility.

> *The Mind/Body Institute*
> UCLA Medical Plaze
> 13547 Ventura Blvd. #642
> Sherman Oaks, California 91423
>
> *The Mind/Body Center for Women's Health at Boston IVF*
> 40 Second Ave. Suite 300
> Waltham, Mass. 02451
>
> *The Mind Body Medical Institute*
> 824 Boylston St.
> Chestnut Hill, Mass. 02467

New Reproductive Alternatives Society
Canadian support group and lobby association for donor conception
families.
email: spratten@nisa.et

Organization of Parents Through Surrogacy (OPTS)
A national, not-for-profit, all volunteer organization with some international members. We provide information, support, networking and
advocacy for families built through surrogate parenting.

PO Box 213
Wheeling, IL
847-394-4116
www.opts.com

RESOLVE, Inc.
(National Infertility Association)
A national support organization which sponsors many seminars and self-help groups. Local chapters are located in most areas. RESOLVE offers many useful publications about the medical and psychological aspects of infertility.
7910 Woodmont Avenue, Suite 1350
Bethesda, MD 20814
301-652-8585
www.resolve.org

Shared Journey
A complete information and support site for those dealing with infertility, adoption, pregnancy loss, or pregnancy after infertility. Interactive features such as hosted message boards and chats.
www.sharedjourney.com

Single Mothers by Choice (SMC)
Organization that offers information and support to single women interested in parenthood
PO Box 1642
Gracie Square Station
New York, NY 10028
Tel. 212-988-0993
http://mattes.home.pipeline.com

www.parentsplace.com
On on-line community, consisting of articles, message boards and chats, devoted to all aspects of fertility, pregnancy and parenting, including egg donation.
www.parentsplace.com

2ofus4now
A religious support network for infertility, adoption, and pregnancy loss.
www.2ofus4now.org

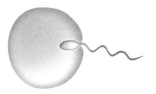

Index

About the Publisher

Perspectives Press Inc.
The Infertility and Adoption Publisher
www,perspectivespress.com

Since 1982 Perspectives Press, Inc has focused exclusively on infertility, adoption and related reproductive health and child welfare issues. Our purpose is to promote understanding of these issues and to educate and sensitize those personally experiencing these life situations, profession-als who work in these fields, and the public at large. Our titles are never duplicative of or competitive with material already available through other publishers. We seek to find and fill niches which are empty.

Currently in print titles from Perspectives Press, Inc. include

For Adults

Perspectives on a Grafted Tree
Understanding Infertility: Insights for Family and Friends
Sweet Grapes: How to Stop Being Infertile and Start Living Again
A Child's Journey through Placement
Adopting after Infertility
Flight of the Stork: What Children Think (and When) about Sex and Family Building
Taking Charge of Infertility
Looking Back, Looking Forward
Launching a Baby's Adoption
Toddler Adoption: The Weaver's Craft
Choosing Assisted Reproduction

PCOS: The Hidden Epidemic
Inside Transracial Adoption
Attaching in Adoption
Adoption Is a Family Affair! What Relatives and Friends Must Know
Having Your Baby through Egg Donation

For Children

The Mulberry Bird: A Story about Adoption
Filling in the Blanks: A Guided Look at Growing Up Adopted
Two Birthdays for Beth
Let Me Explain: A Story about Donor Insemination
Sam's Sister
Borya and the Burps!

About the Authors

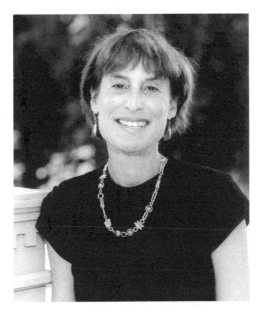

ELLEN SARASOHN GLAZER is a clinical social worker specializing in infertility, adoption, third party reproduction, pregnancy loss and parenting after infertility. She has worked in fertility centers and for adoption agencies and is now in full time private practice in Newton, Massachusetts. Ellen's practice includes in person and telephone counseling and coaching for individuals and couples considering adoption, egg donation and gestational care. She is the author of two books, *The Long Awaited Stork: A Guide to Parenting After Infertility* (Jossey Bass, 1998) and *Experiencing Infertility: Stories to Inform and Inspire* (Jossey Bass, 1998) and the co-author, with Dr. Susan Cooper, of two books, Without Child (Lexington Books, 1988) and *Choosing Assisted Reproduction: Social, Emotional and Ethical Considerations* (Perspectives Press, 1998). Ellen is also a freelance writer and essayist, whose articles have appeared in the Boston Globe, The New York Times and Newton Magazine. She has two daughters, Elizabeth and Mollie Glazer. It was their long awaited arrivals that inspired Ellen's work in the field of reproductive medicine.

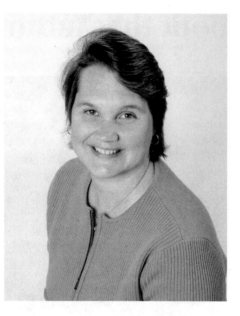

EVELINA WEIDMAN STERLING is a doctoral student in the Department of Sociology at Georgia State University. Her primary research interests include issues related to public health, gender and sexuality. In addition, Evelina holds a Bachelor of Science degree in Biology from the University of Mary Washington and a Master's degree in Public Health from the Department of Health Policy and Management at the Johns Hopkins University School of Public Health. Evelina is a Certified Health Education Specialist. She has spent over 10 years working in the field of public health and health education. Previous positions include working for the American Association for Health Education, Health Resources and Services Administration, Gallaudet University and the American Heart Association. She is currently working part-time as a consultant to various non-profit and government agencies in the areas of program planning, evaluation and health services research. Evelina has written several articles, as well as given numerous presentations, regarding fertility and reproductive health. She is the co-author with Angie Best-Boss of another book, *Living with PCOS—Polycystic Ovary Syndrome* (Addicus Books, 2000). Evelina lives in Atlanta with her husband and two children.